T0211470

Women's Health in Mid-Life
A Primary Care Guide

This book highlights the needs and healthcare concerns of women in their mid life. Women in middle age are often overlooked by medical practitioners. From the end of childbearing to old age, approximately ages 40–65 years, their health needs are complex and changing. This is a time of challenge and opportunity, when the physician and woman working collaboratively can change her health and future. Mid-life healthcare is far more than hormones. Healthy behaviors such as good nutrition and exercise can be promoted, which will result in lower risk and sometimes improved care of heart disease, hypertension, and diabetes. Adequate screening and treatment can prevent diseases and complications. This book performs a critical evaluation of the burgeoning literature on allopathic and complementary medicine and compares it with that of established medical care. Written by 20 primary-care physicians, this book will help family practitioners provide the best possible healthcare for these women.

Dr Jo Ann Rosenfeld is Assistant Professor of General Internal Medicine at Johns Hopkins School of Medicine, and former Professor of Family Medicine at East State Tennessee University. Her editorial responsibilities include being Associate Editor of *BMJ USA*, Associate Editor of *AAFP FP Comprehensive Monograph Course*, and Associate Editor of the Johns Hopkins Advanced Studies in Internal Medicine journal. She is the author of 50 articles on women's health, and three other books on the subject, including *Handbook of Women's Health* (Cambridge University Press, 2001) and *Women's Health in Primary Care* (Lippincott Williams & Wilkins, 1997).

Women's Health in Mid-Life

A Primary Care Guide

Edited by

Jo Ann Rosenfeld

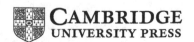

CAMBRIDGE
UNIVERSITY PRESS

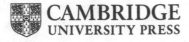

CAMBRIDGE
UNIVERSITY PRESS

Shaftesbury Road, Cambridge CB2 8EA, United Kingdom

One Liberty Plaza, 20th Floor, New York, NY 10006, USA

477 Williamstown Road, Port Melbourne, VIC 3207, Australia

314–321, 3rd Floor, Plot 3, Splendor Forum, Jasola District Centre, New Delhi – 110025, India

103 Penang Road, #05–06/07, Visioncrest Commercial, Singapore 238467

Cambridge University Press is part of Cambridge University Press & Assessment, a department of the University of Cambridge.

We share the University's mission to contribute to society through the pursuit of education, learning and research at the highest international levels of excellence.

www.cambridge.org
Information on this title: www.cambridge.org/9780521823401

First published 2004

A catalogue record for this publication is available from the British Library

Library of Congress Cataloging-in-Publication data
Rosenfeld, Jo Ann.
Women's health in mid-life : a primary care guide / Jo Ann Rosenfeld.
    p.   cm.
Includes bibliographical references and index.
ISBN 0 521 82340 4
1. Middle aged women – Health and hygiene.   2. Primary care (Medicine)   I. Title.
RA778.R619   2004
613'.04244 – dc22   2003060809

ISBN   9780521823401   Paperback

To my mother, Judy Rosenfeld,
who taught me how to write.

Contents

Part III Disease prevention

Part IV Cancer prevention

Contributors

Kathy Andolsek, M. D.
Duke University Medical Center,
Durham, NC, USA

Tracey D. Conti, M. D.
University of Pittsburgh, Pittsburgh,
PA, USA

**Mary-Anne Enoch, M. D.,
M. R. C. G. P**
Laboratory of Neurogenetics,
National Institute of Alcohol Abuse
and Alcoholism, National Institutes
of Health, Bethesda, MD, USA

Margaret Gradison, M. D.
Department of Community and
Family Medicine, Duke University
Medical Center, Durham, NC,
USA

Cathrine Hoyo, M. P. H., Ph. D.
Department of community and
Family Medicine, Duke University
Medical Center, Durham, NC,
USA

Melissa H. Hunter, M. D.
Department of Family Medicine,
University Family Medicine,
Charleston, SC, USA

Victoria S. Kaprielian, M. D.
Department of Community and
Family Medicine, Duke University
Medical Center, Durham, NC, USA

Dana E. King, M. D.
Department of Family Medicine,
University Family Medicine,
Charleston, SC, USA

Diana McNeill, M. D., F. A. C. P
Department of Medicine, Division of
Endocrinology and Metabolism,
Duke University Medical Center,
Durham, NC, USA

Phillippa Miranda, M. D.
Department of Medicine, Division of
Endocrinology and Metabolism,
Duke University Medical Center,
Durham, NC, USA

Tanya A. Miszko, Ed. D., C. S. C. S
VA Medical Center (Atlanta),
Decatur, GA, USA

Cathy Morrow, M. D.
Marine Dartmouth Family Practice
Residency

Gwendolyn Murphy, Ph. D., R. D.
Department of Community and
Family Medicine, Duke University
Medical Center, Durham, NC, USA

Margaret R. H. Nusbaum, D. O., M. P. H.
Department of Family Medicine,
University of North Carolina, Chapel
Hill, NC, USA

Jo Ann Rosenfeld, M. D.
Johns Hopkins School of Medicine,
Baltimore, MD

Ellen Sakornbut, M. D.
University of Iowa

Jeannette E. South-Paul, M. D.
Department of Family Medicine,
University of Pittsburgh, Pittsburgh,
PA, USA

Valerie K. Ulstad, M. D., M. P. H., M. P. A., F. A. C. C.
West Hennepin County Medical
Center, Minneapolis, MN, USA

Anne Walling, M. D.
University of Kansas, Wichita

Introduction

Jo Ann Rosenfeld

The middle ages of women are an often forgotten time and the women are often overlooked in healthcare. No longer in their childbearing and birth control years, and not yet geriatric, the women are frequently ignored or their needs and wishes combined into one homogeneous group. Regularly, healthcare providers address only the women's hormonal needs and minimize discussion of their health and wellbeing. These women, who are from the ages of 40 to 65, are in a variety of situations and circumstances, both medical and social. These ages are a time of change, stress, and opportunity.

Despite the fact that there are more women than men at every age, this time of change is poorly studied and understood for women (Figure 1.1). Many large population studies have not included women, have included only a few women, or have not reported data by gender. Few studies have examined this age group. The change to adolescence, adulthood, and elder has been well examined and researched. Each of these ages has their own specialists (obstetrician/gynecologist or geriatrician). However, the middle ages are often neglected. Menopause is not a disease, a definite time, or a curse. Its needs, challenges, and effects on women's health are not understood well. Familial and social stresses may be challenging or overpowering, as the woman has to redefine herself within society, employment, and her family.

The opportunities for improvement for future health are immense. Women can make lifestyle changes that will profoundly affect their future health, comfort, and length of life. Quitting smoking, improving exercise regimens, and achieving ideal body weight can improve the rest of a woman's life. Treatment of hypertension and diabetes is believed to improve mortality and morbidity. Screening for cancer may improve mortality. Health promotion and disease prevention are possible if each woman is considered an individual and her health needs addressed personally.

The social variations and changes in this age group are immense. The woman can be a new mother, a mother of small children or adolescents, childless, a grandmother living with her husband or family, a widow alone, or a

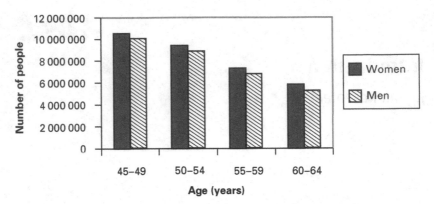

Figure 1.1 Population by age and gender, from US Census 2000.

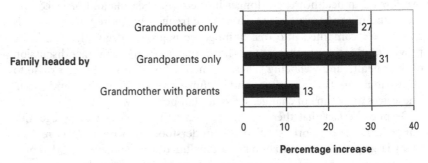

Figure 1.2 Percentage increase in families headed by grandmothers/grandparents 1990–1997. (From Casper, L. M. and Bryson, K. R. Co-resident grandparents and their grandchildren: grandparent maintained families. Population Division, US Bureau of the Census, Washington, DC, March 1998. http://www.census.gov/population/www/documentation/twps0026/twps0026.html. Accessed April 13, 2003.)

grandmother raising small grandchildren. Twenty five million women aged 15–44 in the USA are childless.[1] Approximately 19% of women age 40–44 were childless in 1994 in the USA, almost double the number in 1970.[2]

They can be single, married, divorced, or widowed. The traditional depiction of the aging mother or grandmother with "empty nest" concerns may not be valid. The number of never-married women aged 39 almost tripled from 1970 to 1994, from 5 to 13%.[1] The woman may have husband, mother, grown children, or their children living with her. Women are more likely to be living alone than men. Approximately 14% of women live alone, and this number has doubled from 1970 to 1994.[1] In the past decade, the number of grandmother-headed families has increased tremendously, and those grandparent- or grandmother-headed families are more likely to be in poverty or receiving public assistance (Figures 1.2 and 1.3).[3]

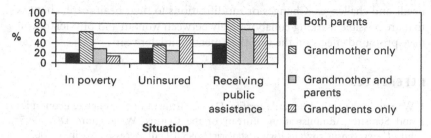

Figure 1.3 Percentage of households with children headed by different groups. (From Casper, L. M. and Bryson, K. R. Co-resident grandparents and their grandchildren: grandparent maintained families. Population Division, US Bureau of the Census, Washington, DC, March 1998. http://www.census.gov/population/www/documentation/twps0026/twps0026.html. Accessed April 13, 2003.)

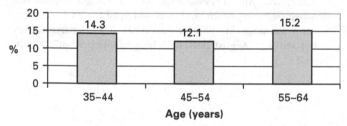

Figure 1.4 Percentage of women, by age, who are uninsured.

Approximately 25% of women of this age are carers of their parents or their spouses' parents. Most of these women are in the workforce as well, at the midpoint or highpoint of their careers. Approximately 57% of all women are in the workforce.[1] They may be secure financially, or recently downsized, fired, widowed, or divorced, or without work or insurance. Approximately 12–15% of US women of this age are medically uninsured (Figure 1.4). They may be comfortable at work or fighting a new boss.

The medical variation in women this age is tremendous. Most women enter this age group in good health, but chronic health conditions often intrude. These women are more likely to be disabled and have disabling arthritis and diabetes.[4] Women are more likely than men to die of heart disease and stroke, but are less likely to die from cancer and lung disease (the latter is due to the greater history of smoking in men and may change over the coming years).[2] The reaction and changes women make to these diseases, illnesses, and disabilities will profoundly affect how their lives progress over the last third of their years.

These women must not be viewed either as "finished" or unimportant simply because they are finished with childbearing and/or approaching menopause, nor must they be considered pre-elderly. They have their own needs and challenges. Changes or modifications to their healthcare, changes that are possible working collaboratively between woman and physician, will have profound effects on the way they meet their later years.

REFERENCES

1 Women in the United States: a profile. US Department of Commerce, Economics and Statistics Administration. Bureau of the Census. Washington, DC. 1995. http://www.census.gov/apsd/www/statbrief/sb95_19.pdf. Accessed April 21, 2003.
2 Record share of new mothers in labor force. Department of Commerce, Economics and Statistics Administration. Bureau of the Census. Washington, DC. October 24, 2000. http://www.census.gov/Press-Release/www/2000/cb00-175.html. Accessed March 1, 2003.
3 Casper, L. M. and Bryson, K. R. Co-resident grandparents and their grand-children: grandparent maintained families. Population Division. US Bureau of the Census. Washington, DC. March 1998. http://www.census.gov/population/www/documentation/twps0026/ twps0026.html. Accessed April 13, 2003.
4 Highlights of Women's Earnings in 2000 (report 952). US Department of Labor, Bureau of Labor Statistics. August 2001. www.bls.gov/cps/cpswom2000.pdf. Accessed April 10, 2003.

Part I

Health promotion

Physical activity and exercise

Tanya A. Miszko, Ed.D., C.S.C.S.

Introduction

For our ancestors, physical activity was ingrained in daily life. In the early 1900s, before automobiles were invented and mass-produced, walking was a common mode of transportation. Today, automobiles are used for leisurely one-mile drives to the local video store or half-mile treks to the grocery store. Improved technology has reduced our physical activity level by making life "easier."

This "easier" way of life has added to increases in cardiovascular disease, hypertension, high cholesterol, osteoporosis, obesity, and diabetes mellitus. In 1999, cardiovascular disease was the leading cause of death for women in the USA. The American Heart Association states that one in five women has some form of blood vessel or heart disease, 5.7 million women have physician-diagnosed diabetes mellitus, and almost half (46.8%) of non-Hispanic white women are overweight; 23.2% are obese. Genetics cannot be ruled out as a contributing factor to these chronic conditions, but it must also not be an excuse.

In addition to increased morbidity, physical inactivity also has an effect on the economy, amounting to $24 billion of US healthcare expenditures.[1] The yearly cost of medical care for a physically active individual is approximately $330 less than that for an inactive person. Furthermore, if inactive people became active, $76.6 billion in year-2000 dollars would have been saved in direct medical costs.[1] Intuitively, these data would be an alarming incentive for health insurance companies to embrace interventions that focus on the prevention of disease; however, that medical paradigm is not yet emphasized. Because medical costs increase around age 45–54 for inactive women, this is a perfect time for women to take charge of their physical, as well as financial, health.[1]

During a woman's middle-aged years, many physiological changes occur, some of which are modifiable. The risk of cardiovascular disease increases.

Regular physical activity can reduce the risk of premature death from coronary artery disease, colon cancer, hypertension, and diabetes mellitus.[2] However, more than 60% of adult Americans are not regularly physically active, 25% of adult Americans are not active at all, and women continue to be less active than men.[2] The World Health Organization states that "age 50 marks a point in middle age at which the benefits of regular physical activity can be most relevant in avoiding, minimizing, and/or reversing many of the physical, psychological, and social hazards which often accompany advancing age."[3] Middle age is an opportune time for the middle-aged woman to make lifestyle changes and take charge of her life.

This chapter will provide scientifically derived information on the proper exercise regimen for the middle-aged woman. Much research is published about the effects of exercise in older (>60 years) and younger (18–25 years) women, but less information is available for middle-aged women (45–60 years). This may be due partially to the plethora of physiological changes that are occurring during those years, especially the changes in the hormonal milieu. This chapter will also briefly address certain medical conditions/diseases pertaining to aging women and how exercise can function as a primary or secondary preventive tool. Available research data will demonstrate that regular physical activity and exercise can improve all aspects of health, spirit, mind, and body.

Benefits of exercise

Case: Hattie is a 55-year-old first-grade teacher. She has had diet-controlled type II diabetes for two years, although her last hemoglobin A1C was 7.8% and her morning fasting blood sugars are running 150–180 mg/dl. She weighs 83 kg. At her regular follow-up, you discuss the effects of exercise and the possibility that it might reduce her sugars and her weight. She shrugs, saying that she is on her feet all day and that should be enough exercise.

A distinction must be made between physical activity and exercise. Physical activity refers to any bodily movement produced by skeletal muscles and that results in energy expenditure, such as mowing the lawn, grocery shopping, and doing household chores.[4] Exercise, on the other hand, is physical activity with the purpose of improving some component(s) of fitness (muscle strength and endurance, cardiorespiratory endurance, body composition, flexibility), such as regular participation in an endurance-training or strength-training program at an intensity that will confer physiological and performance benefits.[2]

Exercise and physical activity can improve most aspects of mental and physical health.[3,5–7] The benefits derived, however, are specific to the type of exercise performed (Table 2.1).

Table 2.1 Benefits of exercise

Resistance training	Endurance training	Yoga	T'ai chi
Increases muscle strength	Increases aerobic capacity	Increases muscular strength and endurance	Reduces fall rate
Increases type II fiber area	Reduces blood pressure	Increases flexibility	Decreases depression
Increases muscle cross-sectional area	Increases bone mineral density	Increases aerobic capacity	Increased positive affect
Increases or preserves bone mineral density	Reduces anxiety (state and trait)		
	Reduces fatigue in cancer patients		

Regular physical activity

Moderate levels of physical activity have significant effects on a woman's health. Burning approximately 150 kilocalories per day or 1000 kilocalories per week leads to a reduction in the risk of coronary heart disease by 50% and of hypertension, diabetes, and colon cancer by 30%.[2] After adjusting for covariates such as age, smoking, alcohol use, history of hypertension, and history of high cholesterol, women who are regularly physically active are 50% less likely to develop type II diabetes (relative risk = 0.54) than women who are not regularly active.[8] Vasomotor and psychosomatic symptoms associated with menopause are also reduced with moderate amounts of activity.[6,9] Examples of moderate levels of physical activity are depicted in Table 2.2.

Regular physical activity can also reduce the risk of colon cancer, the third leading cause of cancer incidence and mortality in the USA. The risk of colon cancer is reduced by 40–50% in highly active people compared with low active individuals.[10] The mechanisms responsible for a reduction in the risk of colon cancer are:

- reduced transit time in the bowel, which decreases exposure to carcinogens;
- reduction in insulin action, which decreases colon mucosal cells;
- increase in prostaglandin F2α, which increases intestinal motility;
- reduction in prostaglandin E2, which increases colon cell proliferation.

The evidence for exercise providing a reduction in the risk of breast cancer, however, is equivocal. In a cohort of 37 105 women who exercised regularly, there was a lower risk of breast cancer compared with those who did not exercise.[11] The Nurses' Health Study suggests that the risk of breast cancer is reduced modestly in physically active women (relative risk = 0.82).[12] Decreased body fat and estrogen levels may be responsible for the reduction in

Table 2.2 Examples of moderate levels of physical activity

Washing a car for 45–60 minutes	Less vigorous, more time
Playing volleyball for 45 minutes	
Gardening for 30–45 minutes	
Wheeling oneself in wheelchair for 30–40 minutes	
Walking 1.75 miles in 35 minutes (20-min mile pace)	
Basketball (shooting baskets) for 30 minutes	
Bicycling five miles in 30 minutes	
Pushing a stroller 1.5 miles in 30 minutes	
Raking leaves for 30 minutes	
Walking two miles in 30 minutes (15-min mile pace)	
Dancing fast (social) for 30 minutes	
Water aerobics for 30 minutes	
Bicycling four miles in 15 minutes	
Jumping rope for 15 minutes	
Shoveling snow for 15 minutes	
Walking stairs for 15 minutes	More vigorous, less time

Sources: US Department of Health and Human Services. Physical activity and health: a report of the Surgeon General. Atlanta, GA: US Department of Health and Human Services, Centers for Disease Control and Prevention; 1996.

breast cancer risk associated with exercise.[13] More research is needed in this area to substantiate exercise's protective effect against breast cancer.

Small increases in physical activity level and subsequently energy expenditure have a positive effect on psychological outcomes and physiological parameters in middle-aged women. Women who increase their level of physical activity by at least 300 kilocalories per week have a smaller reduction in high-density lipoprotein (HDL) cholesterol with advancing age and are less depressed and stressed than those women who remain at their current activity level.[14] Women who are physically active have higher resting metabolic rates and lower body fat, but similar fat-free mass, body mass index, and body weight compared with their sedentary counterparts.[15] These results suggest that physical activity is a component of a healthy lifestyle.

Resistance training

Although resistance training has been proven to alter positively some of the modifiable risk factors for disease (obesity, hypertension, low bone mass, etc.), fewer than 16% of the US population between the ages of 18 and 64 years participate regularly in a resistance-training program.[16] Women who participate in a resistance-training program increase muscle strength and power, alter muscle ultrastructure (type II fiber area), increase or preserve bone mineral density, and improve cardiovascular risk factors for disease.[17,18]

Muscle strength and power are compromised during a woman's middle-aged years because of age-associated changes, including a reduction in type II fiber area and a decreased number of functioning motor units.[19,20] In a sedentary individual, maximal strength is reduced by approximately 7.5–8.5% per decade beginning around age 30 and muscle power is reduced by approximately 35% per decade.[21] This reduction is relative to the remaining strength and power, such that muscle power in a 50-year-old woman is 35% less than it was when she was 40 years old but 35% more than she will have when she is 60 years old. Considering that muscle power is lost at a faster rate than muscle strength after age 65,[21] having a high strength and power base before this age could protect against losses later in life, thus serving as a buffer to functional decline.

Regular participation in a resistance-training program has profound effects on muscle ultrastructure. *Resistance training attenuates the loss in muscle cross-sectional area, type II fiber area, strength, and bone mineral density commonly associated with aging.*[5,22,23] Significant increases in maximum torque, electromyography, maximal strength, and type II mean fiber area have been observed in middle-aged women after participating in an explosive-strength training program.[5] Additionally, motor unit activation is increased, thereby providing evidence for neural adaptations.[24]

Cross-sectional and longitudinal exercise data support the efficacy of resistance training as an effective modality for the prevention and treatment of osteoporosis.[24] A recent meta-analysis demonstrated that resistance training can increase or preserve bone mineral density in pre- and postmenopausal women. With the cessation of exercise, bone mineral density will return to pre-exercise levels at a rate similar to that in age-matched controls.[25] Thus, the continued participation in a resistance-training program is essential for bone health.

Endurance training

Case: Sarah is a 42-year-old bank teller with no cardiac risk factors and who was found to have a fasting total cholesterol level of 299 mg/dl with a low-density lipoprotein (LDL) cholesterol level of 179 mg/dl at a recent screening. After three months of vigorous change of diet to a low-fat diet, she returns for a fasting lipid profile. Total cholesterol has only decreased to 245 mg/dl, with an LDL of 145 mg/dl. She asks what else she can do without starting on pharmocotherapy.

You suggest walking three times a week for 30 minutes *each time* as a form of exercise. She agrees; six months later, she has lost 4.5 kg and her total cholesterol level is 195 mg/dl, with an LDL of 120 mg/dl.

Endurance training can reduce some of the risk factors associated with cardiovascular disease, such as hypertension, high cholesterol, and inactivity.

As little as two to three days per week are required to gain health benefits from a moderate-intensity (50% maximum oxygen consumption) endurance-training program. These health benefits include a reduction in systolic and diastolic blood pressure, total cholesterol, and body mass index, and an increase in HDL cholesterol.[26,27] Brisk walking for three or more hours per week can reduce the risk of cardiac events in middle-aged women (relative risk = 0.65).[28] *Becoming physically active in middle age also reduces the risk of cardiac events.* Exercise can be used as preventive medicine.

Despite the age-associated reduction in aerobic capacity, endurance training can have a positive effect on the cardiovascular system. On average, maximal aerobic capacity declines at a rate of approximately 7.5–9% per decade after age 25.[29,30] Although endurance athletes have a greater absolute rate of decline in aerobic capacity than sedentary women, their relative (ml/kg/min) rate of decline in aerobic capacity is smaller.[31] This may be explained by increases in aerobic capacity, stroke volume, and arterial-venous oxygen difference ($(a-v)O_2$diff), reduction in resting heart rate, improved blood lipid profile, and increased exercise time that is frequently observed after participation in an endurance-training program.[32,33] This indicates that older endurance-trained women have higher aerobic capacities throughout life, thus serving as a physiological reserve against functional decline.

In addition to improvements in the cardiovascular system, endurance exercise also improves a woman's psychological outlook and the skeletal system. Women who exercise regularly are less neurotic, have greater self-esteem, and are more satisfied with life compared with their sedentary counterparts.[34] Weight-bearing activities such as walking increase or preserve bone mineral density by approximately 5%.[35] However, as with resistance training, *the positive effects of exercise are negated when exercise is discontinued or reduced (fewer than three days per week).* Regular exercise has a significant impact on the human body.

Alternative therapies

Alternative therapies, such as yoga and t'ai chi, have also demonstrated positive improvements in health.[36–38] Yoga involves various standing, seated, and supine postures and breathing and relaxation techniques designed to enhance functioning of the various physiological systems by supporting a natural posture. T'ai chi incorporates slow body movements, called forms, that concentrate on balance and body-weight transfers. Young and old men and women have performed yoga and t'ai chi for centuries in Eastern countries. Both have been purported to focus concentration and relax the body.

Yoga practice has been shown to improve muscular strength, endurance, flexibility, and aerobic capacity. In men, evidence suggests that yoga practice reduces sympathetic activity, improves aerobic capacity, reduces perceived exertion after maximal exercise, and reduces heart rate and left-ventricular end-diastolic volume at rest.[39,40] Similar benefits would be expected for women; however, there is a paucity of research dealing with women. Additionally, yoga practice may retard the progression and increase the regression of atherosclerosis in patients with coronary artery disease.[41]

T'ai chi practice improves mood states, range of motion, physical function, and hemodynamic parameters.[32,42,43] Reductions in anger, total mood disturbance, tension, confusion, and depression and an increase in self-efficacy are evident after regular t'ai chi practice.[32] Improvements in self-reported physical function and a reduction in falls is also reported.[37,42,44] Patients suffering from acute myocardial infarction can reduce blood pressure after practicing t'ai chi.[45] T'ai chi is an effective modality for improving several aspects of health.

Empirical scientific evidence has demonstrated the positive benefits of exercise, such as improved strength, reduced anxiety, improved blood lipid profile, and decreased risk of cardiovascular disease. The modality required to obtain these benefits can vary from a structured exercise program (resistance training and walking/running) and alternative therapies (yoga and t'ai chi) to daily physical activity (mowing the lawn and climbing stairs).

Exercise prescription for healthy populations

The type of exercise performed depends on the desired goal. If a woman wants to build muscular strength, then resistance training is appropriate. Endurance training (walking, running, cycling, swimming) is required if a woman wants to improve her cardiovascular health and endurance. Yoga and t'ai chi are therapeutic alternatives to the rigors of strength and endurance training that can reduce stress, increase strength and flexibility, and improve cardiovascular parameters. A certified yoga or t'ai chi instructor should be consulted for more information on the styles of each.

Resistance training

Resistance training is the mode of exercise performed to stimulate the neuromuscular system. Variations of the number of sets, repetitions, rest period, and weight lifted determines the outcome of the training program. Programs designed to increase strength are typically performed at a high intensity (80% of the one-repetition maximum, 1RM) with long rest periods (two to three minutes) and low to moderate volume (one to three sets of eight to ten repetitions), whereas programs designed to promote muscle hypertrophy are performed at a moderate to high intensity (60–80% 1RM) with shorter rest periods (30–60 seconds) and higher volume (three to four sets of ten to 12 repetitions).[46]

Table 2.3 Resistance training exercises

Muscle group	Exercise
Quadriceps and hamstrings	Squat*
	Lunge*
	Leg press*
	Leg curl
	Step-up*
Pectoralis major and minor	Bench press (barbell or dumbbell)*
	Push-up*
	Fly
Lumbar extensors, latissimus dorsi, rhomboids	Lat pull-down*
	Row (seated or dumbbell)*
	Trunk extension
Deltoids	Side lateral raise
	Rear deltoid raise
	Military press (with dumbbells)*
Triceps and biceps	Triceps extension (cable, single-arm, or double-arm)
	Biceps curl (dumbbell or barbell)

*Multi-joint exercises.

In a generally healthy population, resistance training can be performed with exercise machines or with free weights. Examples of resistance-training exercises are provided in Table 2.3. Multi-joint, multi-planar exercises commonly associated with free weights may be more functional because their motor patterns mimic motor patterns of daily tasks.[47]

Machines offer more safety for beginners and isolate muscle groups more so than free weights.[48] However, free weights require the individual to use accessory/stabilizer muscles, as they would naturally in daily life, and improve strength more than training on machines.[48] Free weights also concurrently train balance, strength, and coordination – similar to the demands of daily activities. Household items (rice bags, jugs of water, soup cans, etc.) can also be used for resistance instead of metal weights or a cable system. For an individual with no resistance training experience, machines should be used initially to increase strength so that a progression to free weights can be made safely.

The design of the program is somewhat more of an art than a strict, regimented science. Science provides the basis for sound training principles, but creativity is needed to continually manipulate the training volume, exercise selection, and order of exercise. For general muscle strengthening, approximately two to three sets of eight to 12 repetitions should be performed. A 5% increase in resistance is suggested when 12–15 repetitions can be performed.[49] The exercise prescription can be written for specific combinations of muscle groups (back and hamstrings, chest and arms, etc.), agonist versus antagonist (leg extension versus leg curl, chest press versus seated row), and upper versus lower body (legs on Monday, chest, back, and shoulders on Tuesday, etc.) muscle groups.

Regardless of the design of the program, specific guidelines should be followed. Within each session, individuals should perform large muscle groups (prime movers) before smaller muscle groups (secondary movers) to avoid fatigue of the larger muscles. However, smaller, stabilizing muscles (rotator cuff, hip adductor/abductor, neck muscles, etc.) should not be neglected. If left untrained, these smaller, stabilizing muscles are at risk for injury. The Valsalva maneuver, holding the breath during exertion, should never be performed. To avoid a reduction in venous return to the heart and a significant increase in blood pressure, individuals should exhale on exertion. As always, medical clearance should be sought before beginning an exercise program if an individual has a condition that may be made worse by exercise.

Endurance training

The cardiovascular system is improved most effectively by endurance training. Endurance training involves rhythmic movements of large muscle groups. For example, running/walking, bicycling, swimming, and dancing are effective and common modes of endurance exercise. However, a combination of modalities within an exercise session might provide extra motivation and reduce boredom.

The exercise prescription for endurance training offers variety, similar to resistance training. *The American College of Sports Medicine recommends 20–60 minutes a day, three to five days per week at an intensity equal to 60–90% of age-predicted maximum heart rate ($HR_{max} = 220 - age$).*[50] Intensity and duration are related inversely, such that a reduction in intensity requires an increase in duration. Any of these variables can be manipulated within and between exercise sessions. For example, in a three-days-a-week exercise program, day one = 40 minutes of treadmill walking at 65% HR_{max}, day two = ten minutes of bicycling at 70% HR_{max}, ten minutes of intervals at 90% HR_{max}, then five minutes at 60% HR_{max}, and day three = 20 minutes of swimming at 80% HR_{max}. All three variations can provide health and fitness benefits.

To maximize benefits and reduce the risk of injury, specific guidelines should be followed. The American College of Sports Medicine recommends training large muscle groups. These large muscle groups utilize more oxygen and generate more adenosine triphosphate (ATP) than smaller muscle groups. Thus, *more calories are expended when training larger muscle groups.*

To facilitate energy utilization during training sessions, adequate hydration is essential before, during, and after exercise. Although experts and common practice state that proper warm-up is also advised before stretching, little evidence supports this traditional wisdom.[51] This increases blood flow to the working muscles and increases body temperature, thus reducing the risk of musculoskeletal injuries.

Manipulating certain extraneous factors also reduces the risk of injury. Because the ambient temperature is hottest at midday, outdoor exercises should be performed in the morning or evening, when the temperature is cooler. Loose-fitting, light-colored clothing is appropriate for warmer climates in order to circulate air and facilitate evaporative cooling.[52] In cooler temperatures, however, layers of dark-colored clothing should be worn to trap heat or to be removed as the body temperature rises.[53] The inner layer of clothing should be made from a wicking material that carries moisture away from the body. Proper footwear with a supportive arch and adequate cushioning is also necessary. These guidelines can help to improve performance while reducing the risk of injury.

Exercise prescription for special populations

The athletic woman

Exercise prescription for a female athlete is specific to the demands of the sport. Differences in energy system requirements dictate the intensity and design of the program. Training of anaerobic athletes (sprinters, swimmers, etc.) requires high-intensity, short-duration activities, whereas an aerobic athlete (runner, triathlete, road cyclist, etc.) requires low to moderate intensity for longer durations. Periodized changing-endurance training (sprint drills, hiking, running) is a variation of a typical endurance-training program that can improve athletic and occupational performance in women.[54] The metabolic demand of the sport should match the metabolic demand of the training sessions. Thus, these programs are sport-specific and require assistance from a professional in the field such as a certified strength and conditioning specialist or an exercise physiologist.

The career woman

Women with busy daily schedules can still find time to exercise and take care of their health by manipulating their daily routine. The American College of Sports Medicine has stated that 30 minutes of continuous exercise is not necessary to elicit health benefits; rather, 30 minutes of total accumulated time is required (a minimum of ten-minute bouts).[55] The time commitment is less restrictive, which allows a woman to plan exercise sessions around her work and family schedule. For example, a ten-minute walk in the morning before work, ten minutes of stair-climbing during work, and a ten-minute bike ride or walk after dinner would satisfy the recommendation for 30 minutes per day. The intensity should be in the range of 65–90% of age-predicted maximum heart rate and the exercise should be performed most days of the week.[30]

Strength training should be a component of any exercise program.[45] Whole-body, multi-joint strength-training programs may be beneficial to shorten the time of each session while still gaining benefits. A whole-body, multi-joint strength program performed two to three days per week could include exercises such as a lunge, squat, medicine ball swing, standing dumbbell row, and stability ball dumbbell chest press (refer to the list of resources at the end of this chapter for more information). These exercises can be performed in the home with little equipment and can be adapted to fit any schedule and available space.

Disease considerations

The most common causes of morbidity and mortality in the USA are associated with modifiable risk factors: obesity, sedentary lifestyle, smoking, and poor diet (*source*: www.cdc.gov). *Exercise is important as a preventive measure as well as a treatment option for certain diseases*, combined with a healthy, balanced diet, relaxation practice, and continued supervision/treatment from a physician. Exercise prescriptions can be modified for those people who have a diagnosed disease. Exercise guidelines are given in Table 2.4 for select diseases.

In November 2000, the Centers for Disease Control and Prevention released a report on the health and economic burden of chronic disease.[56] Seventy percent of Americans who die do so of a chronic disease. For women aged 35–64 years old, cardiovascular disease, lung cancer, and breast cancer are the three leading causes of death. One-sixth of the American population has arthritis, the primary disabling disorder. Fifty percent of individuals with osteoporosis cannot walk unassisted and 25% require long-term care. Clearly, there is a need for exercise intervention to help mitigate the effects of aging, to prevent chronic disease, and to enhance quality of life.

Summary

Because of the multitude of physiological changes that start occurring during early middle age, these years are a welcomed opportunity for a woman to directly impact her current and future health. Exercise and physical activity can forestall the age-associated changes (reduced muscle strength, power, aerobic capacity, and bone mineral density) that can lead to dependence and disability. As a minimum, *women (all adults) should be active for at least 30 minutes on most, if not all, days of the week to gain health benefits*. To improve certain aspects of fitness (muscular strength, cardiovascular endurance,

Table 2.4 Exercise guidelines for selected diseased populations

Disease	Fitness parameter	Mode	Frequency	Intensity	Duration
Arthritis	Aerobic capacity	Non-weight-bearing activities, low-impact activities (swimming, cycling)	3–5 days/week	60–80% peak heart rate*	5–10 minutes to begin, then progress to 30–45 minutes
	Muscle strength	Circuit strength training	2–3 days/week	1–2 sets of 3–12 repetitions (start at 3 and progress to 12)	
	Flexibility	Range-of-motion (ROM) exercises	Every day	Slight discomfort, no pain; never bounce	Hold each position for approximately 30 seconds
Diabetes	Aerobic capacity	Walking, cycling	4–7 days/week	50–90% peak heart rate*	20–60 minutes/session
	Muscle strength	Free weights, machines	2–3 days/week	1–2 sets of 8–10 repetitions	
Osteoporosis	Aerobic capacity	Weight-bearing activities (walking, stair-climbing)	3–5 days/week	40–70% peak heart rate*	20–30 minutes/session
	Muscle strength	Free weights, machines	2 days/week	2–3 sets of 8 repetitions	
	Flexibility	ROM exercises, stretching	5–7 days/week	Slight discomfort, no pain; never bounce	Hold each stretched position for approximately 30 seconds
Myocardial infarction	Aerobic capacity	Large-muscle activities	3–4 days/week	40–85% heart rate reserve**	20–40 minutes/session; 5–10 minutes of warm-up and cool-down
	Muscle strength	Circuit training	2–3 days/week	1–3 sets of 10–15 repetitions	
Valvular heart disease	Aerobic capacity	Large-muscle activities	3–7 days/week	60–85% peak heart rate* (resting heart rate + 30 beats after surgery)	20–60 minutes/session
Cancer***	Muscle strength	Machines	2–3 days/week		
	Aerobic capacity	Large-muscle groups (walking, cycling)	3–5 days/week	50–75% heart rate reserve	20–30 minutes/session, continuous

Modified from American College of Sports Medicine. *Exercise Management for Persons with Chronic Diseases and Disabilities.* Champaign, IL: Human Kinetics; 1997.

* From Courneya, K. S., Mackey, J. R. and Jones, L. W. Coping with cancer. Can exercise help? *Phys. Sports Med.* 2000; **28**:49–73.

** Heart rate reserve = ((% intensity)(220 − age − heart rate at rest)) + heart rate at rest.

*** Peak heart rate = maximal heart rate obtained during an exercise test.

flexibility, aerobic capacity, body composition), however, a more vigorous exercise regimen would have to be adhered to.

Regular physical activity and exercise can result in positive improvements in health and fitness. Moderate amounts of physical activity can reduce the risk of certain types of cancer, heart disease, diabetes, and obesity. Resistance training can preserve or increase bone mineral density and increase muscle fiber area, strength, and power. Endurance training can reduce resting heart rate, improve blood lipid profiles, decrease blood pressure, and increase aerobic capacity. T'ai chi and yoga complement these programs by reducing stress, increasing flexibility, reducing falls, and increasing strength. The available evidence suggests strongly that physical activity and exercise can have a positive effect on morbidity and mortality, thus attenuating functional decline and increasing quality of life, which could lead to a more able old age.

FURTHER RESOURCES

Books

Chu, D. *Explosive Power and Strength.* Champaign, IL: Human Kinetics; 1996.

Goldenberg, L. and Twist, P. *Strength Ball Training.* Champaign, IL: Human Kinetics; 2002.

Coulter, H. D. and McCall, T. *Anatomy of Hatha Yoga: A Manual for Students, Teachers, and Practitioners.* Honesdale, PA: Body and Breath.

Videos

Santana, J. C. *Functional Training.* New York: Perform Better; 2001.

Santana, J. C. *The Essence of Stability Ball Training.* New York: Perform Better; 2001.

Johnson, M. *Tai Chi for Seniors: Self Healing Through Movement.* Mill Vally, CA Tai Chi for Seniors; 2001.

Johnson, J. A. (1999). *Power Tai Chi: Total Body Workout.* San Diego, CA: Goldhill Home Media; 1999.

On-line yoga classes available at http://www.yoga4realpeople.com

REFERENCES

1 Pratt, M., Macera, C. A. and Wang, G. Higher direct medical costs associated with physical inactivity. *Phys. Sports Med.* 2000; **28**:204–7.

2 US Department of Health and Human Services. Physical activity and health: a report of the Surgeon General. Atlanta, GA: US Department of Health and Human Services, Centers for Disease Control and Prevention, National Center for Chronic Disease Prevention and Health Promotion; 1996.

3 Chodzko-Zajko, W. J. The World Health Organization issues guidelines for promoting physical activity among older persons. *J. Aging Phys. Act.* 1997; **5**:1–8.

4 American College of Sports Medicine. *Guidelines for Exercise Testing and Prescription*. Philadelphia: Lea & Febiger; 1991.

5 Hakkinen, K., Kraemer, W. J., Newton, R. U. and Alen, M. Changes in electromyographic activity, muscle fibre and force production characteristics during heavy resistance/power training in middle-aged and older men and women. *Acta Physiol. Scand.* 2001; **171**:51–62.

6 Slaven L. and Lee, C. Mood and symptom reporting among middle-aged women: the relationship between menopausal status, hormonal replacement therapy, and exercise participation. *Health Psychol.* 1997; **16**:203–8.

7 Tran, M. D., Holly, R. G., Lasbrook, J. and Amsterdam, E. A. Effects of hatha yoga practice on health-related aspects of physical fitness. *Prev. Cardiol.* 2001; **4**:165–70.

8 Hu, F. B., Sigal, R. J., Rich-Edwards, J. W., *et al.* Walking compared with vigorous physical activity and risk of type 2 diabetes in women: a prospective study. *J. Am. Med. Assoc.* 1999; **282**:1433–9.

9 Ueda, M. and Tokunaga, M. Effects of exercise experienced in the life stages on climacteric symptoms for females. *J. Physiol. Anthropol.* 2000; **19**:181–9.

10 Colditz, G. A., Cannuscio, C. C. and Frazier, A. L. Physical activity and reduced risk of colon cancer: implications for prevention. *Cancer Causes Control* 1997; **8**:649–67.

11 Moore, D. B., Folsom, A. R., Mink, P. J., Hong, C.-P., Anderson, K. E. and Kushi, L. H. Physical activity and incidence of postmenopausal breast cancer. *Epidemiology* 2000; **11**:292–6.

12 Rockhill, B., Willett, W. C., Hunter, D. J., Manson, J. E., Hankinson, S. E. and Colditz, G. A. A prospective study of recreational physical activity and breast cancer risk. *Arch. Intern. Med.* 1999; **159**:2290–96.

13 Singh, M. A. Exercise comes of age: rationale and recommendations for a geriatric exercise prescription. *J. Gerontol. A Biol. Sci. Med. Sci.* 2002; **57A**:M262–2.

14 Owens, J. F., Matthews, K. A., Wing, R. R. and Kuller, L. H. Can physical activity mitigate the effects of aging in middle-aged women? *Circulation* 1992; **85**:1265–70.

15 Gilliat-Wimberly, M., Manore, M. M., Woolf, K., Swan, P. D. and Carroll, S. S. Effects of habitual physical activity on the resting metabolic rates and body compositions of women aged 35 to 50 years. *J. Am. Diet. Assoc.* 2001; **101**:1181–8.

16 National Center for Health Statistics. *Healthy People 2000 Review*. Hyattsville, MD: Public Health Service; 1997.

17 Nelson, M. E., Fiatarone, M. A., Morganti, C. M., Trice, I., Greenberg, R. A. and Evans, W. J. Effects of high-intensity strength training on multiple risk factors for osteoporotic fractures. *J. Am. Med. Assoc.* 1994; **272**:1909–14.

18 Hakkinen, K., Kallinen, M., Izquierdo, M., *et al.* Changes in agonist-antagonist EMG, muscle CSA, and force during strength training in middle-aged and older people. *J. Appl. Physiol.* 1998; **84**:1341–9.

19 Doherty, T. J., Vandervoort, A. A., Taylor, A. W. and Brown, W. F. Effects of motor unit losses on strength in older men and women. *J. Appl. Physiol.* 1993; **74**:868–74.

20 Larsson, L., Grimby, G. and Karlsson, J. Muscle strength and speed of movement in relation to age and muscle morphology. *J. Appl. Physiol.* 1979; **46**:451–6.

21 Skelton, D. A., Greig, C. A., Davies, J. M. and Young, A. Strength, power and related functional ability of healthy people aged 65–89 years. *Age Ageing* 1994; **23**:371–7.

22 Hagberg, J. M., Zmuda, J. M., McCole, S. D., *et al.* Moderate physical activity is associated with higher bone mineral density in postmenopausal women. *J. Am. Geriatr. Soc.* 2001; **49**:1411–17.

23 Layne, J. E. and Nelson, M. E. The effects of progressive resistance training on bone density: a review. *Med. Sci. Sports Exerc.* 1999; **31**:25–30.

24 Sale, D. G. Influences of exercise and training on motor unit activation. *Exerc. Sport Sci. Rev.* 1987; **15**:95–151.

25 Kelley, G. A., Kelley, K. S. and Tran, Z. V. Resistance training and bone mineral density in women. *Am. J. Phys. Med. Rehabil.* 2001; **80**:65–77.

26 O'Hara, R. B. and Baer, J. T. Effect of a culturally based walking program on blood pressure response in African-American women. *Med. Sci. Sports Exerc.* 2000; **32**:S313.

27 Okazaki, T., Himeno, E., Nanri, H. and Ikeda, M. Effects of a community-based lifestyle-modification program on cardiovascular risk factors in middle-aged women. *Hypertens. Res.* 2001; **24**:647–53.

28 McCartney, N., Hicks, A. L., Martin, J. and Webber, C. E. Long term resistance training in the elderly: effects on dynamic strength, exercise capacity, muscle, and bone. *J. Gerontol. A Biol. Sci. Med. Sci.* 1995; **50A**:B97–104.

29 Buskirk, E. R. and Hodgson, J. L. Age and aerobic power: the rate of change in men and women. *Fed. Proc.* 1987; **46**:1824–9.

30 Tanaka, H., DeSouza, C. A., Jones, P. P., Stevenson, E. T., Davy, K. P. and Seals, D. R. Greater rate of decline in maximal aerobic capacity with age in physically active vs. sedentary healthy women. *J. Appl. Physiol.* 1997; **83**:1947–53.

31 Eskurza, I., Donato, A. J., Moreau, K. L., Seals, D. R. and Tanaka, H. Changes in maximal aerobic capacity with age in endurance-trained women: 7-yr follow-up. *J. Appl. Physiol.* 2002; **92**:2303–8.

32 Green, J. S., Stanforth, P. R., Gagnon, J., *et al.* Menopause, estrogen, and training effects on exercise hemodynamics: the HERITAGE study. *Med. Sci. Sports Exerc.* 2002; **34**:74–82.

33 Blumenthal, J. A., Emery, C. F., Madden, D. J., *et al.* Cardiovascular and behavior effects of aerobic exercise training in healthy older men and women. *J. Gerontol. A Biol. Sci. Med. Sci.* 1989; **44**:M147–57.

34 Brown, D. R., Wang, Y., Ward, A., *et al.* Chronic psychological effects of exercise and exercise plus cognitive strategies. *Med. Sci. Sports Exerc.* 1995; **27**:765–75.

35 Dalsky, G. P., Stocke, K. S., Ehsani, A. A., *et al.* Weight-bearing exercise training and lumbar bone mineral content in postmenopausal women. *Ann. Intern. Med.* 1988; **108**:824–8.

36 Lan, C., Lai, J. S., Chen, S. Y. and Wong, M. K. 12-month Tai Chi training in the elderly: its effect on health fitness. *Med. Sci. Sports Exerc.* 1998; **30**:345–51.

37 Li, F., Harmer, P., McAuley, E., *et al.* An evaluation of the effects of Tai Chi exercise on physical function among older persons: a randomized controlled trial. *Ann. Behav. Med.* 2001; **23**:139–46.

38 Tran, M. D., Holly, R. G., Lasbrook, J. and Amsterdam, E. A. Effects of hatha yoga practice on health-related aspects of physical fitness. *Prev. Cardiol.* 2001; **4**:165–70.

39 Konar, D., Latha, R. and Bhuvaneswaran, J. S. Cardiovascular responses to head-down-body-up postural exercise (Sarvangasana). *Indian J. Physiol. Pharmacol.* 2000; **44**:392–400.

40 Ray, U. S., Sinha, B., Tomer, O. S., *et al*. Aerobic capacity and percieved exertion after practice of Hatha yogic exercises. *Indian J. Med. Res.* 2001; **114**:215–21.

41 Manchanda, S. C., Narang, R., Reddy, K. S., *et al*. Retardation of coronary atherosclerosis with yoga lifestyle intervention. *J. Assoc. Physicians India* 2000; **48**:687–94.

42 Li, F., Harmer, P., McAuley, E., Fisher, K. J., Duncan, T. E. and Duncan, S. C. Tai Chi, self-efficacy, and physical function in the elderly. *Prev. Sci.* 2001; **2**:229–39.

43 Van Deusen, J. and Harlowe, D. The efficacy of the ROM Dance Program for adults with rheumatoid arthritis. *Am. J. Occup. Ther.* 1987; **41**:90–95.

44 Wolf, S. L., Barnhart, H. X., Kutner, N. G., McNeeley, E., Coogler, E. and Xu, C. Reducing frailty and falls in older persons: an investigation of Tai Chi and computerized balance training. Atlanta FICSIT Group. Frailty and Injuries: Cooperative Studies of Intervention Techniques. *J. Am. Geriatr. Soc.* 1996; **44**:489–97.

45 Channer, K. S., Barrow, D., Osborne, M. and Ives, G. Changes in haemodynamic parameters following Tai Chi Chuan and aerobic exercise in patients recovering from acute MI. *Postgrad. Med. J.* 1996; **72**:349–51.

46 Starkey, D. B., Pollock, M. L., Ishida, Y., *et al*. Effect of resistance training volume on strength and muscle thickness. *Med. Sci. Sports Exerc.* 1996; **28**:1311–20.

47 Rutherford, O. M., Greig, C. A., Sargeant, A. J. and Jones, D. A. Strength training and power output: transference effects in the human quadriceps muscle. *J. Sports Sci.* 1986; **4**:101–7.

48 Santana, J. C. Machines versus free weights. *Strength Cond. J.* 2001; **23**:67–8.

49 Pollock, M. L., Franklin, B. A., Balady, G. J., *et al*. Resistance exercise in individuals with and without cardiovascular disease. Benefits, raltionale, safety, and prescription: an advisory from the Committee on Exercise, Rehabilitation, and Prevention, Council on Clinical Cardiology, American Heart Association. *Circulation* 2000; **101**:828–33.

50 American College of Sports Medicine. The recommended quantity and quality of exercise for developing and maintaining cardio-respiratory and muscular fitness in healthy adults. *Med. Sci. Sports Exerc.* 1990; **22**:265–74.

51 Herbert, R. D. and Gabriel, M. Effects of stretching before and after exercising on muscle soreness and risk of injury: systematic review *Br. Med. J.* 2002; **325**:468.

52 Gisolfi, C. V. Preparing your athletes for competition in hot weather. GSSI: Coaches' Corner 1996.

53 Pate, R. R. Tips on exercising in the cold. GSSI: Coaches' Corner 1996.

54 Reynolds, K. L., Harman, E. A., Worsham, R. E., Sykes, M. B., Frykman, P. N. and Backus, V. L. Injuries in women associated with a periodized strength training and running program. *J. Strength Cond. Res.* 2001; **15**:136–43.

55 Pollock, M. L., Gaesser, G. A., Butcher, J. D., *et al*. The recommended quantitiy and quality of exercise for maintaining cardiorespiratory and muscular fitness, and flexibility in healthy adults. *Med. Sci. Sports Exerc.* 1998; **30**:975–91.

56 Centers for Disease Control and Prevention. Unrealized prevention opportunities: reducing the health and economic burden of chronic disease. Atlanta, GA: Centers for Disease Control and Prevention; US Department of Health and Human Services; 2000.

3

Nutrition

Victoria S. Kaprielian, M.D., Gwendolyn Murphy, Ph.D., R.D.
and Cathrine Hoyo, M.P.H., Ph.D.

Normal healthy diet

Case: S.K. is a generally healthy 49-year-old woman who presents for a routine annual exam. She complains of occasional hot flushes and asks what she can do about them without taking hormones. She also has a family history of cancer in several relatives, so she wants to know what she should do with her diet to stay healthy.

A healthy diet is a concern of people of all ages. Having traditionally been in charge of feeding the family, women tend to be even more interested. Current dietary recommendations for women in the mid-life years focus in three main areas: caloric balance, fat intake, and calcium.

Balancing intake and output

Perhaps the most important characteristic of a healthy diet is balance – a balance of food types and a balance of intake and output. To maintain a stable weight, one must burn off as much as one has taken in. Therefore, a healthy diet is always connected closely with healthy levels of activity (see Chapter 2 for details on exercise).

Two models that are useful regarding the proper balance of food types are the Food Pyramid and the New American Plate.

The Food Pyramid, developed by the US Department of Agriculture (USDA), illustrates the healthy diet as based on a foundation of plant-based foods, including whole-grain complex carbohydrates and substantial amounts of vegetables and fruits. Meat and dairy products make up a smaller proportion, with fats and sweets being used only sparingly.

The New American Plate, developed by the American Institute for Cancer Research, simplifies this further. This model indicates that two-thirds or more of a dinner plate should consist of vegetables, fruits, whole grains and beans;

one-third or less should be animal protein. Most Americans eat more meat than their bodies can use. A 60–90-g portion (the size of a deck of cards) twice a day is more than adequate protein consumption when eaten with a balanced diet that includes grains, vegetables, and milk.

Limiting fat intake

In the average American diet, approximately 36% of calories come from fat. To reduce the risk of heart disease, the fat content of the diet should be limited to 30% or less. Some have taken this much lower (see Pritikin and Ornish diets, pp. 29). *To control cholesterol levels and heart disease risk, reduction in saturated fat intake is generally recommended.* Modifying the type of fat in the diet to replace saturated fats with polyunsaturated fat will reduce the risk of coronary artery disease.[1] Considering both heart disease and cancer risk, less than 10% of the total calories per day should come from each category of fat (saturated, monounsaturated, polyunsaturated). Providers should recommend use of low-fat dairy products, limited amounts of lean meats, and avoidance of added fats. For cooking, high monounsaturated oils (olive, canola) are preferable.

Adequate calcium

Menopausal women are at increased risk for osteoporosis, especially if they are Caucasian and/or thin. Cigarette-smoking and a positive family history increase the risk. While taking adequate calcium during the bone-building years (before age 30) is essential, calcium intake in later years is still important to slow the bone mineral loss that inevitably happens after menopause.

The best calcium source is dairy products. Three servings (glasses of milk, cups of yogurt, slices of cheese) provide the recommended daily allowance of 1000 mg. Some people feel that an even higher intake of calcium (up to 1500 mg/day) after the age of 50 is essential. Use of low-fat or fat-free dairy products enables one to achieve this without exceeding fat goals.

Many adults have some degree of lactose intolerance and are unable to eat this quantity of dairy products without abdominal discomfort, increased gas, nausea, and diarrhea. Individuals may need to experiment with different foods to assess their own level of tolerance. Whereas a cup of milk contains 11 g of lactose, a cup of yogurt contains only 5 g. Cheese and cottage cheese have high levels of calcium but are much lower than milk in lactose; they are often tolerated by people who are lactose-intolerant. Other options for lactose-intolerant individuals are listed in Table 3.1. Calcium is absorbed better from food than from tablets; taking supplements with meals can help increase absorption.

Vitamin D is needed for optimal calcium absorption and utilization. Milk in the USA is fortified with vitamin D, and people who get their calcium from

Table 3.1 Other options for lactose-intolerant individuals

Taking lactase supplements with ordinary dairy products
Using lactose-reduced or lactose-free dairy products
Using substitutes such as calcium-fortified orange juice and soy milk

Table 3.2 Proposed possible dietary alternatives to hormones

Soy products contain estrogen-like compounds called isoflavones
Extracts of black cohosh contain triterpene glycosides
Red clover contains isoflavones that are similar to those in soy products
Vitamin E

dairy products generally have an adequate intake. Individuals with limited dairy intake and who do not get year-round sun exposure may benefit from supplementation. Many calcium supplements now contain vitamin D as well.

Diet as therapy

Menopausal symptom control

With fewer women taking hormone replacement therapy due to recent evidence, more women are looking for alternatives to control menopausal symptoms, particularly hot flushes. Several possibilities have been promoted for this, with a variety of depth of evidence.

Soy products contain estrogen-like compounds called isoflavones. These are converted in the liver to substances similar to selective estrogen receptor modulators (SERMs) and have both agonist and antagonist activity at estrogen receptors. *Intake of soy protein may therefore be helpful in the short-term (two years or less) treatment of hot flushes associated with menopause* (evidence level C). Soy intake in the longer term may reduce serum cholesterol and protect against osteoporosis (evidence level C). Dietary soy intake may differ in biological activity from isoflavones in supplements (Table 3.2).[2,3]

Extracts of black cohosh contain triterpene glycosides, which have estrogenic activity. Black cohosh may be effective for short-term treatment of vasomotor symptoms (evidence level C). No studies have reported safety or efficacy beyond six months of use.[3] Black cohosh may cause significant gastrointestinal side effects.[2]

Red clover contains isoflavones similar to those found in soy products. There is conflicting evidence as to whether red clover has any effectiveness in reducing menopausal symptoms.[2] Vitamin E has also been suggested as an option for women with a history of estrogen-dependent cancers and who must avoid use of estrogenic substances.[4] Chasteberry (also known as Vitex), evening primrose oil, dong quai, and wild yams have not been shown to have significant effect in reducing menopausal symptoms and should not be recommended for this purpose.[2]

Cancer risk reduction

Many patients are interested in the possibility of reducing cancer risk through diet. The relationship between diet and cancer is controversial and an area of active research. A number of factors are worth considering.

Dietary factors that may increase risk
Alcohol has been associated with cancer of the mouth, pharynx, larynx, breast, esophagus, cervix, and liver. Women should limit intake of alcohol to no more than one drink per day (360 ml beer, 150 ml wine, 30 ml 100-proof spirits). Women who are at high risk for breast cancer may consider not drinking any alcohol. The combination of alcohol and tobacco use increases risk far more than either one alone.

Obesity is associated with increased risk of colon, breast, and endometrial cancers. Avoidance of excessive calorie intake and maintenance of normal body weight reduces this risk.

Randomized clinical trails have shown that high-dose beta-carotene supplements increase the risk of lung cancer in smokers. Rather than taking supplements, people should be encouraged to eat naturally occurring sources of beta-carotene in the form of fruits and vegetables.

Well-designed and conducted cohort studies have shown that meat is associated with colon cancer. Thus, one should avoid excessive consumption of red meats.

Meats cooked at high temperatures (such as broiled or grilled) contain heterocyclic amines. Rather than cooking at high temperatures for long periods, meats should be braised, steamed, poached, stewed, or microwaved. *Nitrates found in preserved meats are associated with colorectal and stomach cancer.* One should reduce the intake of meats preserved by smoke or salt. If preserved meats are eaten, then the meal should also contain vegetables and fruits that contain vitamin C and phytochemicals, which retard the conversion of nitrates to carcinogenic nitrosamines in the stomach.

Pickled foods and foods with high levels of salt have been associated with stomach, nasopharyngeal, and throat cancer. The best advice is to avoid excessive salt and pickled foods.

The foods listed in Table 3.3 have not been shown to be associated with cancer.[5]

Dietary factors that may decrease risk
An association exists between consumption of fruits and vegetables and decreased incidence of lung, oral, esophageal, gastric, and colon cancer.[5] One should eat five or more servings of fruits and vegetables per day. Food sources are superior to

Table 3.3 Foods not found to be associated with an increased risk of cancer

Aspartame
Bioengineered foods
Cholesterol
Caffeine
Fluoride
Food additives
Irradiated foods
Foods contaminated by pesticides and herbicides
Saccharin
Trans-fats

supplements. Tomatoes in particular (with a small amount of added fat) are thought to aid in cancer prevention.

A randomized controlled trial has shown that foods high in calcium help prevent colorectal cancer. Women over 50 years of age should consume at least 1200 mg/day of calcium.[6]

A deficiency of folate is associated with cancer of the colon, rectum, and breast. In the USA, many grain products are now fortified with folate. A diet that includes fruits, vegetables, and enriched grains should provide sufficient intake. Animal studies and one human study have shown that selenium deficiency is associated with lung, colon, and prostate cancer. If selenium supplements are taken, then the maximum dose should be 200 μg/day.[5]

Insufficient water intake is associated with bladder cancer. One should drink eight or more glasses of water per day to dilute bladder carcinogens.

Omega-3 fatty acids (found in fish oils and flax seeds) have been shown to suppress cancer formation in animals; it is theorized that they would do the same in humans, but there are no human studies that support this.

There is insufficient evidence to support the following foods/supplements for reduction of cancer risk: antioxidant supplements (including vitamins A, C, E), garlic, lycopene supplements, olive oil, organic foods, phytochemical supplements, soy products, and tea.[5]

The role of fiber in colon cancer prevention is controversial; at least one well-designed randomized controlled trial found no benefit of fiber supplements for reduction of adenomatous polyps of the colon.[7-9]

Weight concerns

Overweight and obesity

Case: M.B. is a 51-year-old female who presents asking for advice on how to lose weight. She is 160 cm tall and weighs 85 kg (body mass index, (BMI) = 33).

Table 3.4 Conditions in which weight loss is specifically recommended

To lower blood pressure in overweight and obese persons with high blood pressure
To improve plasma lipid levels in overweight and obese persons with dislipidemia
To lower blood glucose levels in overweight and obese persons with type 2 diabetes

She has been overweight all her life; everyone in her family is heavy. She has tried Weight Watchers, the Atkins diet, and several others diets. Sometimes she loses weight, but she always regains it. She wonders whether there's a way for her to really lose weight, or whether it's hopeless at this point in her life.

Obesity is one of the most important public health problems in the USA. The combined prevalence of overweight and obesity (defined as BMI greater than or equal to 25) in American adults is 59%.[10] The prevalence of obesity (defined as BMI greater than or equal to 30) increased 61% between 1991 and 2000, to almost 20% of all USA adults.[10]

Strong evidence supports an association between obesity and increased morbidity and mortality. Recent research has linked excessive weight and body fat to a "dysmetabolic syndrome," which includes diabetes, hypertension, and coronary artery disease.[11]

Little evidence exists from prospective studies on the effect of weight loss by obese individuals on long-term morbidity and mortality. Nonetheless, in developing evidence-based guidelines for the treatment of obesity, a National Heart Lung and Blood Institute (NHLBI) expert panel assumed that, for most adults, the beneficial effects of weight loss exceed the potential risks.[12] Weight loss is specifically recommended in the circumstances listed in Table 3.4 (all evidence level A).

The NHLBI guidelines recommend a two-step process of assessment and management. Treatment is recommended for patients with a BMI of 25–29.9 or a high waist circumference, and two or more risk factors.[10] Patients with a BMI of 30 or more should receive treatment regardless of risk factors. The initial goal for weight loss should be to reduce body weight by 10% from baseline (evidence level A). With success, further loss can be attempted, if warranted, based on further assessment. A combined intervention including caloric reduction, increased physical activity, and behavior therapy is recommended as most effective.

The key to weight control lies in the first concept of the normal healthy diet – balancing intake and output. In order to lose weight, one must burn off more calories than are taken in. If calories in (i.e. dietary intake) are fewer than calories out (energy expenditure through normal body maintenance and exercise), then the result will be weight loss. As long as the body's minimal requirements are met for protein, water, vitamins, and minerals, then reducing calories below maintenance level should allow for safe weight reduction.

This again raises the unbreakable link with activity levels: the less active a person is, the less they can eat without gaining weight. Physical activity is recommended as part of a comprehensive weight-control program because it contributes to weight loss (evidence level A), may decrease abdominal fat (evidence level B), increases cardiorespiratory fitness (evidence level A), and may help with maintenance of weight loss (evidence level C).[10] Encouraging patients to be physically active and to become more fit (no matter what their weight) is more efficient than to tell them to exercise in order to lose weight.

The simplest approach to caloric reduction is reducing portion size. Caloric deficits are additive over time; decreasing intake by only 50 calories per day (the equivalent of half a cookie) will result in loss of 4.6 kg over a year. The NHLBI panel recommended a deficit of 500–1000 kcal/day to achieve a weight loss of 0.5–1 kg per week (evidence level A). Simply taking in a little less at each meal can make a significant impact over time. Combining this with an increase in activity amplifies the effect.

Reducing excessive dietary fat can also help. Fat has more than twice the number of calories per gram of either protein or carbohydrate. By replacing fatty foods with less fatty foods, the number of calories is decreased even without appreciably decreasing the portion size. For example, half a cup of potatoes with one teaspoon of butter or margarine has about 110 calories; without the added fat (butter or margarine), the potatoes have only 65 calories. Reducing dietary fat alone, without reducing total caloric intake, is not sufficient to create weight loss (evidence category A).[10]

There are many other approaches to weight loss that are promoted widely, many promising dramatic results in a short time. Some of the most well known are listed below:

- The Atkins Diet is a restricted-carbohydrate, high-protein, and restricted-fat diet. This diet takes advantage of the ketosis that develops during starvation; the resulting anorexia reduces appetite. However, ketosis can also cause fatigue, constipation, and vomiting. Potential long-term side effects include heart disease, bone loss, and kidney damage. In addition, high-protein, low-carbohydrate diets tend to be low in calcium, fiber, and healthy phytochemicals. The proponents of this diet advise taking vitamin and mineral supplements to replace lost nutrients.
- The Pritikin Diet is a very-low-fat (15% of calories), high-fiber, vegetarian (or nearly vegetarian) diet combined with exercise. It claims to reduce serum cholesterol and prevent or reverse cardiovascular disease.
- The Dean Ornish Diet carries low fat even further, with only 10% of calories being obtained from fat. Again, it claims reduction of serum cholesterol and prevention of heart disease.
- The Grapefruit Diet claims that grapefruit contains a special fat-burning enzyme that is activated when half a grapefruit is eaten for each meal along with small amounts of other food. As with all single-nutrient diets, excessive

reliance on one food type leads to imbalance in nutrient intake, and deficiencies may develop over time. In addition, grapefruit has significant interactions with some prescription medications.

None of these diets has any well-documented evidence supporting its use.

Diet pills

Both prescription and non-prescription substances are marketed with the promise of helping people to lose weight. According to the NHLBI guidelines, weight-loss drugs should be considered as only part of a comprehensive treatment plan for patients with BMI over 30, or over 27 with accompanying obesity-related disease. *Weight-loss drugs should never be used without concurrent lifestyle modification efforts* (evidence level B).

The two drugs approved by the Food and Drug Administration(FDA) for long-term use are sibutramine and orlistat. Sibutramine is an appetite suppressant, working to promote weight loss by decreasing appetite or increasing the feeling of satiety. Orlistat is a lipase inhibitor; it works by reducing the body's ability to absorb dietary fat.

Many over-the-counter medications and dietary supplements are marketed with similar promises. Some pose significant health risks:

• Phenylpropanolamine was previously used in many over-the-counter weight-loss products. It was withdrawn from the US market in 2000 because of findings of increased risk of hemorrhagic stroke.
• Ephedrine-containing products are often marketed for weight loss. They are commonly labeled as "natural" or "herbal" and use common names for herbs as the source of active ingredients (ma huang, Chinese ephedra, Sida cordifolia). Reported adverse events range from tremor and headache to death. Stroke, myocardial infarction, chest pain, seizures, insomnia, nausea, and vomiting, fatigue, and dizziness were among the problems reported. Seven of the eight reported fatalities were attributed to myocardial infarction or cerebrovascular accidents.[13]

Other dietary supplements promoted for weight loss include conjugated linoleic acid, 7-keto-dihydroepiandrosterone (DHEA), and garcinia. There is insufficient evidence to support effectiveness of any of these for weight loss.

Weight-reduction diets alone usually do not result in maintenance of weight loss. Behavior modification, sustainable lifestyle changes, and exercise are usually required to maintain the new lower weight. A program consisting of dietary therapy, physical activity, and behavior therapy should be continued indefinitely (evidence level B).[10]

Eating disorders

Eating disorders are associated most commonly with younger women – teenagers and young adults. Anorexia nervosa rarely persists into later life, but without successful treatment it may be fatal. When anorexia does last into mid life, serious health consequences can arise due to prolonged malnutrition. These include heart failure, liver damage, and hypokalemia-induced arrhythmias.

In contrast, bulimia and binge eating can persist for years and may be associated with obesity. Purging is less common in mature women than in adolescents and may take different forms. Self-induced vomiting is unlikely to be continued into mid life and would likely result in severe dental damage if it were. *Laxative and diuretic abuse may be more likely in this age group.*

Underweight patients are easy to identify and question further about eating habits. Because many bulimics are normal weight or heavier, they are more difficult to recognize. Routine questions may be helpful in identifying patients for more targeted questioning, such as:

• Are you concerned about your weight?
• Do you ever binge or feel out of control when eating?

A positive response should trigger further assessment of intake, purging, exercise, and use of laxatives or diuretics.

Patients with eating disorders can often benefit from counseling, whether or not they are willing to attempt to "cure" their problem. True anorexia nervosa generally requires a multidisciplinary team approach to management. Some women, while not meeting strict criteria for anorexia, maintain an unhealthy fixation on weight and may over-restrict their intake. Providers can work with these patients to identify a healthy body weight and encourage a balanced, varied diet.

Diet and medical problems

Diabetes

Case: A.P. is a 47-year-old woman diagnosed with diabetes five years ago. She recently started on metformin and is tolerating it well. The need to start medication has motivated her to work on losing weight and controlling her disease. She wants to know what she should eat and not eat.

The recommended diet for people with diabetes follows all the same guidelines of a normal healthy diet.[14] The diet should contain carbohydrate, protein, and fat in reasonable proportions. Calories should be at a level that promotes a healthy weight, and the diet should be based on the intake of a variety of foods.

The major nutrient that affects blood sugar levels is carbohydrate in the form of sugar and starch, as found in grains, fruits, vegetables, sweets, and milk. *The total amount of carbohydrate consumed is more important than the source or type (evidence level A).* Sucrose, or table sugar, does not increase blood sugar any more than the same amount of starch, so sucrose can be substituted for other carbohydrates in the diet. There is no evidence to support the avoidance of concentrated sweets as long as total energy and carbohydrate levels are maintained. Non-nutritive sweeteners such as aspartame, saccharin, acesulfame potassium, and sucralose, are safe at normal levels of intake.

Protein, while an insulin stimulant, does not increase blood sugar in the amounts usually eaten. Hyperglycemia can contribute to increased protein turnover. However, since most adults eat much more protein than is required, there is no need for diabetics to increase protein intake beyond usual levels (evidence level B). For those with diabetic nephropathy, reduction of protein intake to 0.8 g per kilogram of body weight may slow the progression of renal disease (evidence level C).

Whereas dietary fat helps to modulate the absorption of glucose, saturated fat and cholesterol should be limited in the diet. Saturated fat in the diet stimulates low-density lipoprotein (LDL) cholesterol production, and people with diabetes are more sensitive than the general population to dietary cholesterol. Less than 10% of calories should come from saturated fats, and dietary cholesterol should be less than 300 mg/day. Some individuals may benefit from lowering intake further (7% saturated fat, 200 mg/day cholesterol) (evidence level A). Intake of trans fatty acids should be minimized (evidence level B).

Both reduced energy consumption and weight loss improve insulin resistance and blood glucose levels. In patients with impaired glucose tolerance, weight loss of 10–15% may be sufficient to hold off frank diabetes. Weight-reduction diets by themselves are unlikely to result in long-term weight loss. Lifestyle changes that include nutritional, behavioral, and exercise components can reduce weight by 5–7% in the long term. Reduced fat and calories, regular physical activity, and provider contact and support are recommended (evidence level A).

Early studies suggested a positive effect of dietary fiber on blood sugar levels.[14] Very large amounts are necessary to confer metabolic benefits, and it is not clear whether these outweigh the side effects of this intake. Individuals with diabetes do not need to consume more fiber than the general population (evidence level B).

Because diabetes may be a state of increased oxidative stress, vitamins may be of benefit. Placebo-controlled trials of antioxidants have failed to show a benefit and, in some cases, have raised concern about adverse effects. B-complex vitamins have been considered in the treatment of diabetic neuropathy, but benefit has not been established. Deficiencies of certain minerals (potassium, magnesium, zinc, chromium) may worsen carbohydrate intolerance. Benefit from chromium supplementation has been reported, but conclusions are limited by methodological issues in the studies. In all, there is no clear evidence of benefit from vitamin or mineral supplementation for women with diabetes, with the exception of calcium for osteoporosis prevention. Routine use of antioxidant supplements is not advised because of questions regarding long-term safety and efficacy (evidence level B).

Treatment of hypoglycemia is best accomplished with oral glucose or glucose-containing food. The addition of fat retards the absorption of the glucose and should be avoided. Adding protein to the treatment does not affect the glycemic response, nor does it prevent subsequent hypoglycemia. Ten grams of oral glucose will raise blood sugar levels by about 40 mg/dl over 30 minutes, and 20 g will raise blood sugar levels by about 60 mg/dl over 45 minutes.[15]

To give tailored information about dietary changes, one must first have a complete diet history. This is accomplished most easily by having the patient complete a three-day record, either at home or while waiting for the doctor. Small meals and snacks are preferable to large meals. Low fat (but not no fat) should be the goal. The New American Plate may be a helpful model. Sometimes, having the patient eat from a smaller plate helps in portion control. Patients should be encouraged to eat more fruits and vegetables but to restrict juice and sweetened drinks to no more than 0.25–0.5 l per day. Monounsaturated fats (such as olive or canola oil) should be used to replace saturated fats in cooking.

Heart disease

C.B. is a 58-year-old woman who presents for hospital follow-up. She is now four weeks after her first heart attack and still stunned that this happened to her. At hospital discharge, she declined cholesterol-lowering medication, saying she really doesn't want more drugs. She asks what she can do with her diet to reduce her risk of another heart attack.

Limitation of dietary fat intake may be helpful in controlling serum lipids and thereby reducing risk of progression of coronary artery disease. The type of fat is important.[1] Epidemiologic and other studies have documented strong correlation between saturated fat intake (as a percentage of calories) and coronary death rates. Replacing saturated fat with unsaturated fat is more effective than simply reducing total fat consumption in lowering heart disease risk.

A strong positive correlation between coronary disease risk and intake of trans fatty acids has been suggested. Avoidance of hard margarines and hydrogenated vegetable fats (often found in baked goods and convenience foods) is advisable. Polyunsaturated fats may have beneficial effects beyond improving lipid profiles. The lowest risk of coronary disease is seen with low intake of trans fats combined with a high proportion of polyunsaturated fats.

Monounsaturated fat intake is associated inversely with risk of heart disease. Coronary death rates are very low in Mediterranean populations that use olive oil as the primary source of fat. Canola oil, nuts, and avocados are other good sources. Omega-3 fatty acids (most commonly found in cold-water fish) prolong bleeding time, increase erythrocyte deformability, and decrease blood viscosity. Epidemiologic evidence links fish consumption to reduced cardio-vascular mortality. Omega-3 fatty acids have been shown to reduce mortality in patients who survived a heart attack within the past three months. In the Nurses' Health Study, women with a higher intake of omega-3 fatty acids had a lower risk of coronary disease.[16] The American Heart Association recommends fish intake (but not fish oil supplements) as part of a heart-healthy lifestyle.

Overall, there is good evidence to support increasing dietary fiber, vegetable, fish, and nut consumption.[17] Dietary intervention trials in general support the benefit of replacing saturated fat with unsaturated fat.

Soy protein intake has been found consistently to induce modest reduction of serum cholesterol. The US FDA and the American Heart Association now agree that 25 g per day of soy protein, in conjunction with a low-fat diet, may reduce the risk of heart disease. Fenugreek, a legume used as a supplement, has also shown cholesterol-lowering effects in preliminary studies.[17]

Antioxidants and folic acid are also potentially protective against coronary disease. The evidence on these, however, is inconclusive:

- *Vitamin E:* observational studies suggest a benefit, but controlled trials have not shown a protective effect against fatal myocardial infarction and are inconsistent regarding the effect on non-fatal myocardial infarction.[18] Doses of 100–800 IU/day may be useful for secondary prevention.
- *Vitamin C:* evidence from observational studies is inconclusive. Only one controlled study has investigated this, with neutral results.[18]
- *Folate:* non-clinical and observational evidence in support is extensive; results from controlled clinical trials have yet to be published. The US food supply is now fortified with folate (0.14 mg of folic acid per 100 g of cereal grain product since 1996).
- *Vitamin B12:* supplementation of B12 with folate consistently lowers homo-cysteine levels, and therefore may be beneficial.[18]
- *Vitamin B6:* in one study, the combination of folate, B12, and B6 reduced the rate of re-stenosis after intervention.[18]
- *Beta carotene:* available evidence weighs against use for this purpose.

While the available evidence is insufficient to recommend use of these vitamins for heart disease prevention, the known safety and low cost of these supplements have led some to recommend them until more evidence is available. Since there is still significant possibility of other protective components in foods that are not included in supplements, a heart-healthy diet, emphasizing fruits and vegetables containing antioxidants and B vitamins, is preferable.

Hypertension

C.C. is a 51-year-old woman with borderline hypertension. She's been success-ful in losing a few pounds, and her pressure today is 138/86 mm Hg. She's concerned because the nurse at work told her she needed to cut out all salt from her diet if she wanted to get her pressure down, but all the salt-free foods she's tried have been awful.

The connection between sodium and hypertension is not as strong as was once believed. The degree of salt sensitivity varies among patients. While moderation in salt intake (e.g. limiting cured meats, high-salt snacks, and processed foods) is advisable for all, strict sodium restriction is unnecessary for most patients. *Current recommendations limit salt intake to no more than 6 g/day (2400 mg or 100 mmol sodium).*[19]

About 40% of hypertensive individuals are salt-sensitive (defined as 10% or greater difference in blood pressure on low-sodium versus high-sodium diet). The major predictors of salt sensitivity are body weight, age, blood pressure, kidney function (creatinine level), and race (African-American). Sodium restriction may be warranted in patients with increasing obesity and blood pressure, although its effect is usually moderate, at best.

Blood pressure is a highly integrated response to interactions among various anions and cations. In particular, high intake of sodium chloride in conjunction with low dietary potassium, calcium, and/or magnesium increases the risk for hypertension.

Epidemiologic studies show an inverse relationship between potassium intake and blood pressure. The higher the sodium, the more effect potassium has on lowering blood pressure. Dietary sources of potassium include milk, fruits, grains, and vegetables. The less processed these foods are, the higher the potassium-to-sodium ratio. For example, potatoes, tomatoes, and milk have high potassium-to-sodium ratios whereas potato chips, ketchup, and cheese have high sodium-to-potassium ratios.

A meta-analysis of randomized controlled trials showed that the effect of calcium on blood pressure is small and inconsistent. However, it may act in conjunction with other nutrients to lower blood pressure. An increase in calcium consumption reduces blood pressure only in those with hypertension. The blood-pressure-lowering effects of magnesium are small and inconsistent. The Nurses' Health Study showed that women with a magnesium intake greater than 300 mg/day had a 23% reduction of risk for developing hypertension compared with women with a magnesium intake of less than 200 mg/day. The average dietary intake of magnesium is 300 mg/day.

The DASH (Dietary Approaches to Stop Hypertension) diet is high in fruits (five servings per day), vegetables (four servings per day), low-fat dairy products (two servings per day), whole grains, poultry, fish, and nuts, with small amounts of red meat. It has been shown to reduce systolic blood pressure by 5.5 mm Hg and diastolic blood pressure by 3.0 mm Hg. When the DASH diet was combined with low sodium intake, systolic blood pressure was reduced by 7.1 mm Hg in normotensive subjects and by 11.5 mm Hg in hypertensive subjects.[20]

Alcohol is a significant pressor agent. Heavy drinkers (more than 3 l of wine/day) have significantly more hypertension than those drinking less than 1 l of wine/day. Alcohol should be reduced to moderate amounts. Those with resistant or difficult-to-treat hypertension should discontinue alcohol intake. Hypertensive patients with optimal blood pressure control may be allowed light to moderate alcohol consumption. For a woman, this means less than 15 ml ethanol (360 ml beer, 150 ml wine, 30 ml 100-proof whiskey) per day, preferably consumed with meals.

Increased body weight, particularly abdominal obesity, is a major factor in blood pressure control. The combined effects of aging and weight gain may affect blood pressure more than either alone. A weight loss of 3.5–4.5 kg results in a reduction of systolic blood pressure of 5–5.8 mm Hg and a diastolic reduction of 3.2–7.0 mm Hg.

Vitamin C, fish oil, fiber, and the amino acid composition of the diet may affect blood pressure, but not as much as those factors listed above.[21] A diet that is high in fruits, vegetables, and low-fat dairy foods, in conjunction with moderation in sodium intake, is likely to improve blood pressure. These measures, coupled with weight loss and exercise, are the best non-pharmacologic treatments for hypertension.

Cancer

J.T. is recovering from a mastectomy for breast cancer and is about to undergo a course of chemotherapy. She's always been thin and is aware that she needs to keep up her intake so she doesn't lose too much weight. The stress has really hurt her appetite, and she's afraid the chemo will make it even more difficult for her to eat.

Malnutrition is the most frequently identified determinant of severity of illness and death among cancer patients.[22] Cancer patients with adequate nutrition have been shown to fare better in general, and specifically have a higher tolerance for side effects related to therapeutic interventions. Many factors determine the severity of side effects, including the type and location of the tumor, and the type, length, and dose of treatment.

Surgery
Pain often leads to anorexia and reduced fluid intake, subsequently causing weakness and fatigue. Excessive pain can also induce nausea, vomiting, and diarrhea, further depleting nutritional resources.

Radiation
While all cells exposed to radiation are affected, most normal cells can recover. The size of the radiation field, the total dose, and the number of treatments may

adversely affect nutritional status indirectly, through loss of appetite, or more directly, through damage to the gastrointestinal tract. Side effects typically start during the second or third week of treatment; most end two to three weeks after completion of therapy.

Chemotherapy

Side effects of chemotherapy include loss of appetite, changes in taste and smell, mouth tenderness or sores, nausea, vomiting, changes in bowel habits, fatigue, leukopenia, and weight gain. Many side effects of chemotherapy dissipate quickly. Their frequency and severity depend on initial nutritional status, type and dosage of chemotherapy, and other drugs and treatments given simultaneously.

Maintaining a balanced dietary intake helps storage of nutrients, decreases risk of infection, and accelerates healing and recovery. This will likely improve tolerance to treatment-related side effects. A diet high in protein will facilitate maintenance of weight and strength, tissue regeneration, and healing. Small and frequent feedings may be tolerated better than large meals. Multivitamin and mineral supplements can be used in addition to food intake. Adequate fluid intake must also be maintained to avoid dehydration. Adding unsaturated fat to a patient's diet may be appropriate if weight gain is desired. Fats are a concentrated calorie source, and the tastes and textures they add to foods may encourage increased intake.

Caloric needs are dependent on body size, age, and the level of physical activity. The formula suggested by the American Cancer Society in 2001 provides a rough guide: assuming light activity, caloric intake for underweight adults should be equivalent to the patient's weight in pounds multiplied by 18. For normal and overweight adults, recommended caloric intake can be estimated by multiplying the patient's weight by factors of 16 and 13, respectively.

Dietary interventions may be helpful in the management of side effects of cancer treatment. Considerations of the diet for the patient with cancer are included in Table 3.5.

Overall, frequent and small meals containing adequate protein and a moderate amount of fat are advisable. Good fluid intake is essential, and a multivitamin supplement may be considered.

Chronic lung disease

S.L. is 58 years old and a smoker since she was 13. She just cut back from two packs a day to one. She's experiencing more frequent acute exacerbations of her chronic bronchitis, and her recovery seems to take longer each time. She is worried that she seems to be losing more and more weight with each bout of bronchitis. She's read that fish oil is supposed to be good for your lungs, and wonders if there's anything she can do with her diet to help.

Table 3.5 Ways to improve diet of patients with cancer

If immune function is compromised, avoid uncooked meats, unpasteurized dairy products, raw vegetables such as sprouts, and herbal nutrient supplements.

Because fever expends considerable energy, adequate intake of carbohydrates, fats, and vitamins should be encouraged, especially during episodes of infection.

During chemotherapy treatments, meat often seems to have a very bad taste and smell for the patient. One way to counteract this is to use fruit or fruit juice when preparing or serving meat.

Dry mouth symptoms can be alleviated by rinsing with a saline mouthwash before meals. Mouthwash can be made from one teaspoon salt and one teaspoon baking soda added to about a liter of water. Commercial mouthwashes and alcoholic and acidic beverages can aggravate an irritated mouth.

For patients with mouth or throat soreness, bland, lukewarm, or cool foods can be soothing. Acidic, spicy, or salty foods may be irritating.

Drinking enough fluids will help to counteract the constipation often caused by analgesics. If the gastrointestinal tract is not too tender, then constipation may be alleviated by high-fiber foods such as whole-grain breads, raw fruit and vegetables, dried fruits, seeds, and nuts.

Diarrhea due to chemotherapy or radiation may be alleviated by a soft diet and avoidance of whole grains, legumes, dried fruit, and raw fruit and vegetables. Limiting intake of high-fat foods may also help.

Patients reporting difficulty in swallowing solids should be advised to drink thick fluids such as soups, high-calorie or -protein drinks, yogurt, ice cream, and milk shakes to meet the patient's nutritional needs.

The primary concern in vomiting patients is dehydration. Frequent fluid intake should be advised. Clear, light, and cool drinks may be tolerated better than icy or hot drinks.

An important aspect of nutrition during chemotherapy is that if the treatment causes an immediate negative gastrointestinal reaction (nausea, vomiting, or diarrhea), food eaten just before treatment may cause an aversion reaction thereafter. It is best, therefore, not to eat a favorite food just before chemotherapy.

One complication of chronic obstructive pulmonary disease (COPD) is malnutrition. Malnutrition, in turn, exacerbates COPD by leading to weakened respiratory muscles and compromised pulmonary function. As a result, COPD patients can become trapped in a cycle in which recurrent pulmonary infections lead to poor intake, and the malnutrition subsequently increases the susceptibility to infection.

Weight loss in COPD patients has been well documented. Reversing undernutrition has proven difficult, and nutritional supplementation programs have received mixed reviews.[23] A study in which supplementation was combined with rehabilitative exercise demonstrated a significant weight gain (albeit in fat mass) in the calorie-supplemented group.[24] Episodic weight loss may result from prolonged or recurrent cytokine production, which occurs during infections and exacerbations.[25]

In one study, short-term nutritional support of COPD patients improved muscle function by 10%–20% without a measurable change in cell mass.[26] Long-term nutrient supplementation improved nutritional status in some patients. Caloric supplements for at least two weeks resulted in improved pulmonary function, respiratory muscle strength, anthropometric measures, and functional exercise capacity. In a study of patients treated with 500–750 kcal/day above regular diet for eight weeks, 19 of 24 had increased weight gain. Lack of weight gain was associated with elevated inflammatory response.[27] Studies among hospitalized patients suggest that increased caloric input (1.7 times the resting expenditure) should balance the caloric input/output equation.[28]

Recent speculations suggest that foods rich in omega-3 fatty acids (found in fish oils, flax seed oil, green leafy vegetables, and olives) may benefit COPD patients therapeutically[29] because the presence of omega-3 fatty acids may displace inflammatory precursors such as arachadonic acid from cell-membrane lipids and lower the product of inflammatory eicosanoids.[28] In one large study, the risk of developing COPD was lower in smokers with a high intake of omega-3 fatty acids compared with smokers with a low intake of omega-3 fatty acids.[30] Daily recommended doses are 1800–3000 mg/day of combined docosahexaenoic acid(DHA) and eicosapentaenoic acid (EPA).[31]

In summary, encouraging increased caloric intake orally or prescribing additional calories parenterally is important. The intake should be adequate in protein, vitamins, and minerals. Carbohydrate should not be restricted, and supplemental omega-3 fatty acids may be beneficial.

Arthritis

N.L. is 55 years old. She's had problems with pain in her joints since her early 40s. Her biggest problem is her knees. It hurts to walk, so she's decreased her exercise and is gaining weight. Ibuprofen helps the pain, but it's starting to irritate her stomach. The man at the healthfood store recommended some supplements with glucosamine and chondroitin, and she asks you if they're worth trying.

There are multiple types of arthritis, with differing pathophysiologies. The nutritional issues vary with the type of joint disease.

The most common type of arthritis responsible for symptoms of the large, weight-bearing joints is osteoarthritis. The most common cause of this "wear and tear" arthritis is obesity. Patients who are overweight or obese, and who complain of pain in the knees and/or hips, should attempt to reduce to a healthy weight. A combination of calorie reduction and a regular pattern of non-impact exercise can be very helpful in reducing symptoms.

Gout is a metabolic disease in which acute joint inflammation is caused by uric acid crystals in synovial fluid. *Dietary strategies that reduce serum uric acid levels can be useful in decreasing the frequency of recurrences.*[32] Urate production for any individual appears to vary directly with body weight; hence, weight loss is recommended. Alcohol intake should be minimized. A low-purine diet can be helpful. Purine-rich foods include beer, shellfish, sardines, yeast, and bacon. Since endogenous urate production is increased with a high-protein diet, excessive protein intake should be avoided. Adequate fluid intake (2–3 l/day) is advisable to promote excretion of uric acid and reduce the formation of urate stones.[32]

Numerous supplements are promoted for help in controlling arthritis pain. Evidence varies as to their safety and efficacy.

Glucosamine appears to be safe and somewhat effective and may stimulate cartilage growth. Taken in doses of 1500 mg/day, glucosamine decreases symptoms of osteoarthritis with similar or fewer side effects than non-steroidal anti-inflammatory drugs (NSAIDs). A recent long-term study showed significantly less joint space loss over three years in patients treated with glucosamine compared with patients treated with placebo.[33] Most studies on glucosamine have involved arthritis in the knee; evidence is less consistent for osteoarthritis in the spine.

Chondroitin is often sold in combination with glucosamine, with a scarcity of evidence. Most of the studies on this, however, have been done on the injectable form, because it is not absorbed well from the gastrointestinal tract.

Omega-3 fatty acids reportedly affect prostaglandin production. Early studies evaluating fish oil in rheumatoid arthritis found modest but statistically significant improvements in a number of symptoms and functional indices. Improvement is generally not seen in less than 12 weeks, and full effect may not be reached until 24 weeks.[34]

Gamma-linoleic acid is found in evening primrose, blackcurrant, and other oils. The evidence for the usefulness of these in treating arthritis symptoms is inconclusive.[35]

Some have suggested that food reactions may contribute to the inflammatory processes in rheumatoid arthritis, and advocate elimination diets as part of a treatment regimen. Most studies, however, have been done on very small groups of patients, many studies being controlled inadequately. Food hypersensitivity appears to be a factor in a small minority of patients at most. Evidence is insufficient to recommend elimination diets for treatment of inflammatory arthritis.[34]

FURTHER RESOURCES

A comprehensive discussion of dietary issues of interest to mid-life women is beyond the scope of this chapter. Recommended resources for reliable information for patients and providers include the following (URLs accessed November 2002):

General dietary information: American Dietetic Association: http://www.eatright.org/
Weight control, diabetes, and other medical disorders: National Institute of Diabetes, Digestive and Kidney Disorders: http://www.niddk.nih.gov/health/ nutrition.htm
Dietary supplements: National Center for Complementary and Alternative Medicine: http://nccam.nih.gov/
Calcium: National Women's Health Information Center: http://www.4woman.gov/ faq/calcium.htm

REFERENCES

1 Hu, F. B., Manson, J. E. and Willett, W. C. Types of dietary fat and risk of coronary heart disease: a critical review. *J. Am. Coll. Nutr.* 2001; **20**:5–19.

2 Benz, J. D. Supplements for menopause. *Prescr. Letter* 2002; **9**:180911.

3 Taylor, M. Use of botanicals for management of menopausal symptoms. ACOG Practice Bulletin 2001, number 28. http://www.acog.org/from_home/publications/ misc/pb028.htm.Accessed October 2002.

4 Pritchard, K. I. Hormone replacement in women with a history of breast cancer. *Oncologist* 2001; **6**:635–62.

5 American Cancer Society. Common questions about diet and cancer. http://www3.cancer.org/docroot/ped/content/ped_3_2x_common_questions_ about_diet_and_cancer.asp?sitearea=ped. Accessed October 2002.

6 Baron, J. A., Beach, M., Mandel, J. S., *et al.* Calcium supplements for the prevention of colorectal adenomas. Calcium Polyp Prevention Study Group. *N. Engl. J. Med.* 1999; **340**:101–7.

7 Schatzkin, A., Lanza, E., Corle, D., *et al.* Lack of effect of a low-fat high-fiber diet on the recurrence of colorectal adenomas. *N. Engl. J. of Med.* 2000; **342**:1149–55.

8 Alberts, D. S., Martinez, M. E., Roe, D. J., *et al.* Lack of effect of a high-fiber cereal supplement on the recurrence of colorectal adenomas. *N. Engl. J. Med.* 2000; **345**:1156–62.

9 Michels, K. B., Giovannuci, E., Joshipura, K. J., *et al.* Prospective study of fruit and vegetable consumption and incidence of colon and rectal cancers. *J. Nat. Cancer Inst.* 2000; **92**:1740–52.

10 National Heart, Lung, and Blood Institute. Clinical guidelines on the identification, evaluation, and treatment of overweight and obesity in adults: the evidence report. NIH Publication no. 98–4083. September 1998.

11 Ramlo-Halsted, B. A. and Edelman, S. V. The natural history of type 2 diabetes: implications for clinical practice. *Prim. Care* 1999; **26**:771–89.

12 Lyznicki, J. M., Young, D. C., Riggs, J. A. and Davis, R. M. Obesity: assessment and management in primary care. *Am. Fam. Physician* 2001; **65**:2185–96.

13 Adverse events associated with ephedrine-containing products – Texas, December 1993–September 1995. *Morb. Mortal. Wkly Rep.* 1996; **45**:689.

14 American Diabetes Association. Position statement: evidence-based nutrition principles and recommendations for the treatment and prevention of diabetes and related complications. *Diabetes Care* 2002; **25**(supp 1):S50–60.

15 Cryer, P. E., Fisher, J. N. and Shamoon, H. Hypoglycemia (technical review). *Diabetes Care* 1994; **17**:734–55.

16 O'Mara, N. B. Fish and fish oil and cardiovascular disease. *Prescr. Letter* 2002; **9**:180510.

17 Gavagan T. Cardiovascular disease. *Prim. Care* 2002; **29**: 32–38.

18 Pearce, K. A., Boosalis, M. G. and Yeager, B. Update on vitamin supplements for the prevention of coronary disease and stroke. *Am. Fam.* Physician 2000; **62**:1359–66.

19 Keevil, J., Stein, J. H. and McBride, P. E. Cardiovascular disease prevention. *Prim. Care* 2002; **29**:66–96.

20 Appel, L. J., Moore, T. J., Obarzanek, E., *et al.* A clinical trial of the effects of dietary patterns on blood pressure. DASH Collaborative Research Group. *N. Engl. J. Med.* 1997; **336**:1117–24.

21 Whelton, P. K., He, J., Appel, L. J., *et al.* Primary prevention of hypertension: clinical and public health advisory from the national high blood pressure education program. *J. Am. Med. Assoc.* 2002; **288**:1882–8.

22 Rock, C. L. and Demark-Wahnefried, W. Nutrition and survival after diagnosis of breast cancer: a review of the evidence. J. *Clin. Oncol.* 2002; **20**:3302–16.

23 Ferreira, I. M., Brooks, D., Lacasse, Y., *et al.* Nutritional support for individuals with COPD: a metaanalysis. *Chest* 2000; **117**:672–8.

24 Schols A. M., Soeters P. B., Mostert. R., et al. Physiologic effects of nutritional support anabolic steroid in patients with obstructive pulmonary disease: a placebo-controlled randomized trial. *Am. J. Respir. Crit. Care Med.* 1995; **152**:1268–74.

25 De Godoy, I., Donahoe, M., Calhoun, W. J., *et al.* Elevated TNF production by peripheral blood monocytes of weight losing COPD patients. *Am. J. Respir. Crit. Care Med.* 1996; **153**:633–7.

26 Fiaccadori, E., Coffrini, E., Ronda, N., *et al.* A preliminary report on the effects of malnutrition on skeletal muscle composition in chronic obstructive pulmonary disease. In Ferranti, R. D., Rampulla, C., Fracchia, C. and Ambrosino, N. (eds.). *Nutrition and Ventilatory Function.* Verona, Italy: Bi and GI Publishers; 1992.

27 Schols, A. M. W. J., Slangen, J., Volovics, L., *et al.* Weight loss is a reversible factor in the prognosis of chronic obstructive pulmonary disease. *Am. J. Respir. Crit. Care Med.* 1998; **157**:1791–7.

28 Berry, J. K. and Baum, C. L. Malnutrition in chronic obstructive pulmonary disease: adding insult to injury. *AACN Clin. Issues* 2001; **12**:210–19.

29 Schwartz, J. Role of polyunsaturated fatty acids in lung disease. *Am. J. Clin. Nutr.* 2000; **71**(supp):393–6S.

30 Allen, J. The therapeutic use of fish oil.*Prescr. Letter* 1997; **4**:130624.

31 Smit, H. A., Grievink, L., Tabak, C. Dietary influences on chronic obstructive lung disease and asthma: a review of the epidemiological evidence. *Proc. Nutr. Soc.* 1999; **58**:309–19.

32 Cleland, L. G., Hill, C. L., and James, M. J. Diet and arthritis. *Baillieres Clin. Rheumatol.* 1995; **9**:771–85.

33 Reginster, J. Y., Deroisy, R., Rovati, L. C., *et al.* Long-term effects of glucosamine sulfate on osteoarthritis progression: a randomized, placebo-controlled clinical trial. *Lancet* 2001; **357**:251–6.

34 Darlington, L. G. Dietary therapy for arthritis. *Rheum. Dis. Clin. North Am.* 1991; **17**:273–85.

35 Barre, D. E. Potential of evening primrose, borage, black currant, and fungal oils in human health. *Ann. Nutr. Metabol.* 2001; **45**:47–57.

4

Psychosocial health promotion of mid-life women

Cathy Morrow

Introduction

The promotion of health in women during the mid-life years requires a knowledge base beyond the traditional biomedical one. This base extends considerably the boundaries with which many primary care providers are familiar, moving into psychological, economic, sociologic, and political realms. *A context for understanding the psychosocial issues that may enhance or detract from the quality of a given woman's life is critical to the respectful and thoughtful care that best serves the woman in need.* Appreciation of the developmental issues facing mid-life woman as they age and their particular relational context is critical to the provision of good medical care.

No woman's psychosocial health can be assessed or promoted in a vacuum. Gender expectations, socialization, caring, multiple roles, economic demands, perceived and actual supports, and ethnicity and race impact healthy functioning. Experienced providers appreciate the power of these issues on the perception and experience of wellbeing and recognize that time and attention paid to these matters is not wasted. Indeed, the relational work of provider–patient can itself be a powerful tool in the cause of health promotion.

A dilemma confronts the practitioner committed to evidenced-based medicine in the arena of psychosocial health and change. Unfortunately, there is no "evidence base" for such complex, intertwined issues of culture, race, class, identity, socialization, and gender roles, and their intersection with social, economic, and political realities. Data available from epidemiological, sociologic, and psychological studies are presented in this chapter to provide context from which the provider might go on to explore and understand the particular psychosocial issues confronting a given woman. This background knowledge base is, arguably, useful regardless of the particular concern and, potentially, essential in the interests of genuine health promotion.

Developmental issues for the mid-life woman

Women in the USA are presented with two predominantly negative scripts of the mid-life experience. One script is of a medicalized focus on menopause as a time of transition from a healthy, estrogen-rich time of life to the stage of inevitable health decline, with an attendant increased risk of heart disease and osteoporosis. The other readily available scenarios are social descriptions of an empty nest, abandonment for the woman, or that of a useless, used-up "fertility has-been."[1] Both of these views are in contrast with the repeated observations that women feel better about menopause, and themselves, after having traversed it.[2,3] Considerable sociocultural variation in attitude toward the experience of menopause exists.[4,5] Yet, *overall, women have positive associations with mid life as a time to take stock and renew.* Primary care providers have the opportunity to explore these beliefs with their patients and educate them about what is actually known about wellbeing during mid life.

The primary task of mid life, according to the Eriksonian model,[6] is for generativity to win out over stagnation or self-absorption. While this stage has been described in terms of raising and caring for children, the process is symbolic of an ability to look beyond one's own needs to the wellbeing of others, marked by a concern for future generations and the ability to give without expectations of reciprocity. Generative activities may include teaching, mentoring, writing, social activism, or contributing to society in any number of ways. Stagnation is the opposite – caring for no one and being self-absorbed. The Ericksonian model is rooted in a paternalistic world view, as are virtually all of the developmental models.

Women in this culture, however, are typically confronted with very different challenges. Socialized to be the carer in any group and stressed because many women are employed outside of the home, mid-life women have their greatest problems concerning overextension. Women are socialized to multi-task and to be the "care experts," often at the expense of other aspects of their own wellbeing. Thus, the focus of providers' work with mid-life women may be to support them in pulling back from their habitual and socially sanctioned roles to allow them to take time for themselves. Women often need to be given permission to rebalance their time and energy to allow more time for introspection and the self-knowledge that will lay the foundation for change and adaptation to inevitable transitions ahead.

Health behaviors and self-care

The opportunity for mid-life women is to make lifestyle changes that will have significant effect on the development of physical disease, such as diabetes, osteoporosis, osteoarthritis, and coronary artery disease. In addition, many of these same behaviors will have a positive impact on life experience.

Women know which actions promote wellbeing and disease prevention. One study of women aged 49–55 found that there is a belief that changing health behaviors, such as smoking, diet, and physical activity, will reduce their risks of cardiovascular disease and osteoporosis.[7] Lists of reported self-care behaviors include everything from the well-documented effects of nutrition, physical activity, and social interactions to less studied behaviors such as solitude.[8]

Unfortunately, knowledge does not necessarily translate into action, and there are many social factors that constitute barriers to such self-care. One of the most persistent associations with non-participation in healthy behaviors is low socioeconomic status, again burdening this already at-risk group.[9] While most literature on health behaviors and self-care reports on white, middle-class women, one study that looked intentionally at physical inactivity in an ethnically and racially mixed population found multifaceted barriers, ranging from care-giving role demands to specific attributes of one's neighborhood.[10]

Physical activity is an excellent marker of health behaviors because it is well established to be beneficial in many domains and, in theory, has no barriers to access. While providers can not change the patients' demographics, we can support general behaviors and activities specific to mid life that have been shown to enhance wellbeing with a sensitive eye toward the realities of the individual woman's life.

Self-knowledge

The process of taking stock or life review is a normal and integral part of the activities of mid life.[11] This ongoing transformation of one's identity in response to experience becomes more favorable through the lifespan; this kind of reflection can have a positive effect.[12]

Many different terms are applied to self-knowledge in the social science literature, each of them capturing a different aspect. Self-concept includes learned beliefs, attitudes, and opinions that a person holds to be true about themselves. This is the basis for motivated behavior.[13] Self-concept is linked closely to self-esteem, which refers to how one feels about or values oneself. A third concept is identity, which is the process of making meaning out of one's experience.[14]

Encouraging patients to find time to explore the arena of self can be very powerful at mid life. Techniques such as journaling or self-help books can be offered. *Longitudinal evidence has found that an individual who uses life review to first set goals and then make desired life changes is likely to experience greater wellbeing.*[15]

Body image is part of one's self-concept and continues to be a significant issue for women in mid life. Commonly associated with body image is an unhealthy preoccupation with physical appearance and, in particular, weight; this is the plague of many young women and teens. However, how this issue is handled in middle-aged and older women is inconsistent. While dieting and excessive concern about weight in the old can be associated with poor nutritional status, a healthy investment in one's appearance can be associated with higher self-esteem and life satisfaction.[16]

A different and, for many, a new dimension in one's relationship to one's body is predictable in mid life; that is the experience of physical limitations or vulnerability. The years between 40 and 65 are the time when most women will first experience physical restrictions and discomfort. *Visual changes and the experience of musculoskeletal pain are early and predictable reminders of the aging of women's bodies.* One study in Sweden, which interviewed middle-aged individuals (53–63 years old) at intervals over the subsequent 24 years showed that 21.8% had musculoskeletal pain at every interview, a percentage that was more persistent and severe in women than men.[17] While women live longer than men, their risk of chronic disease is greater.

Social roles

The interaction between self-concept and social roles (paid worker, parent, spouse or partner) is less important than might be expected but is significant for single women and women who are employed full-time.[18] Women with paid employment have better health status.[19] However, the literature on multiple roles is approached from a gendered set of assumptions. Because woman's primary role throughout the ages has been the primary homemaker and nurturer, the effect on women of being in the workplace was initially studied from the perspective of "role strain" or an assumption that the impact was negative. Eventually, the opportunity for multiple roles to provide opportunities to promote growth and functioning has also been acknowledged and explored.[20]

In addition, there has been an acknowledgement that the home is not a "stress-free sanctuary."[21] Work based on the National Survey of Midlife Development in the United States (MIDus) has looked at a more ecological model that considers the potential for both negative and positive "spillover" to occur in both directions, family on work and work on family.[22] The specific attributes of jobs, such as sense of control, hours worked per week, job pressures, and supports at work, and specific attributes of family life and the life situation of the individual all contribute to the relationship. For women in particular, the strongest association was a positive spillover from work to family.

Exploring the specific meaning of work to one's patients is essential. Helping to identify both the stresses and opportunities for growth, and how those features interact with personal or family demands and resources, is important.

In a follow-up study, positive spillover from work to family was associated with better physical and mental health.[23] The interaction and significance of multiple roles for women are complex, and positive role attributes outweigh the stressful ones.[24] Most women do not work "out of choice," but have the same financial need for employment as men.[25] Increasingly, some women are forgoing the roles of partner, mother, and homemaker and making their occupation the focus of their life.

Generational identity

Considering life roles and other aspects of a woman's mid life in the context of her generational cohort is important. Sociocultural expectations for women have changed dramatically from the experiences of women who are part of the pre-boomer or "silent generation" (born before and during World War II) to baby boomers (born between 1946 and 1964). Seventy-six and a half million women were born in the USA during that period, creating the largest demographic cohort in the country.[26]

Significant changes have resulted in women arriving at mid life better educated, more assertive, and with a realistic expectation of a longer life and a greater sense of the importance of their work and personal level of achievement.[27] The changes brought about by the women's movement and other dramatic cultural changes of the 1960s and 1970s have benefited and stressed women in multiple ways, including forcing them to critically define and create new identities. As is always true, these positive opportunities are more available to women of affluence, majority status, and heterosexual identity.

Relational theory

A relational theory of women's development, described by several authors,[28–30] provides an excellent anchor from which to understand the challenges that may face the mid-life woman as she ages. This theory holds that a woman's development must be understood in the context of attachment, relationship, and mutuality. *Autonomy is achieved through connection to others, rather than through separation or detachment.* Those forces that serve to foster continued connectedness, even in the face of loss, will, thereby, promote health and wellbeing. Concomitantly, those forces that sever connection, such as those frequently associated with aging, may lead to illness. Yet, the specific meaning of these "losses" must be kept in perspective; the converse also may well be true. With some disconnections, there is new found independence, freedom, or potential for change that was previously unexplored.

Family structure and care-giving

The multiple developmental issues confronting the mid-life woman must be understood simultaneously within the relational contexts in which the majority of women live. The mid-life years extend across a spectrum of time that may encompass a broad section of the human lifecycle. In aggregate, the ages from 40 to 65 may include mothering an infant child (7.9/1000 live births in 2000 were to women aged 40 years or older[31]) and/or partner loss (14.8% of adult women in the USA in 2000 lived alone)[32]. The new mother at age 40 has substantially different concerns than the 60-year-old confronting a serious illness in a partner.

Though the lifecycle stage may range widely across the mid-life age span, the status and roles of women in modern Western culture are remarkably similar in terms of social construct. Over 90% of women in the USA marry at least once in their lifetime.

Despite a divorce rate of 50%, 75% of those who divorce remarry, though remarriage rates are lower for African-American and Hispanic women compared with European American women.[33] Despite increases in the number of women who choose childlessness, the rate of bearing at least one child is 90% and an additional 4% of the population adopt children.[34]

In 2000, 80% of adult women lived with relatives, including a partner and their children. Approximately 54% of women are married. One-third of the 80% live with their children but without a spouse or partner. Single motherhood, whether resulting from choice, divorce, separation, death, or never marrying, is remarkably common in the USA, comprising 12% of the nationwide adult female population. The composition of US households has been relatively stable in the years between 1995 and 2000.[35]

Women have substantial roles as care-givers for family members, with a disproportionate burden falling on lower-income women. Overall, approximately 26% of US families currently have elder parent care responsibilities, and this number is expected to increase substantially to roughly 60% over the next decade.[36] In 1998, 9% of women were caring for a disabled or sick relative, with 43% providing more than 20 hours per week. Fifty two percent of those had incomes of less than $35 000 per year, while only 29% of those with incomes greater than $35 000 had such responsibilities. Lower-income women were also significantly more likely to live with the relative for whom they were providing the care.[37]

There were more than 2.4 million grandparents primarily responsible for their grandchildren's care in the USA in 2000; 62% of these carers were grandmothers. *Grandparents raising grandchildren are more likely to be in poor health, have multiple chronic health problems, and be clinically depressed than those without this additional burden.*[38]

Relational aging

The many roles women fulfill in the family and culture may transition over the mid-life years. There is no distinct orderly sequence for this series of transitions, because they are dependent upon the individual woman's life circumstances. Shifting demographics in modern Western culture have altered norms for ages of partnering, marriage, childbearing or choosing not to have children, and entering or leaving the workplace. As a woman enters the mid-life years, she may progress in orderly fashion through several transitions of job stabilization or promotion, launching children, menopause, caring for aging parents and caring for an aging partner. However, there may be significant mixing of these lifecycle events at any one given period of time.

Clearly, *the collision of several major life transitions into a concentrated period of time puts the woman at risk for many stress-related symptoms, such as fatigue, irritability, mood swings, sleeplessness, weight changes, and generally poor self-care.* Prolongation of these stressors may increase the likelihood of genuine anxiety and depressive disorders and medical illnesses that require medical and/or psychological intervention. Anticipatory guidance by the provider sensitive to the multiplicity of roles and transitions facing a given woman may prevent serious negative outcomes or at least support more intentional coping strategies. Reminders about self-care are important. Perhaps more important is the respectful line of inquiry about the transitions that a given woman is facing, and empathic listening with genuine interest may be the best intervention of all.

Aging children

The "empty nest syndrome" is a period of transition that is well described and with several hundred websites devoted to the idea.[39, 40] However, there is little scientific evidence to support the notion that such a syndrome exists. Although traditionally defined as feelings of sadness, grief, depression, and loss as children prepare to accomplish their own developmental task of leaving home, most women accomplish this transition with little long-term negative effect. Feelings of loss, fear for the child's safety, and anxiety about the child's adaptation to their new life are quite common. Many women describe this transition as a bittersweet time, proud of their children's accomplishments and abilities to move on into adulthood but grief for the ending of this phase of their own life and reminded, inevitably, of their own aging.

Women who have been engaged intensely in their children's lives may experience a sense of having less meaning in their life, particularly if they do not have meaningful work, supportive partners, and connections to community supports and involvements that absorb them.[41]

Ideas about the impact of "empty nests" are embedded deeply in the culture and in the highly socialized views of women. Norms for the age of departure of children, reasons for departure, and connectedness post-departure are influenced strongly by the socioeconomic, ethnic, and individual family system from which the young adult departs. The assumptions that women's children leave home to go to college are held by many healthcare providers, yet the reality for women and their families may be quite different.

Similarly, assumptions about the departure of children as a loss, though encountered frequently, may be quite inaccurate. In an Australian study of more than 400 women over nine years, in the first year after the last child departed there was overall improvement in women's positive mood and sense of total wellbeing, reduction in negative mood, and reduction in the number of "daily hassles."[42] Many women describe this period as a time of new found independence and freedom, with fewer responsibilities and an opportunity for exploring different life options. The quality of relationship between mother and child will impact this transition as well, with evidence of those who have developed and subsequently maintain good relationships transitioning with the least distress on all sides.[43]

External stressors in any given woman's life may affect this time of transition. Single mothers who have been the sole parent of a leaving-home child may find this period of time particularly intense and painful. Women who depend on their child's presence for substantial income through child support, social security, or other benefits may be at special economic risk. Handicapped or chronically ill women may depend on the presence of children for some measure of physical support and care, complicating the normal leave-taking process. Women who have been victims of domestic violence or abuse, or who live with an alcoholic or abusive partner, may depend on the presence of children as buffers, leaving them more vulnerable. Mother and child may be at risk in any of these circumstances. Provider knowledge of family structure and supports, well in advance of expected normative departures, can facilitate helpful referrals for resources, supports, and the psychological readiness needed on the part of the mother to allow for this critical letting go.

The reverse phenomenon – the return of the adult child to the home – may be a more stressful and difficult adaptation for mid-life women. Known in popular culture as "boomerang kids,"[44] there is a trend of higher numbers of children aged 25–34 living at home, though data are limited and more likely to be reported in popular lay literature than studied. Predictors of a child returning home after leaving previously are change in marital status such as divorce, pursuing further educational opportunities, financial constraints, and initial reason for leaving home.[45] Though the stressors inherent in adapting to the returned presence of an adult child seem obvious, in the Australian study the only negative finding was a trend toward reduced frequency in sexual activity; no mood changes were found.[42] The individual circumstances of the family leading to a boomerang child will be most relevant in anticipating positive or negative health effects for a given woman.

Aging parents

Between seven million and 52 million people are involved in formal and informal care-giving to disabled adults, elderly parents and friends, depending on criteria and definitions of care-giving. Seventy-five percent of the providers of this care are women. Studies examining men in care-giving roles also show that even in settings with higher rates of male involvement, women spend 50% more time providing care. The average age of women providing family care ranges from 43 to 46 years.[46] The *burden of care provision for family members (and friends) beyond the child-raising years falls squarely and heavily on the backs of mid-life women.* Many social and cultural expectations perceive care-giving as an extension of child rearing and assume, without inquiry, that this is a task falling naturally to women, particularly in certain ethnic groups. Asian-Americans provide care for parents at the highest rates (42%), with Hispanic (34%) and African-Americans (28%) in the middle, and Caucasian Americans (19%) at the lowest rates; the person most likely to be providing care is a daughter.[47]

Women in mid life providing care to elderly parents or friends have a significantly higher risk of depression and anxiety, and struggle with feelings of being overwhelmed, worried, frustrated, and sad.[48] Care-givers use prescription drugs for depression, insomnia, and anxiety at approximately two to three times the rate of the general population.[49] About 50% of care-givers provide care without any outside assistance, and only 10–20% of family care-givers use formal services through agencies.

Care-giving is not a short-term proposition: the average duration of care is 4.5 years. Despite the grimness of the statistics, care-givers also describe overwhelming feelings of love, being valued and appreciated, and proud of the work they are doing. Successful care-giving relationships correlate with strong social support and networks, mutuality of support and shared care-giving with partners or spouses, good family communication, role flexibility, higher income, good health on the part of the care-giver, and ongoing community and church/spiritual involvement.[50,51] *The ability to acknowledge vulnerability and request help is key to successful care-giving.* Isolation may heighten risks for declining mental and physical health on the part of care-givers. Rural and poor women with less access to resources will be at higher risk than their more resource-rich counterparts.[52]

The provider concerned with health promotion will recognize the health hazards inherent in significant care-giving responsibility. Knowledge of community resources, respite care alternatives, and ongoing reassessment of the burdens and costs of such care should be offered to the mid-life woman.

Recognition that risks to the woman's health will differ, depending on her individual vulnerability, resources, and ability to seek help when needed, is essential. Concerns about her own aging and mortality may surface during the period of care-giving and may intersect with some of the more traditional mid-life developmental tasks, such as mid-life review, assessment of accomplishments and goals, and career stabilization or change. The care-giving role may overwhelm a given woman and impair her ability to accomplish these or other personal tasks of value. Helping to provide a supportive framework and assisting in solution-finding is essential. *An important role for primary providers in these settings may be permission-giving: the encouragement and support to say no, to ask others for help, to admit that the burden is too large, or simply to take a day off.*

Aging partner/spouse

Many of the same principles and challenges inherent in care-giving apply, regardless of whether the cared-for person is a disabled child, a parent, or a partner or spouse. The aging of a partner and the development of serious illness, dementia, or diminished functioning from previously high levels can pose particular stresses for women. Increased financial vulnerability, loss of quality of relationship with a beloved companion, recognition of one's own mortality and potential for illness, shift in relationship from one of equity to dependence, and many other changes within the relationship and the larger community can disturb a woman's equilibrium substantially. Uncertainty, anxiety, and fear about the future may become more dominant themes. Genuine financial changes such as loss of an income can put aging partners at major financial risk. If the woman has other significant caring responsibilities, then illness in a partner can become overwhelming. Women in households where alcohol, abuse, or mental illness prevail, or where the woman is the primary breadwinner, will be particularly vulnerable.[53]

Potentially, the mid-life woman confronting the serious illness of her partner is at high risk for depression, anxiety, substance abuse, and worsening of her own health. Yet, studies do not report uniformly that all care-givers decline in wellbeing. Increased expressions of tenderness toward the care-giver, preserved sexual relations, and limited change in the overall atmosphere of a marriage have been reported even three to five years after the onset of dementia in a partner.[54]

For most mid-life women, partners of similar age will not experience disabling illnesses requiring ongoing caring; rather, they will confront normal aging health declines in concert with each other. Relationships that are defined by strong support, affection, problem-solving, mutuality, caring, and shared life values will thrive and often strengthen through mid-life years.[55] Focus on the relationship, family, friends, and community may become more predominate as work and career issues are stable or deemed less critical.

Attitudes about care-giving and care-giving roles are embedded deeply in the socialized narratives of the women who provide care. Providers trained in a dominant Western medical culture, in which autonomy is valued highly and dependency seen as a negative burden, must be cautious to recognize that in a multicultural world, other values of family and relationship may prevail. It should be appreciated that the level of stress or satisfaction derived from a caring experience will depend upon, to a greater or lesser extent, the extent of socialization provided by the carer's culture, the life narrative, and the unique family dynamics.[56] Exploring with a woman her ideas and understanding about caring roles with interest rather than judgment, and listening empathically rather than "problem-solving", may facilitate the woman's health and growth in the face of caring challenges.

Conclusion

This chapter, given its interest in health promotion, has focused on the challenges and stresses confronting women in mid life in hopes of facilitating the identification of risk factors that may impair health. However, it must be emphasized that, for many women, the mid-life years will be a period of significant pleasure. Freed of the demands of raising children, and with more time to explore personal interests, hobbies, and community involvement or embark on new educational or work-related pursuits, many women experience the mid-life years as genuinely positive and regenerative. Factors that have been identified as predictive of feelings of wellbeing in mid life include stable finances, having a confidante or group of women friends, good health, high self-esteem and low self-denigration, goals for the future, a positive life narrative, and positive mid-life role models.[57] This particular study examined white women in New York City and may well not be generalizable to women whose cultural narrative does not focus as sharply on individual success and achievement. Women of cultural backgrounds with strong focus on family and community, rather than individual autonomy, may be more likely to have ongoing strong social supports and, in fact, enjoy status and respect as aging women, rather than traditional perceptions of loss and diminishing value dominating. The primary provider caring for the wellbeing of aging women can facilitate these positive cultural views by their own approach and respect for the numerous psychosocial issues that are central to health.

Implications for work with mid-life women

The medical orientation of training has been to approach life stages that are marked by biological events, such as birth and menopause, as pathological

Table 4.1 Psychosocial factors to explore when caring for mid-life women

Assess life stage as opposed to chronological age
Explore beliefs about mid life
Identify care-giving roles and their meanings
Appreciate the multiple spheres of work (home, job, community, etc.) and how each
    one brings rewards and stressors
Review self-care behaviors (exercise, diet, social supports, rest, spirituality,
    reflection)

processes that need to be diagnosed and treated rather than from a stance of observation, coaching, and support. The current generation of mid-life women is the group that revolutionized the practices consistent with what we know about the importance of relationships for women in development and health. Supporting women in adopting behaviors and attitudes that have been associated with greater health and longer life can take place best in the context of a provider–patient relationship, which includes the frequent discussion of psychosocial features of that woman's life experiences. We may be in the midst of an equally profound change in the content of healthcare in mid life. The ready availability of medical information to the public on the Internet only reinforces this transformation. As literature grows, revealing the significance of the patient-centered approach to health outcomes,[58,59] providers have a mandate to employ patterns of communication that are empowering and elicit the patients' ideas and opinions. This model of working with patients is in concert with literature on motivating change and even more significantly consistent with what we know about the importance of relationships for women in development and health.

Supporting women in adopting behaviors and attitudes that have been associated with greater health and longer life can take place best in the context of a provider–patient relationship that includes the frequent discussion of psychosocial features of that woman's life experience (Table 4.1).

REFERENCES

1 McQuaide, S. Women at midlife. *Social Work* 1998; **43**:21–31.
2 Dennerstein, L., Smith, A. and Morse, C. Psychological well-being, mid-life and the menopause. *Maturitas* 1994; **20**:1–11.
3 Avis, N. E. and McKinlay, S. M. A longitudinal analysis of women's attitudes toward the menopause: results from the Massachusetts Women's Health Study. *Maturitus* 1991; **13**:65–79.
4 Sampselle, C. M., Harris, V., Harlow, S. D. and Sovers, M. Midlife development and menopause in African American amd Caucasian women. *Health Care Women Int.* 2002; **23**:351–63.

5 Adler, S. R., Fosket, J. R., Kagawa-Singer, M., *et al.* Conceptualizing menopause and midlife: Chinese American and Chinese women in the US. *Maturitas* 2000; **35**:11–23.

6 Erickson, E. H. *Childhood and Society*. New York: WW Norton & Company, Inc., 1959.

7 Hunter, M. S. and O'Dea, I. Perception of future health risks in mid-aged women: estimates with and without behavioral changes and hormone replacement therapy. *Maturitas* 1999; **33**:37–43.

8 Hartweg, D. L. Self-care actions of healthy middle-aged women to promote well-being. *Nurs. Res.* 1993; **42**:221–7.

9 Calnan, M. Patterns in preventive behavior: a study of women in middle age. *Soc. Sci. Med.* 1985; **20**:263–8.

10 King, A. C., Castro, C., Wilcox, S., Eyier, A. A., Sallis, J. F. and Brownson, R. C. Personal and environmental factors associated with physical inactivity among different racial-ethnic groups of U.S. middle-aged and older-aged women. *Health Psychol.* 2000; **19**:354–64.

11 Stewart, A. J. and Ostrove, J. M. Women's personality in the middle age. Gender, history and midcourse corrections. *Am. Psychol.* 1998; **53**:1185–94.

12 Demo, D. H. The self-concept over time: research issues and directions. *Ann. Rev. Sociol.* 1992; **18**:303–26.

13 Huitt, W. Self-concept and self-esteem. http://chiron.valdosta.edu/whuitt/col/regsys/self.html.

14 Kegan, R. *In Over Our Heads*. Cambridge, Ma: Harvard University Press; 1994.

15 Stewart, A. J. and Vandewater, E. A. "If I had to do it over again . . .": midlife review, midcourse corrections, and women's well-being in midlife. *J. Pers. Soc. Psychol.* 1999; **76**: 270–83.

16 Weiller, F. D. Facing middle age: women, aging and the loss of youthful physical appearance. *Diss. Abstr. Int. B: Sci. Eng.* 2000; **61**:1115.

17 Brattberg, G., Parker, M. G. and Thorslund, M. Longitudinal study of pain from middle age to old age. *Clin. J. Pain* 1997; **13**: 144–9.

18 Gearhart, J. M. Self-concept in adult women: a multidimensional approach. *Diss. Abstr. Int. A: Humanities Soc. Sci.* 1996; **56**:3769.

19 Sleeper, L. A., Waclawiv, M. A. and Follmann, D. A. Multiple roles for middle-aged women and their impact on health. In M.G. Ory and H. R. Warner (eds.). *Gender, Health and Longevity*. New York: Springer; 1990. pp. 204–23.

20 Barnett, R. C. *Toward a Review of the Work/Family Literature: Work in Progress*. Boston: Wellesley College Center for Research on Women; 1996.

21 Baruch, G. K., Biener, L. and Barnett, R. C. Women and gender in research on work and family stress. *Am. Psychol.* 1987; **42**:130–36.

22 Grzywacz, J. G. Reconceptualizing the work-family interface: an ecological perspective on the correlates of positive and negative spillover between work and family. *J. Occup. Health Psychol.* 2000; **5**:111–26.

23 Grzywacz, J. G. Work–family spillover and health during midlife: is managing conflict everything? *Am. J. Health Promot.* 2000; **14**:236–43.

24 Krant, G. and Oestergren, P. O. Common symptoms in middle aged women: their relation to employment status, psychological work conditions and social support in a Swedish setting. *J. Epidemiol. Comm. Health* 2000; **54**:192–9.

25 Gannon, L. R. *Women and Aging: Transcending the Myths*. New York: Routledge; 1999. p. 26.

26 Jacobson, J. M. *Midlife Women: Contemporary Issues*. Boston: Jones and Bartlett; 1995.

27 Woods, N. F. and Mitchell, E. S. Women's images of midlife: observations from the Seattle Midlife Women's Health Study. *Health Care Women Int.* 1997; **18**:439–53.

28 Gilligan, C. A. *Different Voice: Psychological Theory and Women's Development*. Cambridge, MA: Harvard University Press; 1982.

29 Candib, L. *Medicine and the Family*. New York: Basic Books; 1995, pp. 18–36

30 Surrey, J. L. The self-in-relation: a theory of women's development. In A. G. Kaplar, J. B. Miller, I. Stiver, *et al. Women's Growth in Connection: Writings from the Stone Center*. New York: Guilford Press; 1991. pp. 51–66.

31 US Department of Health and Human Services, Health Resources and Service Administration, Maternal and Child Health Bureau. *Women's Health USA 2002*. Rockville, MD: US Department of Health and Human Services; 2002. p. 54.

32 US Department of Health and Human Services, Health Resources and Service Administration, Maternal and Child Health Bureau. *Women's Health USA 2002*. Rockville, MD: US Department of Health and Human Services; 2002. p. 18.

33 Lasswell, M. Marriage and family. In S. G. Kornstein, and A. H. Clayton (eds.). *Women's Mental Health*. New York: Guilford Press; 2002. pp. 515–16.

34 US Bureau of the Census. Statistical Abstract of the United States; 117th edn. Washington, DC: US Government Printing Office; 1997.

35 US Department of Health and Human Services, Health Resources and Service Administration, Maternal and Child Health Bureau. *Women's Health USA 2002*. Rockville, MD: US Department of Health and Human Services; 2002. p. 18.

36 The Sandwich Generation. www.sandwichgeneration.com/pages/lectures.htm. Accessed October 10, 2002.

37 US Department of Health and Human Services, Health Resources and Service Administration, Maternal and Child Health Bureau. *Women's Health USA 2002*. Rockville, MD: US Department of Health and Human Services; 2002. p. 22.

38 US Department of Health and Human Services, Health Resources and Service Administration, Maternal and Child Health Bureau. *Women's Health USA 2002*. Rockville, MD: US Department of Health and Human Services; 2002. p. 22.

39 www.sandwichgeneration.com/pages/lectures.htm. Accessed October 13, 2002.

40 Webber, C. and Delvin, D. Empty-nest syndrome. www.netdoctor.co.uk/womenshealth/features/ens.htm Accessed October 13, 2002.

41 McQuaide, S. Women at midlife. *Soc. Work* 1998; 43:21–31.

42 Dennerstein, L., Dudley, E. and Guthrie, J. Empty nest or revolving door? A prospective study of women's quality of life in midlife during the phase of children leaving and re-entering the home. *Psychol. Med.* 2002; **32**:545–50.

43 www.psychologytoday.com/htdocs/prod/ptoarticle/pto-19960301-000003.asp. Accessed October 16, 2002.

44 www.psychologytoday.com/htdocs/prod/ptohome/home.asp. Accessed January 5, 2003.

45 Gee, E. M., Mitchell, B. A. and Wister, A. V. Returning to the parental "nest": exploring a changing Canadian life course. *Can. Stud. Popul.* 1995; **22**:121–44.
46 Family Caregiver Alliance. Selected caregiver statistics. www.caregiver.org/factsheets/selected_caregiver_statistics.html. Accessed October 20, 2002.
47 Family Caregiver Alliance. Selected caregiver statistics. www.caregiver.org/factsheets/selected_caregiver_statistics.html. Accessed October 20, 2002.
48 Chentsova-Dutton, Y., Schucter, S., Hutchin, S., *et al.* The psychological and physical health of hospice caregivers. *Ann. Clin. Psychiatry* 2000; **12**:19–27.
49 Family Caregiver Alliance. Selected caregiver statistics. www.caregiver.org/factsheets/selected_caregiver_statistics.html. Accessed October 10, 2002.
50 Pohl, J. M., Given, C. W., Collins, C. E. *et al.* Social vulnerability and reactions to caregiving in daughters and daughters-in-law caring for disabled aging parents. *Health Care Women Int.* 1994; **15**:385–95.
51 Leiberman, M. A. and Fisher, L. The impact of chronic illness on the health and well being of family members. *Gerontologist* 1995; **35**:94–102.
52 Cannuscio, C. C., Jones, C., Kawachi, I., *et al.* Reverberations of family illness: a longitudinal assessment of informal caregiving and mental health status in the Nurses' Health Study. *Am. J. Publ. Health* 2002; **92**:1305–11.
53 Vaillant, G. E., Meyer, S. E., Mukamal, K. and Soldz, S. Are social supports in late midlife a cause or a result of successful physical ageing? *Psychol. Med.* 1998; **28**:1159–68.
54 Eloniemi-Sulkava, U., Notkola I. L., Hamalainen, K., *et al.* Spouse caregivers' perceptions of influence of dementia on marriage. *Int. Psychogeriatr.* 2002; **14**:47–58.
55 Berardo, D. H. and Berardo, F. M. Quality of life across age and family stage. *J. Palliat. Care* 1992; **8**:52–5.
56 Davenport, D. S. Dynamics and treatment of middle generation women: heroines and victims of multigenerational families. In M. Duffy (ed.). *Handbook of Counseling and Psychotherapy with Older Adults.* Washington, DC: John Wiley & Sons; 1999. pp. 267–80.
57 McQuaide, S. Women at midlife. *Soc. Work* 1998; **43**:21–31.
58 Kaplan, S. H., Greenfield, S. and Ware, J. E., Jr. Assessing the effects of physician –patient interactions on the outcomes of chronic disease. *Med. Care* 1989; **27** (3 suppl):S110–27.
59 Stewart, M. A. What is a successful doctor–patient interview? A study of interactions and outcomes. *Soc. Sci. Med.* 1984; **19**:167–75.

5

Sexual health

Margaret R. H. Nusbaum, D.O., M.P.H.

Case: a 50 year-old woman presents for her wellness exam. She has no chronic illnesses or allergies, and she is on no medications. She is married, has five children, and has not worked outside of the home since she was married at age 22. Her review of systems is remarkable for tearfulness and occasional feelings of "nervousness." The youngest, and last of her five children to leave home, leaves for college in ten days.

Importance

Sexuality and sexual health are some of the least scientifically studied areas of health and human interaction, and the sexual health of mid-life women is no exception.

Sexuality is much more then sexual behavior. Sexuality is an important part of one's health, quality of life, and general wellbeing. Sexuality is an integral part of the total person, affecting the way each individual – from birth to death – relates to herself, her sexual partner(s), and every other person.[1] This time of life can and should be a tremendously positive time for women in regards to sexual health. How a woman successfully navigates sexual health risks depends on the complexity of how she defines herself and her sexuality in relationship to aging, menstruation, childbearing capability, success with overcoming challenges of her past, and the quality of intimate partnership(s). Risks to sexual health can include unplanned pregnancy, the physiologic changes of transition into and through menopause and with aging, the increased probability of chronic illness and its medical and surgical treatment, abuse in any form, and sexually transmitted infections.

Table 5.1 Women's sexual function, by age

Sexual Dysfunction	Age range (years)			
	40–44	45–49	50–54	55–59
Pain during sex	12.5%	10.3%	7.4%	8.7%
Sex not pleasurable	15.7%	15.4%	15.3%	16.4%
Unable to orgasm	20.8%	18.8%	20.2%	21.8%
Lacking interest in sex	36.0%	33.7%	30.2%	37.0%
Anxiety about performance	10.9%	8.8%	7.8%	4.4%
Climax too early	6.9%	7.1%	9.6%	7.6%
Trouble lubricating	15.9%	22.6%	21.4%	24.8%

Source: Laumann, E. O., Gagnon, J. H., Michael, R. T., and Michael S. *The Social Organization of Sexuality: Sexual Practices in the United States.* Chicago: University of Chicago Press; 1994.

Epidemiology

A study of women aged 40–59 found that the prevalence of specific sexual dysfunctions ranged from 4.4 to 36%[2] (Table 5.1).[2] There was a reduction of frequency of coitus with age. Thirty-seven percent of women aged 25–29 reported coitus two to three times a week and masturbation weekly, whereas fewer than 5% and 2.4% of women aged 55–59 reported those behaviors, respectively.[2]

For genders, for same-sex, and opposite-sex couples, the value of and participation in sexual activity within a relationship appears relatively stable with increasing age. Whatever the individual's and couple's interest and level of activity early on in the relationship, it continues relatively stable with increasing age.

Women's sexual concerns change with age. A primary care patient-based survey of approximately 1200 women revealed that women aged 55 years and older were significantly less likely than younger women to be concerned about body image and having painful intercourse. They were more likely to report concerns about their partner having sexual difficulties and report that they "never had orgasm" when compared with women between ages 45 and 54, and even more so compared with women under age 45.[3] In this same study, approximately 60% of women younger than age 45 (63%, $n = 629$) and aged 45–54 (66%, $n = 169$) reported having sexual desires that differed from their partners.

For women, availability of a willing and able partner is the key to maintaining sexual activity.[4] As with most areas of sexual health, studies are lacking. This chapter will review the sexual health of mid-life women, presenting results from available studies.

Developmental tasks

Case: a 54-year-old woman presents with a nine-month history of amenorrhea, hot flushes, difficulty sleeping, and "edgy" mood. She reports that her mother, sisters, and friends have shared with her how difficult going through the "change" had been for them. She has read about recent study results raising concerns regarding hormone replacement therapy and cardiovascular risks, but she has also heard that hormones can help to reduce the signs of aging. She is divorced and had "launched" her final child from home this past summer. She has enjoyed rearranging the house but is not sure how she will spend her time as she gets closer to finishing this project.

Two stages of psychosexual developmental tasks are described for women aged 40–65, giving this time of life the potential for tremendous personal growth. The first psychosexual developmental task of middle adulthood is identified as generativity versus stagnation. Cessation of employment or childrearing may be followed by volunteer work or return to school. During the early years of mid life, there is potential for growth in self-identity. As changes in gender roles and relationship structures continue, there is increasing awareness that both men and women have the same needs for love and belonging.

In a Danish study aimed at exploring whether women have any positive experiences in relation to the menopause, a questionnaire was sent to a random sample of 51-year-old women.[5] Of 393 women who answered an open-ended question, the total number of replies with a positive content was 268. Concrete positive descriptions included relief that menstruation had ceased, with its associated problems, and the possibility of personal growth and freedom to concentrate on the women's own requirements.[5]

The meaning of menopause varies cross-culturally.[6,7] *Menopausal women do not agree that they become less sexually attractive with age than younger women, and hold a much more positive view of aging and menopause than do younger, premenopausal women.*[6,7] In a study of approximately 1200 female patients aged 18–88 in primary care, women under age 45 (80%, $n = 632$) reported concerns about feeling that they lacked sexual appeal. Fewer women aged 45–54 (74%, $n = 171$), and an even lower proportion of women over 55 (54%, $n = 363$), reported this concern.[8]

The second psychosexual developmental task for later adulthood is defined as ego integrity versus despair. The woman must accept her self-worth, adjusting to both physical and psychosocial changes. This includes her capability to develop a sense of continuity of past, present, and future, and to transcend bodily changes. Failure to accomplish this is to experience a sense of "nothingness" and loss known as despair. This is more difficult for women who value their appearance over their accomplishments. Mid-life crises revolve around losses in critical life exchange values – physiological changes in a society that values youth and beauty.

Lifecycle changes

Mid life includes the possibility of a range of lifecycle changes: late parenthood to the last of the children leaving the home; potentially tumultuous hormonal changes as the woman transitions from premenopause to perimenopause and finally menopause; the beginning of the geriatric age range; and onset of chronic illness and partner health problems.

Problems with the partner

Decreased sexual interest and sexual dissatisfaction were found among 65% of women aged 40–60 ($n = 100$) who had had an acute myocardial infarction versus 24% in a control group ($n = 100$) of same-age women hospitalized for other reasons. The most common causes for sexual dissatisfaction were premature ejaculation or erectile dysfunction in the husband.[9]

Psychosocial issues

A qualitative study of 11 women during mid life, exploring their sense of confusion, found that most notable were their comments about negative societal views of aging and lack of health-related information on physical and physiological changes of midlife.[10] *The most relevant factors influencing a woman's quality of life during the menopausal transition are her previous emotional and physical health, her social situation, her experience of stressful life events (particularly bereavements and separations), and her beliefs about the menopause.*

There are considerable cultural differences in the reporting of vasomotor symptoms, which may be explained by the meaning ascribed to them, the value of older women in societies, and dietary, lifestyle, and genetic differences. Those who seek medical help for menopausal problems report more physical and psychological problems. These women are more likely to be under stress and to hold particular beliefs about the menopause.

These personal and social issues must be addressed in their own right and should not be attributed automatically to menopause. Clinical psychologists and counselors, ideally working as part of the team, can help women and couples to clarify the nature of the problems and to explore solutions. In contrast to childbirth, preparation for the menopause has been neglected in the development of services.[11]

The Midlife Women's Health Survey, examining the beliefs of 280 mostly white, married, highly educated, mid-life women, found that women whose sexual response had changed in the past year (40%) reported more decrements than increases in sexual response. When asked how they accounted for these changes, women referred most often to the physical and emotional changes of menopause and to life circumstances, and less often to their relationships with their partners. Most of the decrements were explained by physical events related to menopause, whereas most of the increases were explained by life circumstances.[12]

The Massachusetts Women's Health Study II was a study of 200 women transitioning through the menopause who were not hormone replacement therapy (HRT) users, who had not had a surgical menopause, and who had partners. It examined associations among menopause status, various aspects of sexual functioning, and the relative contributions of menopause status and other variables to various aspects of sexual functioning. The women were classified as pre-, peri-, or postmenopausal, according to menstrual cycle characteristics and measures of estradiol, estrone, and follicle-stimulating hormone. Menopause status was related significantly to lower sexual desire, a belief that interest in sexual activity declines with age, and women's reports of decreased arousal compared with when in their forties. However, factors such as health, marital status (or new partner), mental health, and smoking had a greater impact than menopause status on women's sexual functioning.[13]

The empty nest

In a study on depression, anxiety, and the empty nest syndrome in 222 perimenopausal and menopausal women with a mean age of 47.7 years (102 of whom were at menopause), disturbed attitudes toward sexuality were the main factors associated with emotional symptoms.[14] Depending on how the woman has defined herself in relationship to her children, the time when children leave the home can provide greater time for her to pursue self-interests and to put greater emphasis on her relationship with her partner. With single women, it may be a time to think about establishing a relationship again. *The greater complexity to her definition of self, the less negative impact the "empty nest" will have on her sexual identity.* Additionally, the quality of the relationship might be tested at this stage. If she and her partner sacrificed their relationship to raise their children, then they will need to become reacquainted with each other.

Family planning and family structure

For pre- and perimenopausal women, contraception is still needed to prevent unplanned pregnancy. HRT, estrogen with or without progesterone, and oral contraceptive agents can suppress testosterone levels, decreasing sexual interest. Supplementation of androgens, dihydroepiandrosterones (DHEAs), and testosterone has been associated with enhanced sexual interest.[15–18]

Hormonal fluctuations

Women have more erratic fluctuations in their hormonal status compared with men. Estrogens and progesterone rise to high levels during pregnancy, only to drop abruptly postpartum as prolactin levels elevate. Perimenopause is now recognized as a unique physiological entity, with dropping levels of estrogen and an even greater loss of progesterone as ovulation becomes inconsistent. The perimenopausal state can last years before menopause. Based on the results of small studies, the perimenopausal state appears to have unique, albeit perhaps transient, effects on sexual health and functioning.

An interview survey of 124 perimenopausal women found that the age group centering around 49 years did not have sexual difficulties in desire, response, or satisfaction in their sexual life, whereas a subset of women with very low estradiol levels tended to have reduced coital activity.[19] In a study of 43 perimenopausal women who kept daily records of menstrual cycles and sexual activity, a negative association was found between hot flush ratings and regularity of sexual intercourse at both time points. Frequency of sexual intercourse and level of plasma estradiol were higher, and hot flush ratings were lower in "early" perimenopausal women who were still having cycles at least once every 30 days, as compared with "late" perimenopausal women who were cycling less often. *A close association exists between increasing irregularity of menstrual cycles, hot flushes, declining estradiol levels, and declining frequency of intercourse during the perimenopause.*[20]

A longitudinal study of 39 women, followed from perimenopausal state until one year or more postmenopausal, found that these women had a significant decrease in frequency of sexual intercourse and fewer sexual thoughts or fantasies. They suffered more from lack of vaginal lubrication during sex and were less satisfied with their partners as lovers after menopause. While estradiol and testosterone levels showed significant declines, testosterone showed the most consistent association with coital frequency.[20]

A cross-sectional telephone survey of 2001 randomly selected Australian-born women aged between 45 and 55 years found variables relating to changes in sexual interest over the prior year. Despite 31% reporting a decline in sexual interest, most (62%) reported no change.[21] Decline in sexual interest was associated significantly and adversely (more so than age) with natural menopause.

DHEA was shown to be the only hormone associated positively with general wellbeing in a study of 141 women aged 40–60.[22] Estrogens and progesterone suppress androgens, making the absence of these hormones in menopause a more favorable physiology for sexual desire. Surgical menopause, when ovaries have been removed, has an abrupt change in hormonal status and causes more significant symptoms.[23]

Beginning in the mid thirties, more than one-third of American women undergo total abdominal hysterectomy with bilateral oopherectomy (TAH/BSO). Hysterectomy is the second most common surgical procedure in women in the USA after cesarean section, with more than 600 000 occurring yearly.[24] Ovarian blood supply is reduced post-hysterectomy, leading to earlier menopause (approximately four years earlier) for women who have undergone hysterectomy without oopherectomy when compared with physiologic menopause.[25] Women who have undergone TAH/BSO or chemical menopause via chemotherapy may experience more intense menopausal symptoms given the more abrupt change compared with natural menopause.[26] Pharmacotherapy or herbal therapy might assist the women through symptomatic menopause and enhance sexual desire. Hormonal supplementation, often with added androgens, can offset perimenopausal symptoms and enhance sexual interest.

Additionally, as ovarian production of hormones decreases, vaginal lubrication can be affected and contribute to dyspareunia, decreased intensity of sexual arousal, and, with decreased androgens, decreased intensity of orgasm. Over-the-counter sexual lubricants, such as Astroglide™, Replens™, and KY Jelly™, can be very helpful. Vaginal estrogen (cream or ring) can offset dyspareunia from vaginal dryness not responsive to lubricants. Vaginal atrophy associated with decreasing physiologic hormones is exacerbated by disuse. For aging women who enjoy vaginal intercourse in their sexual relations, suggesting sexual aides during periods of prolonged illness of a partner or lack of an available partner can offset vaginal atrophy associated with disuse and additionally give her permission to attend to her sexual needs.

For women who choose oral contraceptive agents or HRT, addition of androgens, DHEAs, or testosterone can help offset lowered androgen levels and enhance sexual interest.[17,25]

Body image

How a woman defines her sexuality in relationship to her uterus and ovaries, menstrual cycle, and/or fertility status can affect the intensity of her grief reaction, to menopause body image, and self-esteem. How she adapts to wrinkles and other visible changes of age – such as reframing "age spots" as "experience spots" – can determine how she transitions through ego integrity versus despair.

Additional challenges include the clear existence of agism in our culture. Sexuality is not just for the young. In women's literature, women who have passed the age of childbearing are wise women – "crones" – sought out for words of wisdom by younger generations of women. There is nothing in biology that warrants the prevalent image of sexless, neutered, loveless aging. For many aging people, sexual desire, physical love, and sexual activity continue to be integral parts of their lives, and intimacy is expressed, in addition to intercourse, through closeness, touching, and body warmth. In essence, caring and gentleness in loving activities may be more important. Cessation of sexual activity is not associated with menopause, and many women, freed from the risk of conception, seek intercourse and report heightened sexual satisfaction.

Hysterectomy can generate an emotional crisis for women and their partners, based on how they view their sexuality and their definition of womanhood in relationship to their uterus and ovaries.[25] Worries about changes of sexual response, pain with sexual intercourse, or body image changes can lead to sexual difficulties for the couple. However, for women who have undergone hysterectomy because of abnormal bleeding or pain, sexual desire, enjoyment, and activity increase post-hysterectomy.[27]

Decreased muscle tone and reduced flexibility associated with aging can reduce intensity of orgasm and sometimes require changing sexual positions to reduce pain. These can be managed through lifestyle changes such as daily exercise and stretching and resistance training.

Relationships

The quality of a woman's relationship is a most important aspect of a women's sexual response cycle.[28] The physical, emotional, and sexual satisfaction of the relationship enhance sexual interest and arousal.

This can be a potentially turbulent time for women in heterosexual relationships. Extra-relationship affairs are reportedly highest in the thirties and forties, with contributors including a need to reconfirm sexual identities, relieve sexual boredom, companionship, improved sexual experiences, revenge, changing needs, and mental or physical impairment in a partner that stifles their full participation in a relationship. For women born between 1933 and 1942, 2.4% report extramarital affairs. Approximately 20% of those born between 1943 and 1952 and 14.5% of those born between 1953 and 1962 report extramarital affairs.[2]

Women in this age group underestimate their risk for sexually transmitted infections, including human immunodeficiency virus (HIV), and this represents one of the more rapidly growing demographics for sexually transmitted infections and HIV. According to the Centers for Disease Control (CDC), 14% of all individuals living with HIV are over 50. Acquired immunodeficiency syndrome (AIDS) cases among individuals over the age of 50 have increased 22% since 1991, making heterosexuals aged 50 years and older one of the fastest growing AIDS demographics. In Florida, USA, 25% of all HIV cases occur in older heterosexuals.[28]

Table 5.2 Medical conditions that affect desire

Hypothyroidism
Parkinson's disease
Hyperprolactinemia
Chronic renal failure
Severe COPD/CHF
Alcoholism
Liver disease
Depression
Chronic fatigue
Fibromyalgia

Data from Nusbaum, M. R. H. *Sexual Health.*
Monograph 267 Leawood, KS: American Academy
of Family Physicians; 2001.

Chronic illnesses

With age comes the increasing probability of chronic illness and medications
and/or surgery to treat these illnesses. Many medications can have a negative affect on the sexual reaction cycle (SRC) (Tables 5.2 and 5.3) by affecting
vascular, hormonal, or neurological aspects of the SRC. Obesity, diabetes,
tobacco, alcohol, drugs, osteoarthritis, and lower-back pain can require shifting in sexual positions for greater comfort.[29] Although sexual activity can be
demanding, there are very few medical prohibitions to sexual activity.

Management of sexual concerns

Decreased sexual desire

Sexual desire is that which causes one to be receptive to or initiate sexual
activity. For women, the quality of the relationship and the emotional and
physical satisfaction she receives from that relationship appear to be critical
elements.

Desire requires androgens such as testosterone and DHEAs, neurotransmitters, and the sensory system. Starting in the twenties, there is a progressive decline of physiologically available androgens for both men and women,
which can contribute to decreased sexual interest. Interest in sexual activity can be disrupted by psychosocial, physiological, physical, environmental,
and cultural factors. Fatigue, depression, side effects from medications, self-
esteem, and body image concerns can all interfere with sexual interest. Addressing relationship issues through counseling, supplementing androgens,
treating depression, and assessing medication side effects are all important.

Table 5.3 Medications that affect desire

Anti-androgens
Anti-arrhythmics
Anticancer agents
Cholesterol-lowering agents
Stimulants
Anticholinergics
Antihistamines
Antihypertensives
Antivirals
Corticosteroids
Diuretics
Hormones
Neuroleptics
Recreational illicit drugs
Opiates
Psychotropics
Sedative-hypnotics

Data from Nusbaum, M. R. H. *Sexual Health.* Monograph 267.
Leawood, KS: American Academy of Family Physicians; 2001.

Table 5.4 Taking a sexual history

Ask her to describe the problem
Ask her when she first noticed the problem and the course of the problem
Ask her what she believes to be the cause of the problem
Ask her what she has tried to help resolve the difficulty
Ask her what her expectations and goals are

Data from Nusbaum, M. R. H. *Sexual Health.* Monograph no. 267.
Leawood, KS: American Academy of Family Physicians; 2001.

More important for good sexual desire is attending to scheduling the time and setting the environment for sexual activity, using the senses to the fullest, and incorporating seduction.

The diagnosis of chronic illness and/or its medical and surgical treatment can disrupt sexual desire. The patient may have a misunderstanding that sexual activity is prohibited, such as following myocardial infarction.[30] Table 5.2 lists some common disease processes and Table 5.3 some medications that can interfere with sexual desire.

A general history and a sexual problem history can be helpful for clarifying the timeline, identifying possible etiologies, and developing approaches for management.[29] Table 5.4 describes taking a sexual problem history.[31] Although

Table 5.5 Antidotes for psychotropic-induced decrease in sexual interest

Drug	Dosage
Yohimbine	5.4–16.2 mg 2–4 hours before sexual activity
Buproprion	100 mg when required or 75 mg three times daily
Amantadine	100–400 mg when required or daily
Methylphenidate	5–25 mg when required
Dextroamphetamine	5 mg sublingually 1 hour before sexual activity
Sildenafil	50–100 mg when required

the woman is not likely to identify relationship issues as being etiologic without some prompting, her history of the course of the problem, attempts to resolve it, and what she believes to be the cause can be helpful in management approaches.

Because the quality of the relationship is pivotal in the sexual response cycle for women, *poor or declining quality of relationship can negatively affect desire and subsequently arousal.* Clarify the quality of the relationship and the woman's level of attraction to her partner, recommending counseling for less-than-satisfactory relationships. Assess the couple's investment in time and setting the environment conducive to sexual encounters – for example, expecting spontaneous sexual encounters on the night that grandchildren are sleeping over can be unrealistic. Assess medications for potential negative impact.

Consider discontinuing, substituting, or reducing the dosage of medications that could be contributing. Selective serotonin reuptake inhibitors (SSRIs) are very successful for treating depression and anxiety, but unfortunately they can negatively affect the sexual response cycle. Drug holidays from SSRIs can be effective, but more so for paroxetine than fluoxetine or sertraline, which have longer half-lives. Small studies show benefits to rescue agents,[30,32] such as amfebutanone(buproprion), methylphenidate, amantadine, and dextroamphetamine. Sildenafil[33] and yohimbine can enhance sexual desire by enhancing arousal (Table 5.5).

Serum hormone-binding globulin (SHBG) lowers physiologically available androgens. Increasing age and exogenous hormones raise SHBG. Exogenous hormones, specifically estrogens and progesterone, lower available androgen levels by raising SHBG and thus negatively affecting sexual desire. Should a woman require oral contraceptives, using lower estrogen compounds with androgenic progesterones (levonorgestrel, norgestrel, desogestrel), such as Alesse[TM], Loestrin[TM], or Mircette[TM], may restore her sexual interest. Adding DHEAs 25–75 mg/day as a supplement or substituting a barrier method for contraception are other options. Additionally, should a woman require HRT to offset perimenopausal symptoms that affect her quality of life, then adding androgens (either methyltestosterone or DHEAs supplements) to HRT may offset negative sexual health affects.

Other critical components – sensuality – touch, scents, music, romanticizing the environment – and seduction – committing the time, the intrigue, and foreplay to the relationship in general – and the sexual aspects of the relationship specifically are essential. Pubococcygeal exercises (see Table 5.6) can be helpful for urinary control, blood flow to the perineum, and, thus, sensation of arousal, and can be helpful for all sexual difficulties.

Decreased arousal and/or plateau

Arousal and plateau aspects of the sexual response cycle (SRC) require an intact vascular system, cyclic guanosine monophosphate (cGMP), and, probably, adequate androgen levels. Because this phase of the SRC includes muscular tension, some degree of muscle tone contributes to the sensation of heightened tension that occurs in this phase. As vaginal lubrication and penile erection are equivalent phases of the SRC, the clinician should be aware of medications, illnesses, and physiological changes that affect men's SRC in order to understand women's arousal difficulties. Changes in women's arousal are not readily noticeable to the woman or her partner until a fairly significant change has occurred; penile erectile difficulties are likely noted at a much earlier threshold, since penetrative sex requires a much greater degree of vasocongestion compared with the level of vagocongestion required for receptive vaginal sex.

As with increasing erectile difficulties with age alone, there are age-related changes in vaginal lubrication for women. Sildenafil is beneficial to women experiencing arousal difficulties during perimenopause and should be considered a treatment option.[33] Additionally, nitric oxide – required for cGMP and subsequent vasocongestion – is believed to be androgen-sensitive, heightening the possible benefits of androgen supplementation to enhance arousal.

Because erectile difficulty is an endothelial dysfunction and a harbinger of chronic illness, such as lipid disorder, glucose intolerance, hyperinsulinemia, and cardiovascular disease, arousal difficulties in women should be considered a similar indication and evaluated similarly.[34]

Arousal difficulties leading to delayed vaginal engorgement, reduced vaginal lubrication, pain with intercourse, and decreased vaginal, clitoral, and orgasmic sensation can be caused by or exacerbated by athlerosclerotic disease.[35] Screening laboratory testing should include lipid profile, glucose with or without insulin levels, thyroid stimulating hormone (TSH), and androgen levels (DHEAs and free testosterone).

Lifestyle changes are critical and should include moderation of alcohol intake, exercise, smoking cessation, weight loss, and stress management. Medications that can be discontinued or reduced in dosages should be changed (Table 5.7). Additionally, just as psychotropic agents can significantly reduce

Table 5.6 Pubococcygeal (PC) muscle exercises

Starting out	To recognize the muscles that you want to exercise, next time you are urinating stop the flow of urine midstream. This is the muscle you want to exercise. Urinate a bit more, and then stop the stream again. Initially, you might want to practice these exercises sitting on the toilet or laying in the bed. Once you have identified the PC muscle squeeze that you need to do, you can move on to the three types of exercises below.
Rapid squeeze	Do a rapid succession of quick squeezes and quick relaxing. A slower version is squeeze as you inhale, relax as you exhale. Do not hold your squeeze or breath.
Ten-second hold	Tighten the muscle as you inhale. Squeeze as hard as you can and hold for a count of ten seconds. Relax as you exhale, bearing down gently as if you are having a bowel movement.
Long, slow squeeze	Squeeze slowly, gradually tightening your squeeze over a count of ten seconds. Then, slowly, relax the squeeze over a count of ten seconds. Imagine that your muscle is an elevator that must stop for a second at every floor, until reaching the tenth floor and then back down to the first floor. Each "floor" is a gradual tightening or release of the PC muscles. Vaginal weights are available through health magazines for more advanced exercising
Daily goal	Start with threes: three quick squeezes, three-second squeezes for the hold, three "floors" for the long squeeze, and three of each type of squeeze. You might feel sore at first. This is not a muscle we are accustomed to exercising. Each week, double the number of each type of squeeze and double the number of seconds that you hold the longer squeezes. Aim for a minimum of ten of each type, a total of 30 squeezes a day. Build up to ten-second squeezes and 100 total squeezes a day. Need a reminder? Try to do a couple of squeezes every time you need to stop for a traffic light. Who knows, the person across from you might be doing the same exercises! Other convenient times might be while you are on the phone, at the computer, or watching TV. Be patient: it may take a month or two to notice changes.

Source: (Nusbaum, M. R. H. *Sexual Health.* Monograph no. 267. Leawood, KS: American Academy of Family Physicians; 2001.

Table 5.7 Examples of medications less offensive
to the sexual response cycle

Angiotensin-converting enzyme inhibitors
Buproprion
Alpha-blockers
Nefazodone
Trazodone

sexual interest, they can produce a secondary effect on arousal. Medications that shorten plateau, such as cyproheptadine and buproprion, can be beneficial to offset psychotropic-induced sexual difficulties and may be therapeutic for orgasm difficulties.

Many excellent sexual lubricants are available over the counter, such as Astroglide™, Replens™, and Slippery Stuff™. These can offset changes in vaginal lubrication brought about by age or chronic illnesses and/or their medical treatment and can enhance sensuality in general. Additionally, topical estrogens in the form of vaginal creams, such as Premarin™, or vaginal rings, such as Estring™, can help reduce vaginal-insertion discomfort brought about by atrophy of the vaginal mucosa.

Difficulties with orgasm

Difficulties with orgasm are related most often to lack of understanding of what sort of sexual stimulation is required, difficulty communicating this need to one's partner, or lack of the partner's initiative to provide this stimulation. Additionally, medications, most notably psychotropic agents, can prolong arousal, making orgasm very difficult to attain. Androgen deficiency is believed to contribute to the higher threshold required for orgasm and the lower intensity for orgasm.[14]

Exploring the woman's desire and arousal phases, including quality of her relationship, is important because sexual health comorbidities are likely. Supplementation of androgens should be undertaken if needed. The woman should be encouraged to enhance her self-awareness about what sensual and physical stimulation she requires for orgasm through self-stimulation. An excellent reference is the book *Becoming Orgasmic.*[36]

Long-term relationships

Lack of spontaneity, routine, and attention to matters other then sexual relationships can add particular challenges to long-term relationships. The earlier erotic nature of the newness of the relationship becomes replaced by a predictable and less prioritorized sexual exchange. Responsibilities of paying bills, concerns about health, and caring for children, grandchildren, or aging parents can take priority over the time the couple has to spend with each other. *Quality of life, satisfaction with the relationship, and longevity are associated positively with sexual activity within a committed relationship.*[37] Couples should be encouraged to regard their sexual life a priority; scheduling time and privacy for themselves separate from other life responsibilities is essential. Encourage couples to maintain erotic levels through seduction, touch, and massage outside of and in addition to sexual exchange, use of sensuality such as pleasing scents, music, and lubricants to enhance sexual exchange and intimacy.

Lesbian couples

Five to nine percent of the US male population and 4% of the female population is gay.[2] Homophobia is prevalent in medical schools and healthcare settings and contributes to the differences observed in lesbian and gay men's health arising from this differential treatment.[38, 39] Research is limited regarding healthcare needs of women who have female partners. What little research does exist frequently suffers from small sample size and sampling errors.[40] Convenience sampling with participants drawn from gay bars, bath-houses, gay community centers, and other areas known to have concentrations of lesbian and gay people are not likely to be representative of the larger lesbian and gay male populations, nor the relevant patient populations. The body of research documenting lesbian health needs is even more limited than that for gay men.

Lesbian families, like heterosexual families, take many forms. Couples may be childless or they may have children from previous relationships/marriages or from alternative insemination. Similar to heterosexual and gay-male couples, lesbian couples may be long-term monogamous, serially monogamous, or even "open" to other partners outside the primary relationship. Commitment and areas of conflict do not differ between heterosexual (money, sex, work, family demands, etc.) and lesbian couples. Social support networks, community, friendships, and family, however, are a much more critical impact in terms of support, or lack thereof, given our current society's reluctance to legitimize same-sex couples through, for instance, support for legal marriage and healthcare benefits for partners. Perhaps having to work hard all their lives to establish positive social networks in the face of social prejudice and the necessity to develop more complex aspects to their lives, lesbian women may be better able to cope with stressors of aging.[41]

Rates of violence and abuse do not differ for lesbian women. However, support groups specific to lesbian needs may be lacking in specific communities. Alcohol and substance abuse and eating disorders may be more prevalent among lesbian women.[41] These issues can be equally as problematic for lesbian couples as they are for heterosexual couples. Little is known about lesbian or bisexual sexual health concerns. One might readily surmise that sexual concerns and difficulties do not differ from those of heterosexual women,

Table 5.8 Causes of female genital pain

Vulvar pain	Vaginal pain	Deep dyspareunia
Vulvitis	Inadequate lubrication	Pelvic inflammatory disease
Vulvovaginitis	Vaginal infection	Pelvic/abdominal surgery
Vulvovestibulitis	Irritants	Adhesions
Herpes	Urethritis	Endometriosis
Urethritis	Episiotomy	Pelvic tumors
Atrophic vulvitis	Radiation vaginitis	Irritable bowel syndrome
Inadequate lubrication	Sexual traumas	Urinary tract infections
Topical irritants	Vaginismus	Positional

Source: Butcher, J. ABC of sexual health: female sexual problems II: sexual pain and sexual fears. *Br. Med. J.* 1999; **318**:7176.

except that they have the added strain of societal prejudice for same-sex coupling.

Sexual pain syndromes

Pain during sexual activity can vary from pain with initiation of intercourse to deep dyspareunia (Table 5.8). Sexual pain syndromes are associated with a history of abuse. Clinicians should screen for this history and provide suggestions for individual and couple therapy to support the woman as she tries to reconcile her past.

Vestibulitis, a painful condition of the vaginal introitus, can be reproduced on examination by light touching of the introital area, particularly between 3 and 6 o'clock, with a cotton swab. Dyspareunia can result from decreased vaginal lubrication; it is typically described as burning sensation or pain on initiation of penetration. Sexual lubrications can be very helpful to manage this.

Deep dyspareunia can result from cervical, uterine, or adnexal pathology. A pelvic examination and further assessment by pelvic ultrasonography and gynecologic referral can help discern the etiology and direct treatment.

Vaginismus can be primary or can result from sexual pain syndromes. It is associated most commonly with sexually restrictive cultures, religions, and history of abuse. Women typically have not been able to use tampons, undergo pelvic examinations, or experience vaginal intercourse because of spasm of the pubococcygeal (PC) muscles. Vaginismus can be treated by heightening the patient's awareness of her body and recommending step-wise vaginal insertional activities. Starting with attention to the PC muscle exercises, the woman can be instructed to perform muscular squeezing and pay most attention to the sensation of PC muscle relaxation after the squeeze. Recommending the use of mirrors to become comfortable looking at and touching her external genitalia can help her to become more comfortable with her body. *Becoming Orgasmic*[36] is an excellent reference; it includes illustrations of variation in the appearance of women's external genital anatomy.

Once the woman has accomplished this step successfully, the next step is progressive vaginal insertion. Several options exist for vaginal insertion, including syringes (starting from purified protein derivative (PPD) syringes and progressing to 60-ml syringes), candles (beginning with tiny candles and progressing to larger candles, which can be warmed in a microwave), vaginal dilators of progressive size (which can be purchased in a medical supply store), and, most readily available, fingers. Any of these options can be used in progressive steps and under the woman's control.

Discuss the woman's options to determine which she is most comfortable with. Use of fingers can readily transfer to partner's fingers and, for male partners, the penis. Many couples describe this process as anxiety provoking but also very erotic. Initially, the woman starts her homework solo. With lots of sexual lubrication, have her practice touching her genitalia and inserting one finger into her vagina. Once she is comfortable with this step, have her progress to inserting two fingers. She moves on to the next step once she is comfortable.

The next step is to incorporate her partner. This can be uncomfortable for both parties, but it can also initiate a lot of intimate discussion about sexuality and sexual activity between partners. The woman's partner should give her total control over these steps. Initially, she and her partner should simply look and touch each other's external genitalia. Once she feels ready to try, she takes her partner's well-lubricated finger and inserts it into her vagina. She might want to talk, hug, or kiss or be kissed by her partner during this exercise just for reassurance and emotional support. The next step is to insert two of her partner's well-lubricated fingers. For male partners, the final step would be her control over insertion of the well-lubricated penis. Once she feels she is ready, she gradually relinquishes control to her partner. Clinicians should present her the option of inserting the vaginal speculum herself during her pelvic examination. This allows her to control the angle, the speed, and the position for examination should she choose this option.

Summary

Although decline in sexual activity is reported for aging women, in general women are no less interested in sexual activity as they age, but they and their sexual partners are affected more often by chronic illness and changes in physiology. Sexual difficulties remain common for mid-life and older women, including increase in difficulty for single women to find consistent partners in their age group. Clinicians are encouraged to raise the topic of sexual health and to assist mid-life women as they make their transitions through menopause, and with aging partners, supporting this phase of life as a prime period and the notion that these women are valued for their history and wisdom and unique beauty that mid life and beyond has to offer.

FURTHER RESOURCES

American Association of Sex Educators, Counselors and Therapists: http://www.aasect.org
Sexuality Information and Education Council of the US: http://www.siecus.org
Gay and Lesbion Medical Association (GLMA): http://www.glma.org
AARP/Modern   Maturity   Sexuality   Study: http://research.aarp.org/health/mmsexsurvey_1.htm

REFERENCES

1 Renshaw, D. C. Sexology. *J. Am Med. Assoc.* 1984; **252**:2291–6.
2 Laumann, E. O., Gagnon, J. H., Michael, R. T. and Michael, S. *The Social Organization of Sexuality: Sexual Practices in the United States.* Chicago: University of Chicago Press; 1994.
3 Nusbaum, M. R. H., Helton, M. R. and Ray, N. The changing nature of women's sexual health concerns through the midlife years. *Ann. Fam. Med.*, submitted.
4 Malatesta, V. J. Sexuality and the older adult: an overview with guidelines for the health care professional. *J. Women Aging* 1989; **1**:93–118.
5 Hvas, A. [Positive experiences in connection with menopause.] *Ugeskr. Laeger* 2002; **164**:2614–17.
6 Avis, N. Perception of the menopause. *Womens Eur. Menopause J.* 1996; **3**:80–84.
7 Locke, M. Menopause: Lessons from anthropology. *Psychosom. Med.* 1998; **60**:410–19.
8 Nusbaum, M. R., Hamilton, C. and Lenahan, P. Sexual health care needs of midlfe women. *J. Women Health Gend. Based Med.*, submitted.
9 Abramov, L. Sexual life and sexual frigidity among women developing acute myocardial infarction. *Psychosomat. Med.* 1976; **38**:418–25.
10 Banister, E. M. Women's midlife confusion: "why am I feeling this way?". *Issues in Ment. Health Nurs.* 2000; **21**:745–64.
11 Hunter, M. S. Predictors of menopausal symptoms: psychosocial aspects. *Baillieres Clin. Endocrinol. Metab.* 1993; **7**:33–45.
12 Mansfield, P., Koch, P. B. and Voda, A. M. Midlife women's attributions for their sexual response changes. *Health Care Women Int.* 2000; **21**:543–59.
13 Avis, N., Stellato, R., Crawford, S., Johannes, C. and Longcope, C. Is there an association between menopause status and sexual functioning? *J. Am. Geriatr. Soc.* 1972; **20**:151–8.

14 Huerta, R., Mena, A., Malacara, J. M. and Diaz de Leon, J. Symptoms at peri-menopausal period: its association with attitudes toward sexuality, life-style, family function, and FSH levels. *Psychoneuroendocrinology* 1995; **20**:851–64.

15 Bancroft, J. Endocrinology of sexual function. *Clin. Obstet. Gynaecol.* 1980; **7**:253–81.

16 Basson, R. Androgen replacement for women. *Can. Fam. Physician* 1999; **45**:2100–107.

17 Davis, S. The clinical use of androgens in female sexual disorders. *J. Sex Marital Ther.* 1998; **24**:153–63.

18 Warnock, J., Bundren, J. C. and Morris, D. W. Female hypoactive sexual disorder: case studies of physiologic androgen replacement. *J. Sex Marital Ther.* 1999; **25**:175–82.

19 Cutler, W., Garcia, C. R. and McCoy, N. Perimenopausal sexuality. *Arch. Sex. Behav.* 1987; **16**:225–34.

20 McCoy, N., Culter, W. and Davidson, J. M. Relationships among sexual behavior, hot flashes, and hormone levels in perimenopausal women. *Arch. Sex. Behav.* 1985; **14**:385–94.

21 Dennerstein, L., Smith, A. M., Morse, C. A. and Burger, H. G. Sexuality and the menopause. *J. Psychosomat. Obstet. Gynecol.* 1994; **15**:59–66.

22 Hackbert, L. and Heiman, J. R. Acute dehydroepiandrosterone (DHEA) effects on sexual arousal in postmenopausal women. *J. Womens Health Gend. Based Med.* 2002; **11**:155–62.

23 Levine, S. *Sexuality in Midlife*. New York: Plenum Press; 1998.

24 Cawood, E. and Bancroft, J. Steroid hormones, the menopause, sexuality and well-being of women. *Psychol. Med.* 1996; **26**:925–36.

25 Garth, D., Cooper, P. and Day, A. Hysterectomy and psychiatric disorder: I. Levels of psychiatric morbidity before and after hysterectomy. *Br. J. Psychiatry* 1980; **140**:335–42.

26 Rhodes, J., Kjerluff, K., Laugenberg, P. and Guzinski, G. Hysterectomy and sexual functioning. *J. Am. Med. Assoc.* 1999; **282**:1934–41.

27 Basson, R., Berman, J., Burnett, A., *et al.* Report of the international consensus development conference on female sexual dysfunction: definitions and classifications. *J. Urol.* 2000; **163**:888–93.

28 AIDS Action. What's New. www.aidsaction.org. Accessed January 3, 2003.

29 Nusbaum, M. R. H., Hamilton, C. and Lenahan, P. Health issues and sexuality. *Am. Fam. Physician* 2003; **67**:347–54.

30 Woodrum, S. T. and Brown C. S. Management of SSRI-induced sexual dysfunction. *Ann. Pharmacother.* 1998; **32**:1209–15.

31 Annon, J. S. *The Behavioral Treatment of Sexual Problems*, Vol. 1. Oahu, Hawaii: Enabling Systems Inc.; 1974.

32 Nurnberg, H., Lauriello, J., Hensley, P. L., Parker, L. M. and Keith, S. J. Sildenafil for sexual dysfunction in women taking antidepressants. *Am. J. Psychiatry* 1999; **156**:1664.

33 Caruso, S., Intelisano, G., Lupo, L. and Agnello, C. Premenopausal women affected by sexual arousal disorder traeted with sildenafil: a double blind, crossover, placebo-controlled study. *Br. J. Obstet. Gynaecol.* 2001; **108**:623–8.

34 Andersson, K. E. and Wagner, G. Physiology of penile erection. *Physiol. Rev.* 1995; **75**:191–236.
35 Goldstein, I., Lue, T. F., Padma-Nathan, H., Rosen, R., Steers, W. D. and Wicker, P. A. Oral sildenafil in the treatment of erectile dysfunction. *N. Engl. J. Med.* 1998; **338**:1397–404.
36 Heiman, J. R. and LoPicolo, J. *Becoming Orgasmic: A Sexual and Personal Growth Program for Women.* New York: Prentice Hall; 1988.
37 Palmore, E. Predictors of the longevity difference: a 25-year follow up. *Gerontologist* 1982; **22**:513–18.
38 O'Hanlan, K., Cabaj, R., Schatz, B., Lock, J. and Nemrow, P. A review of the medical consequences of homophobia with suggestions for resolution. *J. Gay Lesbian Med. Assoc.* 1997; **1**:25–39.
39 Harrison, A. Primary care of lesbian and gay patients: educating ourselves and our students. *Fam. Med.* 1996; **28**:10–23.
40 Deevey, S. Lesbain health care. In: C. I. Fogel and N. F. Woods (eds.). *Women's Health Care: A Comprehensive Handbook.* Thousand Oaks, CA: Sage Publications; 1995. pp. 189–206.
41 Nusbaum, M. R. H. *Sexual Health.* Monograph no. 267 Leawood, KS: American Academy of Family Physicians; 2001.

6

Alcoholism, nicotine dependence, and drug abuse

Mary-Anne Enoch, M.D., M.R.C.G.P.

Case: Mrs A., a middle-aged, smartly dressed woman who prided herself on her homemaker skills, came to see her family practitioner, Dr B., complaining of tiredness, depressed mood, anxiety, disturbed sleep, and weight gain. Dr B. knew that her husband, a well-known local politician, had recently left her for a younger woman, so he tactfully avoided that subject, asking instead after her grown children who lived out of state. After questioning Mrs A. about her symptoms, Dr B. concluded that she might be hypothyroid, depressed, anemic, or all three, and ran the appropriate tests. Several visits later, after normal test results and a failed trial of antidepressants, Dr B. was feeling baffled until Mrs A. finally broke down in tears and revealed the cause of her symptoms. She had been a heavy drinker in her youth but had managed to stop when she had decided to have children. However, the recent stress and humiliation of her husband's desertion and subsequent loss of self-esteem, social status, and role in life had been too much for her and she had taken to comforting herself during her long and empty days at home by drinking. Although she made great efforts to hide her drinking problem, she had now reached the point where she could no longer control her urge to drink and was frightened and desperate for help but feared the social stigma of being labeled an alcoholic.

Introduction

Mid life is a vulnerable time for women, both for the development of problem drinking and alcoholism and for the manifestation of the medical consequences of long-term addiction to alcohol and tobacco. The unique problems that mid-life women face are threefold:
- The sense of loss particular to this age, the end of childbearing capabilities, the slipping away of youth, children leaving home, marriage/partner break-up, etc., may precipitate the onset of self-medicating problem drinking and alcoholism.

- The biological effects of menopause-related hormonal changes on the hypothalamic-pituitary-adrenal axis may increase stress and anxiety and hence vulnerability to problem drinking.
- Medical sequelae such as cirrhosis of the liver or cancer are likely to emerge at this age in the women who have been abusing alcohol and tobacco for a decade or two.

In many societies worldwide, people drink alcohol to relax, feel good, and facilitate social interactions. The regular consumption of small amounts of alcohol has been shown to have health benefits. However, for many individuals, there is a dark side because they become addicted and are unable to keep within safe limits of consumption.

Alcoholism is one of the most common mental disorders. In the USA, the lifetime prevalence of alcohol dependence, the severe form of alcoholism, is 20% in men and 8% in women, and that of alcohol abuse is 12% in men and 6% in women.[1] The UK 1999 General Household Survey showed that at any one time, more than 4% of adults are currently drinking alcoholics. The lifetime prevalence of alcoholism in the UK is likely to be the same as in the USA.

For a variety of reasons, problem drinking and alcoholism often go undiagnosed, particularly in women and the elderly.[2] The rate of screening for alcohol consumption in healthcare settings remains lower than 50%.[3] All too often, patients are treated symptomatically for alcohol-related conditions without recognition of the underlying problem.[2] Some patients may withhold information, perhaps because of shame or fear of stigmatization. In general, *women, particularly mid-life and older, experience more social disapproval of alcohol and other drug abuse than men.* This may account for both the tendency for mid-life women to drink in secrecy at home and the lower rates of alcoholism in women.

Nicotine is the other major addictive drug. In the 1990s, 19% of all deaths in the USA were tobacco-related, whereas alcoholism and other drug dependence accounted for only 6%. Social disapproval of smoking is not gender-specific in Western societies, and this may account for the fact that similar percentages of men (31%) and women (27%) are nicotine-dependent. Other addictions are less common. The prevalence of drug dependence in men and women is 9% and 6%, respectively, and that of drug abuse is 5% in men and 3% in women.[1] Although the evidence is not readily available, drug dependence and abuse are more prevalent in younger than older women. In addition, 11% of men and 8% of women report using psychotherapeutic agents (such as benzodiazepines) in a non-prescribed manner.

The main focus of this chapter will be on alcoholism and smoking, because these are the most prevalent addictive disorders in middle-aged women and are most commonly seen and treated in family practice.

Comorbidity with other psychiatric disorders

Alcoholism is complicated by the fact that, particularly in women, it is often accompanied by other psychiatric disorders; therefore, a holistic approach is required for treatment. Comorbid conditions include tobacco use, drug abuse, major depression, anxiety disorders, bulimia nervosa, and antisocial personality disorder (ASPD).[4] Alcohol problems predict the subsequent use of tranquilizing drugs in older women.[5] Severe alcoholism, impulsivity, and suicidal tendencies also tend to coexist but are more likely to group in men.[6] ASPD and antisocial symptoms are more prominent in male alcoholics, whereas in women alcoholism is often associated with anxiety (particularly social phobia) and affective disorders.[4] Major depression is much more common in women than in men, and many studies have shown that *antecedent depression is a risk factor for problem drinking.* In women, there is a strong relationship between depression and smoking; depressed individuals are more likely to smoke and are less successful at smoking cessation.[7]

Alcoholism and smoking often go together: 80–90% of alcoholics smoke cigarettes, as compared with 30% of the general population. Seventy percent of alcoholics are heavy smokers (more than a pack a day) compared with 10% of the general population.[8] Women who are regular smokers are five to six times more likely to be alcoholic compared with women who are non-smokers. Among smoking alcoholics, the initiation of regular cigarette smoking typically precedes the onset of alcoholism by many years.[8] The high comorbidity may be caused by the fact that either drug may increase the positive (rewarding) effects and/or reduce the negative (aversive) effects of the other. Some acute effects of nicotine may antagonize the negative effects of acute alcohol consumption (cognitive impairment, psychomotor function).

Genetic and environmental risk factors

The development of addiction to alcohol and other drugs is a complex process involving many factors, including genetic, environmental, and gene–environment interactions.[9]

Genetic factors

Inheritable vulnerability factors for addiction can be classified broadly into three categories. First, having certain heritable personality traits may predispose an individual to seek out and consume large quantities of alcohol (self-medication) and, therefore, increase their chances of becoming addicted. Neuroticism and anxious temperament have been associated with alcoholism in women but not men.[10,11] Neuroticism is also associated strongly with the development of nicotine withdrawal in women.[12] On the other hand, men with impulsive, novelty-seeking personalities are more likely to seek out pleasure-inducing substances.

Second, a heritable differential response to the effects of alcohol is associated with alcoholism vulnerability. A lower response to the sedating effects of alcohol has been shown in both men and women to be associated with a fourfold increase in the risk for alcoholism over time.[13]

Finally, genetic variation in neurobiological pathways may mean that some individuals are more vulnerable to the development of permanent neurological changes, manifest by a pattern of craving and loss of control over drug consumption.

Large, well-constructed, population-based twin studies have shown that the heritability (the genetic component of interindividual variation in vulnerability) of alcoholism is around 50–60%.[10,14,15] *More severe alcoholism may have a greater genetic component.* Although there is no gender difference in the heritability of alcoholism,[10,15–18] the genes that are involved in alcoholism vulnerability overlap only partially in men and women.[17] Although the heritability of nicotine dependence is the same in men and women (approximately 70%), only half the genes are shared.[19]

Alcohol, cocaine, opiates, and nicotine dependencies co-occur. Approximately 70% of alcoholics are heavy smokers, compared with 10% of the general population. This raises the possibility that there are both shared and substance-specific components to the heritability of alcoholism and other drug addictions. However, the results of large twin studies suggest that inheritance of addiction to alcohol, opioids, cocaine, and cannabis is largely independent.[20]

The strongest evidence for shared as well as specific addiction vulnerability is between alcohol and nicotine. In both men and women, *there is considerable genetic overlap between genes for alcoholism and nicotine addiction, particularly for heavy smoking and heavy drinking.* Approximately 50% of the genetic effects for nicotine dependence are shared with alcoholism, whereas 15% of the genetic effects for alcoholism are shared with nicotine dependence.[19]

Although alcoholism, major depression, and anxiety disorders often occur together in women, there is not much overlap in the genes underlying these disorders. Seventy-five percent of the genetic liability to alcoholism is disease-specific, and only small genetic components for alcoholism load on to a genetic factor common to major depression and generalized anxiety disorder as well as a factor common to phobia, panic, and bulimia nervosa.[21]

Environmental factors

Stress is considered to be a major component in the initiation and continuation of drug use as well as relapse. Smokers often state that they smoke more when stressed, partly because cigarette smoking is anxiolytic. Stress frequently provokes smoking relapse.

Emotional trauma and impaired social circumstances are also vulnerability factors for problem drinking in women. Women are more likely than men to self-medicate with alcohol; they often attribute the start of their problem drinking to a traumatic life event and the continuance of heavy drinking to stressors.[22]

Never married, divorced, and separated women are generally the heaviest drinkers and have the highest rates of drinking-related problems. More women alcoholics are separated or divorced or are likely to have an alcoholic spouse, compared with men alcoholics.[22] Partnership dissolution may be a risk factor for increased drinking in women who are not problem drinkers; obversely, in women who are already drinking heavily, separation or divorce can lead to a reduction in problem drinking, perhaps due to stress resolution.[23] Heavy drinking in women is associated with a lack of social roles, non-traditional jobs, rapid acculturation in ethnic minority women, adverse childhood experiences, and poor interpersonal relationships.[24]

Analyses of large national surveys of women's drinking habits found that the prevalence of childhood sexual abuse in the community was 15–26%,[25] and was associated with a fourfold increase in the lifetime prevalence of alcoholism and other drug abuse, depression, anxiety, and sexual dysfunction.[26,27] Among women drug users, 70% report childhood sexual abuse and more than 80% had at least one parent addicted to alcohol or drugs.[28]

Problem drinking in mid-life women is associated with marital disruption, children leaving home, and not having employment outside the home. Other risk factors are a failure to adapt to aging, heavy spousal drinking, drinking alone at home, and abuse of prescribed psychoactive drugs.[29] Perimenopause is a time of increased psychological and physical vulnerability for some individuals, which may be related to concurrent changes in the reactivity of the hormonal stress system.

Age and drinking patterns in women

Younger women (aged 21–30 years) drink the most and tend to engage in heavy episodic drinking, which can lead to severe adverse behavioral or social consequences. Drinking in mid life and older women is characterized by frequent light or moderate drinking.[23] Nevertheless, a substantial number of older women develop alcohol-related problems.

Drinking patterns and ethnicity

Abstention (approximately 50%) is higher among African-American and Hispanic than Caucasian women. Although Caucasian women drink more over time and per occasion, the proportion of heavy drinkers is the same in each group.[30] A survey of 64 500 African-American women aged 21–69 years from across the USA, enrolled in the Black Women's Health Study, found that the prevalence of current drinking was highest among women aged 40–49 years.[31]

As in men, the prevalence of heavy drinking and alcoholism in Caucasian women is highest in the young (aged 18–29 years) and decreases continuously with age, but in African-American women the prevalence rises to a high point in the 30–64 age group before declining.[30] Abstention and light drinking patterns may be more determined by cultural, social, and historical characteristics than are problem drinking and alcoholism.[30]

Definitions

The ceiling for low-risk alcohol use (advocated by the US government) is one standard drink per day and no more than three drinks per occasion for women, and two standard drinks per day and no more than four drinks per occasion for men. In the USA, the standard drink is 12 g of ethanol (equivalent to one 360-ml bottle of beer (4.5%), one 150-ml glass of wine (12.9%), or 45 ml of 80-proof distilled spirits). In the UK, the standard drink (unit) is 8 g of ethanol, and the ceiling for safe daily drinking is set at three to four units for men and two to three units for women. A meta-analysis of cohort studies evaluating the relationship between alcohol consumption and death from all causes found that the relative risk of death (due to cirrhosis, cancer, and injury) increased significantly in women consuming two to three U.S. standard drinks per day compared with four for men.[32]

In some individuals, problem drinking progresses into alcoholism. *The essential features of addiction are loss of control over consumption, compulsion to obtain the next stimulant, and continuation of abuse despite knowledge of negative health and social consequences.*[2] Prolonged heavy drinking may lead to long-lasting or permanent neurobiological changes, the essence of addiction, leading to craving and a loss of control over consumption. Tolerance and dependence are caused by neuroadaptations.

Medical consequences of long-term alcoholism

Harmful effects

The principal harmful effects of heavy drinking include liver pathology (hepaptitis, hepatoma, cirrhosis), neurological complications, and cancers of the mouth, larynx, oesophagus, and breast. Medical sequelae are likely to start to present in middle age in those alcoholics and smokers who started drinking and smoking in their youth.

Women achieve higher blood alcohol concentrations than men after the consumption of equivalent doses per body weight. The most likely explanation for this is that there is a lower volume of distribution of alcohol in women because the solubility of alcohol is greater in water than in fat and women tend to have proportionally more fat and less body water than men. The higher blood alcohol concentration may cause greater organ toxicity than in men. *Women tend to present with more severe liver disease* (particularly alcoholic hepatitis) and do so after drinking less and over a shorter period of time than men. Women are more likely than men to die from cirrhosis.[33] Women's brains may well be more sensitive to the deleterious effects of alcohol. One study has shown that alcoholic women show greater (reversible) gray and white matter brain shrinkage than alcoholic men, and that this may be caused by differences in neuronal molecular responses; however, these results are controversial.[34]

Many studies report that moderate to heavy alcohol consumption increases the risk for breast cancer.[35] A meta-analysis involving more than 150 000 women with and without breast cancer showed an increased relative risk of breast cancer of 1.32 (95% CI 1.19–1.45) for an intake of 35–44 g of alcohol per day. The relative risk increased by 7.1% for each additional 10 g/day alcohol-intake.[36] The investigators concluded that if the observed relationship is causal, then about 4% of the breast cancers in developed countries are alcohol-related. A prospective cohort study of approximately 45 000 postmenopausal women has shown that the relative risk is doubled when alcohol consumption is combined with hormone replacement therapy.[37] In contrast, smoking has little or no independent effect on the risk of developing breast cancer.[36]

The multiple harmful effects of cigarette consumption are well known and will not be discussed further here. However, the effects of alcohol and cigarette smoking are synergistic in the development of oral, laryngeal, pharyngeal, and esophageal cancers.

Beneficial effects of alcohol consumption

Before the age of 60, breast cancer is a more important cause of death than heart disease. Later on, the risk of heart disease exceeds that of breast cancer, so the benefits of moderate drinking are more apparent. *The consumption of at least one drink a day by mid-life and elderly women is associated with a 20% reduction in the risk of cardiovascular disease compared with non-drinkers.*[38] Like men, women appear to experience a U-shaped relationship between alcohol consumption and coronary artery disease.

Treatment

The treatment options that a family physician may discuss with a patient will depend on the severity of the alcohol problem, the presence of comorbid medical and psychosocial problems, the patient's motivation to change, and the patient's gender. The genders differ in the causes and consequences of alcoholism and in comorbidity, communication styles, levels of self-esteem, interpersonal relationships, and societal roles. Mixed-gender treatment groups are usually composed primarily of men and may, therefore, ignore women's issues. For all these reasons, women might do better in integrated women-oriented treatment approaches (bearing in mind that women alcoholics are not themselves a homogeneous group; they may differ in age, ethnicity, experience of abuse, symptom severity, etc.).

The treatment of women alcoholics includes three unique concerns, including:[39]

• related women's biological issues (reproduction, menopause);
• psychological issues associated with alcoholism more commonly in women than in men, such as past sexual or physical abuse, poor self-esteem, guilt, and shame;
• psychiatric comorbidity and multiple substance abuse.

Treatment programs for women do exist, but research on the impact of these services on both access and outcome is lacking.[40] One controlled study of 200 women demonstrated that women alcoholics treated in a specialized women's unit of a psychiatric hospital showed better control of alcohol consumption and social adjustment than women treated in a mixed unit.[41]

Because of both increased comorbidity and the way that women articulate and rationalize their drinking problems, women are more likely than men to seek treatment in health and social service facilities than in alcoholism and chemical dependency services. However, the cultural constraints against the admission of a drinking problem (even to themselves) for middle-aged women are huge. Unlike men, women often view their heavy drinking as a coping mechanism and not a problem. The most frequent reasons given by women for seeking treatment are depression, alcohol-related medical problems, interpersonal problems with spouse, partner, or children, and, especially among mid-life women, the "empty nest" syndrome.[42] Therefore, it may take longer for mid-life women's alcohol abuse to be recognized and treated.

Treatment of problem drinking: the use of brief intervention in family practice

The family physician can play a key role in recognizing problem drinking and can often intervene successfully, particularly in the early stages. Several formal screening instruments for problem drinking/alcoholism are available.[2] Brief intervention is a short-term, counseling strategy based on motivational enhancement therapy that concentrates on changing patient behavior and increasing patient compliance with therapy. It is designed for health professionals who are not specialists in addiction.[43]

Brief intervention involves:
1 Reviewing with the patient the quantity and frequency of current drinking and their personal causes of excessive drinking.
2 Advising the patient to reduce or stop drinking and making them aware of their personal risks for alcohol-related problems.
3 Discussing with the patient whether, or when, they will reduce or stop drinking and emphasizing their personal responsibility.
4 Suggesting coping mechanisms, behavior modification, and self-help groups (e.g. Alcoholics Anonymous).
5 Establishing a drinking goal and the setting up of a drinking diary.

For brief intervention to be successful, the physician must encourage self-motivation and optimism and be non-judgmental and supportive. *Brief intervention has been shown to be effective for helping socially stable problem drinkers to reduce or stop drinking, for motivating alcohol-dependent patients to enter long-term alcohol treatment,* and for treating some alcohol-dependent patients in whom the goal is abstinence. It is generally necessary to have only four or fewer sessions, each ranging from a few minutes to an hour depending on the severity of the patient's alcohol problem.[43] It is not known whether this kind of intervention is equally effective in men and women and at all ages.

Treatment of alcohol dependence and abuse

A formal diagnosis of alcoholism can have enormous personal implications for a patient. Therefore, assessment should be detailed.[2] Alcohol abuse and dependence have a variable course characterized by periods of remission and relapse. There are three components to alcoholism: (i) physiological dependence (symptoms of withdrawal), (ii) psychological dependence (alcohol used as self-medication), and (iii) habit (the incorporation of drinking into the framework of daily living).

Alcohol dependence is treated in two stages: withdrawal and detoxification, followed by further interventions to prevent relapse.

Immediate treatment: detoxification – the control of alcohol withdrawal syndrome

In heavy, chronic drinkers, withdrawal symptoms begin 6–48 hours after the last drink, peak within 24–48 hours, and gradually resolve within five to seven days. The severity of withdrawal symptoms increases with each withdrawal episode. Severe withdrawal (grand mal convulsions, delirium tremens) occurs in 2–5% of heavy-drinking chronic alcoholics. With treatment, mortality is about 1%, death usually being caused by cardiovascular collapse or concurrent infection.

Benzodiazepines are used widely for treatment of withdrawal, because they greatly reduce symptoms and the risk of seizure. However, benzodiazepines are sedating, produce cognitive impairment, are addictive, and may interact additively with alcohol. An alternative approach is to use non-sedating, non-addictive, anticonvulsant agents such as carbamazepine and valproic acid, which have been used successfully for many years in Europe.[44] However, these drugs have hematological side effects and liver toxicity, so patients have to be medically screened before use. Alcoholics should be admitted to hospital for detoxification if they are likely to have severe, life-threatening symptoms or if they have serious medical conditions, suicidal or homicidal tendencies, or disruptive work or home situations.

Sustained treatment: prevention of relapse

There is considerable evidence that long-lasting neurobiological changes in the brains of alcoholics contribute to the persistence of craving. At any stage during recovery, relapse can be triggered by internal factors (craving for alcohol, depression, and anxiety) or external factors (environmental triggers, social pressures, life events, taking drugs, and narcotics). *Depression is associated with relapse in women but not in men.* For both sexes the severity of alcoholism is a predictor of relapse, but for women a measure of psychological functioning and social networks are predictive of outcome. Married men are less likely to relapse after treatment. For women, being married contributes to relapse in the short term.[45] Alcoholic women appear to receive less support from family and friends than do non-alcoholic women, both in childhood and adulthood.[42] The development of new, fulfilling social roles and an effective social support network (such as through Alcoholics Anonymous or Women for Sobriety) are important aspects of alcoholism treatment for women.

The main elements of treatment for alcoholism are still psychosocial. These methods concentrate on helping patients to understand, anticipate, and prevent relapse. Relapse rates are still very high. However, promising pharmacotherapeutic agents are emerging that can be used as adjuncts to psychosocial treatments.

Behavioral treatment approaches

No one behavioral approach has been shown to produce better results than another; therefore, patient preference, cost considerations, and availability of treatment will determine which approach is taken.

Alcoholics Anonymous, Women for Sobriety, and 12-step facilitation therapy

Alcoholics Anonymous (AA) is a worldwide spiritual program that addresses people from all social strata. Group members share their experiences in a confidential environment and provide each other with help and support in order to maintain sobriety. AA and similar self-help groups follow 12 steps that alcoholics should work through during recovery. There are women-only AA groups. Twelve-step facilitation (TSF) is a formal treatment approach incorporating AA and similar 12-step programs.[46]

Women for Sobriety (WFS) is a rapidly expanding worldwide organization of women for women. The purpose is to help women recover from all aspects of addiction (physiological, mental, and emotional) through the discovery of self, gained by sharing experiences, hopes, and encouragement with other women in similar circumstances. The WFS "New Life" program starts by accepting alcoholism as a disease, getting rid of negative thoughts (guilt, shame), creating and practicing a new, positive view of self, using new attitudes to enforce new behavior patterns, and making efforts to improve relationships and identify life's priorities.

Cognitive-behavioral therapy and motivational enhancement therapy
The aim of cognitive-behavioral therapy (CBT) is to teach patients, by role play and rehearsal, to recognize and cope with high-risk situations for relapse and to recognize and cope with craving.[47] Motivational enhancement therapy (MET) is used to motivate patients to use their own resources to change their behavior and has been found to be most effective in those with high levels of anger.[48]

Pharmacotherapy of alcohol addiction

Only 30–60% of alcoholics maintain at least one year of abstinence with psychosocial therapies alone. This is not much of an improvement over the more than 20% of alcoholics who achieve long-term sobriety without active treatment. More effective therapies are clearly needed.

Pharmacotherapeutic agents are emerging that can complement psychosocial treatments. More research needs to be done to determine which therapies are most effective in which alcoholic subtypes and whether there are gender differences in treatment response.

Anti-craving medications
The most promising medications are the opioid antagonist, naltrexone, and acamprosate, a glutamate antagonist, which have been shown to exert modest effects on the reduction of alcohol consumption.[49] These drugs, either used separately or in combination (currently being tested), are likely to be the beginning of pharmacotherapies targeting multiple neurotransmitters. Further studies are needed to identify subgroups of alcoholics who may be the most responsive to these drugs.

Several studies have shown that naltrexone (50 mg four times daily), also used in the post-detoxification treatment of heroin addicts, reduces alcohol consumption in both men and women alcoholics. Its use is effective when combined with psychosocial treatment in reducing relapse rates.[50,51] A recent preliminary study has found that taking naltrexone two hours before an anticipated high-risk situation reduces alcohol consumption in early problem drinkers, particularly women.[52] Acamprosate, used extensively in Europe and now being tested in the USA, is safe and well tolerated and may almost double the abstinence rate among recovering alcoholics.[53]

Aversive pharmocotherapy

Disulfiram (Antabuse™), a drug with a moderate record of adverse effects, including hepatotoxicity, blocks the metabolism of acetaldehyde and causes the very unpleasant flushing reaction if taken with alcohol. Outcomes with disulfiram are improved when the drug is taken under supervision. Patients must be cognizant of the possibility of severe reactions, including vomiting and even death, if alcohol is ingested while disulfiram is used.

Pharmacotherapy for comorbid conditions

Depression and anxiety can precipitate alcohol abuse but can also be a result of heavy drinking. It is important to take a careful history in order to identify the primary problem. Fluoxetine (Prozac™), a serotonin reuptake inhibitor, has been found to be effective in decreasing both depressive symptoms and the level of alcohol consumption in depressed alcoholics.[44]

Pharmacotherapy of nicotine addiction

The acute effects of smoking (calmness, alertness, increased concentration) can be positively reinforcing, whereas nicotine withdrawal symptoms (depressed mood, insomnia, irritability, anxiety, poor concentration, weight gain) are negatively reinforcing.[49] Pharmacotherapy is an integral part of the treatment of nicotine dependence but is most effective with concurrent behavioral therapy. Both nicotine-replacement therapies and bupropion (Zyban™) double long-term smoking cessation rates and have, therefore, been recommended as first-line therapy by the Agency for Healthcare Research and Quality. Nicotine-replacement therapies (Food and Drug Administration (FDA)-approved), include 2- or 4-mg nicotine polacrilex gum, the nicotine patch, nicotine nasal spray, and the nicotine inhaler.[49]

The choice of therapy can be tailored individually, depending on patient preference, side effects, or the presence of other medical conditions. Sustained-release bupropion is an antidepressant medication.[49] Another antidepressant, nortriptyline, has been shown recently to be efficacious for smoking cessation.

Although nicotine-replacement therapies and bupropion significantly increase smoking cessation rates, many smokers still relapse. The one-year quit rate remains low. There are limited or no research data regarding the success of smoking cessation therapies specific to gender or ethnicity. Further research needs to be done on treating specific populations with comorbid diseases.

Treatment of alcoholic smokers

Alcohol consumption may be a risk factor for smoking relapse, partly because alcohol may increase craving for cigarettes. Likewise, smoking cues may promote craving for alcohol. Most alcoholic smokers state that they want to stop alcohol first and then cigarettes. However, a substantial minority try both treatments simultaneously. It is not known which approach is the most efficacious.

Conclusion

Detecting and treating alcohol problems in mid-life women can be both challenging and complex because of the secrecy, the layers of comorbidity, and the frequent undercurrent of (often suppressed) past adverse life events, particularly childhood sexual abuse. Nevertheless, family physicians are in a good position to diagnose and treat problem drinking because most adults visit their primary care physician at least once every two years and women in particular usually consult their physicians more frequently. In addition, there is often a trusting doctor–patient relationship, built up over years. Screening for alcohol problems needs to become routine in the same way that screening for smoking is now widespread. However, it may be harder for physicians to diagnose drinking problems in mid-life women, partly because this is a group that they may assume to be low risk, partly because they may feel uncomfortable asking about a condition with a built-in social stigma, and partly because many middle-aged women prefer to keep their problem a secret. This stigma may be erased over time with the aging of the current cohort of young women, amongst whom heavy drinking is socially acceptable. A holistic treatment approach needs to be taken, including management of comorbid conditions, counseling for previous emotional trauma, teaching of coping skills, and the development of support networks, for example through AA and WFS.

FURTHER RESOURCES

Alcoholics Anonymous: www.alcoholics-anonymous.org
Find local groups in telephone directory under "Alcoholism" or call 212 870 3400 (USA), 0845 769 7555 (UK)
  Women for Sobriety: www.womenforsobriety.org
  Tel. 1 800 333 1606 (USA)
Center for Substance Abuse Treatment: Tel. 1 800 662 HELP (USA) for information about local US treatment programs
  National Institute on Alcohol Abuse and Alcoholism: www.niaaa.nih.gov

Public Information Office 301 443 3860 (USA)
National Clearinghouse for Alcohol and Drug Information: www.health.org
    Tel. 1 800 729 6686 (USA)
Institute of Alcohol Studies (UK): www.ias.org.uk
    Tel. 020 7222 4001 (UK)
Al-Anon (for spouses/partners) and Alateen (for children of alcoholics):
www.al-anon.alateen.org
    Tel. 1 800 344 2666 (USA)

REFERENCES

1 Kessler, R. C., McGonagle, K. A., Zhao, S., *et al.* Lifetime and 12-month prevalence of DSM-III-R psychiatric disorders in the United States: results from the National Comorbidity Survey. *Arch. Gen. Psychiatry* 1994; **51**:8–19.

2 Enoch, M.-A. and Goldman, D. Problem drinking and alcoholism: diagnosis and treatment. *Am. Fam. Physician* 2002; **65**:441–8, 449–50.

3 Fleming, M. F. Strategies to increase alcohol screening in health care settings. *Alcohol Health Res. World* 1997; **21**:340–47.

4 Kessler, R. C., Crum, R. M., Warner, L. A., *et al.* Lifetime co-occurrence of DSM-III-R alcohol abuse and dependence with other psychiatric disorders in the National Comorbidity Survey. *Arch. Gen. Psychiatry* 1997; **54**:313–21.

5 Graham, K. and Wilsnack, S. C. The relationship between alcohol problems and use of tranquilizing drugs: longitudinal patterns among American women. *Addict. Behav.* 2000; **25**:13–28.

6 Brown, G. L., Kline, W. J., Goyer, P. F., *et al.* Relationship of childhood characteristics to cerebrospinal fluid 5-HIAA in aggressive adults. In C. Chagass (ed.). *Biological Psychiatry*. New York: Elsevier; 1985. p. 177.

7 Perkins, K. A. Sex differences in nicotine versus non-nicotine reinforcement as determinants of tobacco smoking. *Exp. Clin. Psychopharmacol.* 1996; **11**:199–212.

8 National Institute on Alcohol Abuse and Alcoholism. Alcohol and tobacco. *Alcohol Alert* 1998; **39**:1–4.

9 Enoch, M. A. and Goldman, D. Genetics of alcoholism and substance abuse. *Psychiatr. Clin. North Am.* 1999; **22**:289–99.

10 Heath, A. C., Bucholz, K. K., Madden, P. A. F., *et al.* Genetic and environmental contributions to alcohol dependence risk in a national twin sample: consistency of findings in women and men. *Psychol. Med.* 1997; **27**:1381–96.

11 Enoch, M.-A., Harris, C. R. and Goldman, D. Sex differences in the role of anxious temperament in alcoholism and mood disorders. *Fam. Med.*, submitted.

12 Madden, P. A., Bucholz, K. K., Dinwiddie, S. H., *et al.* Nicotine withdrawal in women. *Addiction* 1997; **92**:889–902.

13 Schuckit, M. A., Smith, T. L., Kalmijn, J., *et al.* Response to alcohol in daughters of alcoholics: a pilot study and a comparison with sons of alcoholics. *Alcohol Alcohol.* 2000; **35**:242–8.

14 Heath, A. C. Genetic influences on alcoholism risk. A review on adoption and twin studies. *Alcohol Health Res. World* 1995; **19**:166–71.

15 Kendler, K. S., Heath, A. C., Neale, M. C., Kessler, R. C. and Eaves, L. J. A population-based twin study of alcoholism in women. *J. Am. Med. Assoc.* 1992; **268**:1877–82.

16 Kendler, K. S., Neale, M. C., Heath, A. C., Kessler, R. C. and Eaves, L. A twin-family study of alcoholism in women. *Am. J. Psychiatry* 1994; **151**:707–15.

17 Prescott, C. A., Aggen, S. H. and Kendler, K. S. Sex differences in the source of genetic liability to alcohol abuse and dependence in a population-based sample of U.S. twins. *Alcohol Clin. Exp. Res.* 1999; **23**:1136–44.

18 Prescott, C. A. and Kendler, K. S. Genetic and environmental contributions to alcohol abuse and dependence in a population-based sample of male twins. *Am. J. Psychiatry* 1999; **156**:34–40.

19 Hettema, J. M., Corey, L. A. and Kendler, K. S. A multivariate genetic analysis of the use of tobacco, alcohol and caffeine in a population-based sample of male and female twins. *Drug Alcohol Depend.* 1999; **57**:69–78.

20 Goldman, D. and Bergen, A. General and specific inheritance of substance abuse and alcoholism. *Arch. Gen. Psychiatry* 1998; **55**:964–5.

21 Kendler, K. S., Walters, E. E. and Neale, M. C. The structure of the genetic and environmental risk factors for six major psychiatric disorders in women. *Arch. Gen. Psychiatry* 1995; **52**:374–83.

22 Lex, B. W. Gender differences and substance abuse. *Adv. Subst. Abuse* 1991; **4**:225–96.

23 Wilsnack, S. C., Wilsnack, R. W. and Hiller-Sturmhofel, S. How women drink: epidemiology of women's drinking and problem drinking. *Alcohol Health Res. World* 1994; **18**:173–80.

24 Wilsnack, S. C. and Wilsnack, R. W. Drinking and problem drinking in US women. Patterns and recent trends. *Recent Dev. Alcohol.* 1995; **12**:29–60.

25 Vogeltanz, N. D., Wilsnack, S. C. and Harris, T. R. Prevalence and risk factors for childhood sexual abuse in women: national survey findings. *Child Abuse Negl.* 1999; **23**:579–92.

26 Winfield, I., George, L. K., Swartz, M. *et al.* Sexual assault and psychiatric disorders among a community sample of women. *Am. J. Psychiatry* 1990; **147**:335–41.

27 Wilsnack, S. C., Vogeltanz, N. D., Klassen, A. D. and Harris, T. R. Childhood sexual abuse and women's substance abuse: national survey findings. *J. Stud. Alcohol* 1997; **58**:264–71.

28 Winfield, I., George, L. K., Swartz, M. and Blazer, D. G. National Institute on Drug Abuse. Capsules. *Women and Drug Abuse* 1994; **6**:2.

29 Gomberg, E. S. Risk factors for drinking over a woman's lifespan. *Alcohol Health Res. World* 1994; **18**:220–27.

30 Caetano, R. Drinking and alcohol-related problems among minority women. *Alcohol Health Res. World* 1994; **18**:233–41.

31 Rosenberg, L., Palmer, J. R., Rao, R. S. and Adams-Campbell, L. L. Patterns and correlates of alcohol consumption among African-American women. *Ethn. Dis.* 2002; **12**:548–54.

32 Holman, C. D., English, D. R., Milne, E. and Winter, M. G. Meta-analysis of alcohol and all-cause mortality: a validation of NHMRC recommendations. *Med. J. Aust.* 1996; **164**:141–5.

33 Day, C. P. Who gets alcoholic liver disease: nature or nuture? *J. R. Coll. Physicians Lond.* 2000; **34**:557–62.

34 Wuethrich, B. Does alcohol damage female brains more? *Science* 2001; **291**:2077–9.

35 Smith-Warner, S. A., Spiegelman, D., Yuan, S. S., *et al.* Alcohol and breast cancer in women: a pooled analysis of cohort studies. *J. Am. Med. Assoc.* 1998; **279**:535–40.

36 Hamajima, N., Hirose, K., Tajima, K., *et al.* Alcohol, tobacco and breast cancer – collaborative reanalysis of individual data from 53 epidemiological studies, including 58,515 women with breast cancer and 95,067 women without the disease. *Br. J. Cancer* 2002; **87**:1234–45.

37 Chen, W. Y., Colditz, G. A., Rosner, B., *et al.* Use of postmenopausal hormones, alcohol, and risk for invasive breat cancer. *Ann. Intern. Med.* 2002; **137**:798–804.

38 Thun, M. J., Peto, R., Lopez, A. D., *et al.* Alcohol consumption and mortality among middle-aged and elderly U.S. adults. *N. Engl. J. Med.* 1997; **337**:1705–14.

39 Beckman, L. J. Treatment needs of women with alcohol problems. *Alcohol Health Res. World* 1994; **18**:206–11.

40 Smith, W. B. and Weisner, C. Women and alcohol problems: a critical analysis of the literature and unanswered questions. *Alcohol. Clin. Exp. Res.* 2000; **24**:1320–21.

41 Dahlgren, L. and Willander, A. Are special treatment facilities for female alcoholics needed? A controlled 2-year follow-up study from a specialized female unit (EWA) versus a mixed male/female treatment facility. *Alcohol. Clin. Exp. Res.* 1989; **13**:499–504.

42 Gomberg, E. S. Women and alcohol: use and abuse. *J. Nerv. Ment. Dis.* 1993; **181**:211–19.

43 Fleming, M. and Manwell, L. B. Brief intervention in primary care settings. *Alcohol Res. Health* 1999; **23**:128–37.

44 Myrick, H., Brady, K. T. and Malcolm, R. New developments in the pharmacotherapy of alcohol dependence. *Am. J. Addict.* 2001; **10** (supp):3–15.

45 Schneider, K. M., Kviz, F. J., Isola, M. L. and Filstead, W. J. Evaluating multiple outcomes and gender differences in alcoholism treatment. *Addict. Behav.* 1995; **20**:1–21.

46 Humphreys, K. Professional interventions that facilitate 12-step self-help group involvement. *Alcohol Res. Health* 1999; **23**:93–8.

47 Longabaugh, R. and Morgenstern, J. Cognitive-behavioral coping-skills therapy for alcohol dependence. *Alcohol Res. Health* 1999; **23**:78–85.

48 DiClemente, C. C., Bellino, L. E. and Neavins, T. M. Motivation for change and alcoholism treatment. *Alcohol Res. Health* 1999; **23**:86–92.

49 Kranzler, H. R., Amin, H., Modesto-Lowe, V. and Oncken, C. Pharmacologic treatments for drug and alcohol dependence. *Addict. Dis.* 1999; **22**:401–23.

50 O'Malley, S. S. Opioid antagonists in the treatment of alcohol dependence: clinical efficacy and prevention of relapse. *Alcohol Alcohol. Suppl.* 1996; **1**:77–81.

51 Anton, R. F., Moak, D. H., Waid, L. R., *et al.* Naltrexone and cognitive behavioral therapy for the treatment of outpatient alcoholics: results of a placebo-controlled trial. *Am. J. Psychiatry* 1999; **156**:1758–64.

52 Kranzler, H., Tennen, H., Armeli, S., *et al.* Targetted naltrexone for early problem drinkers. *Alcohol. Clin. Exp. Res.* 2001; **25**(supp):144A.

53 Sass, H., Soyka, M. and Mann, K. and Zieglgansberger, W. Relapse prevention by acamprosate. Results from a placebo-controlled study on alcohol dependence. *Arch. Gen. Psychiatry* 1996; **53**:673–80.

7

Depression and anxiety

Anne Walling

Case: "I am turning into a big fat lump that just lies around eating, sleeping and feeling sorry for myself all the time!" This sudden outburst during a visit for a "routine pap smear" is completely out of character for Marie, a 44-year-old divorced schoolteacher who is usually smartly groomed, articulate, and vivacious. Tactful questioning reveals about a four-week history of excessive sleeping and feelings of fatigue, low stamina, and worthlessness. She has been snacking excessively and has gained about six pounds. Marie admits to severe "blues" during her freshman college year and after the births of her children, but she "toughed it out." This time, she does not have the energy or will to continue her daily activities and she has called in sick for the first time ever as she "just could not face doing a mediocre job for the class."

Introduction and epidemiology

Up to 30% of women seen in primary care clinics suffer from a depressive illness, compared with an estimated 19% of male patients.[1,2] In the general population, approximately one-quarter of all women but only 10% of men suffer from depression at any time during the lifespan. This gender difference begins in adolescence and continues until the sixth decade.[3] As individuals, women generally carry a greater burden of illness in depression than men. Depression is more likely to begin at an earlier age in women[4] and to follow a pattern with more severe, chronic, and recurrent illness with greater functional impairment and more comorbid conditions than in male patients.[5]

Depression ranks fourth on the World Health Organization (WHO) Global Burden of Illness scale and is expected to reach second place by 2020. Because of the heavy caring and professional responsibilities of middle-aged women, depression in this group has a particularly significant impact on society. Approximately 40% of middle-aged women are "sandwich carers," responsible for both dependent children or grandchildren and elderly relatives.[6] A depressive illness in such a carer can have profound effects on the health and functioning of multiple others.

Etiology of gender differences

Several theories have been proposed to explain the gender differences in depression. Biologically based theories focus on gender differences in brain function, especially in neurotransmitter and neuroendocrine systems, and in the neuropsychological effects of reproductive hormones. Psychosocial theories emphasize the low social status of women, role stress, and victimization. Gender differences in the prevalence and manifestations of depression probably result from a combination of biological, environmental, social, and other factors. A family history of mood disorders and other factors linked strongly to depression, such as poverty, victimization, and childhood adversity,[7] are more common in depressed women than in men with the same diagnosis.[2,5]

In a predisposed individual, life events can trigger depression. *Women are more likely than men to report a stressful life event in the six months prior to a major depression and may be more vulnerable to developing depression after stressors.*[5] Many mid-life women face a cluster of potential triggers, such as divorce, relationship issues, loss or illness of parents, retirement/employment issues, concerns over adolescent and adult children, financial stress, domestic violence, and health concerns, including menopause.[6]

Clinical presentation

The presentation of depression in a middle-aged woman may be complex and/or difficult to recognize. A high index of suspicion is required. Women often are reluctant to view themselves as depressed, do not directly complain of a depressed mood, or are hesitant to discuss emotional concerns. Depression may also be masked by physical or vegetative features that are more prominent than mood symptoms. Depressed women commonly present with non-specific complaints of tiredness, low energy, malaise, poor sleep, or vague pain syndromes. "Atypical," yet common, symptoms of depression in women include increased appetite, weight gain, and increased sleep.

Some women maintain high levels of functioning and an external appearance of normalcy in spite of profound inner distress and significant disturbances in energy, sleep, or appetite. Depression remains underdiagnosed and undertreated, in part because of the stigma against mental illness and misconceptions about depression by both physicians and patients.

Three-quarters of depressed women initially consult primary care physicians.[6] They may present with a wide range of physical or emotional symptoms, or a combination of both. A depressed woman may also present with no

Table 7.1 Gender differences in depression

Factors	Difference in women compared with men
Lifetime prevalence	Doubled
Age at onset	Younger
Family history	More common
Triggered by life stressor	Stronger relationship/greater vulnerability
Seasonal pattern	Three times more common
"Atypical" symptoms*	More common
Number of symptoms	Increased
Duration of episodes	Extended
Chronic/recurrent pattern	More common
Severity/functional impairment	Increased
Comorbid psychiatric conditions	Anxiety and eating disorders increased
	Alcohol and substance abuse decreased
	Dependent personality increased
	Antisocial, obsessive-compulsive disorder decreased
Associated medical conditions	Thyroid, rheumatological, migraine
Suicide	More attempts but less successful

*Weight and appetite increase, excessive sleep, psychomotor retardation, anxiety/ somatization.

overt symptoms during a routine physical exam, and may disclose depressive symptoms only if she feels safe and confident that the physician can provide effective help. Physicians are five times more likely to recognize depression if psychiatric symptoms are mentioned early in the interview and if no physical illness is detected.[8] Awareness of gender differences in depression can facilitate diagnosis (Table 7.1). Women may present at certain times, such as premenstrually, during perimenopause, and during exogenous hormone therapy, because of hormonal triggers of depression. Women tend to have a more chronic pattern of depressive illness than men and to express more symptoms of appetite/weight changes, sleep disturbances, psychomotor retardation, guilt, panic, anxiety, and somatization (especially pain syndromes).[9]

Both the presentation and the prognosis of depression may be complicated in women by the higher rates of comorbid psychiatric and medical conditions. Women are more likely than men to attempt suicide, but men are four times more likely to die by suicide because they tend to use more lethal methods.

The spectrum of depressive illnesses

In primary care, most women presenting with depressed mood (dysphoria) have major depressive disorder (MDD),[1] but the spectrum of depressive illness includes adjustment disorder with depressed mood, dysthymia, bipolar affective disorder, premenstrual dysphoric disorder, mood disorder because of a general medical condition, and substance-induced mood disorder.

Major depressive disorder

MDD has been reported in more than 20% of women aged 40–60 years who attended an inner-city primary care practice.[1] By definition, symptoms must last for at least two consecutive weeks, be a significant change in usual functioning, and directly impair ability to conduct normal activities. A classic MDD presentation in a middle-aged woman is of fatigue interfering with managing housework/cooking/family responsibilities, loss of interest in hobbies and activities, gradual neglect of friends, and increasing social isolation. Physical symptoms of fatigue, malaise, pain, and vague physical complaints are also common. Some women express dysphoria more as irritability than as overt sadness.

History and screening

Although several formal screening and assessment tools are available to detect and/or quantify depression, recent guidelines recommend use of two simple questions:[10]

Over the last two weeks have you felt:
1 Down, depressed, or hopeless? (depressed mood)
2 Little interest or pleasure in doing things? (anhedonia).

In primary care, these questions may be as effective as longer screening tools.[11] Any positive response should trigger more detailed questioning for symptoms of depression. Primary-care physicians have high reliability in diagnosing MDD using semi-structured interviews (Table 7.2).[12]

Several validated and reliable screening tools are available,[12] such as the Beck Depression Inventory[13] (and the shorter Beck Depression Inventory for Primary Care[14]), the Zung Self-Rating Depression Scale, and the Hamilton Rating Scale for Depression. Physicians should use the tool with which they feel most comfortable; all appear to give comparable results.[12] The US Preventive Services Task Force (USPSTF) found good evidence that screening for depression improves the accuracy of diagnosis and contributes to effective treatment and decreased morbidity if systems are in place to ensure effective treatment and follow-up (grade B recommendation).[15]

The diagnosis of MDD depends on history supported by observation of the patient's general appearance, language, and demeanor. Change from normal appearance and function is particularly important. Open-ended, unhurried, and non-judgmental questions encourage patients to reveal symptoms. Specific, closed-ended questions can then be used to delineate symptoms, provide

Table 7.2 Establishing the diagnosis of major depression by interview

Symptom	Suggested questions
Dysphoria	How has your mood been over the last two weeks? Do you feel depressed, down, or blue? When did you last feel happy or well?
Anhedonia	Have you lost interest in your usual activities? Do you get less pleasure from things? When was the last time you had fun?
Appetite/weight change	Are you eating more or less than usual? Is your weight increasing or decreasing?
Sleep disturbance	Are you sleeping more or less than usual?
Psychomotor change	Do you feel slowed down or restless and fidgety?
Energy decrease	Are you as energetic as usual?
Guilt/worthlessness	Do you feel guilty or blame yourself for things?
Indecisiveness/concentration	Are you having more trouble than usual in concentrating or making decisions?
Suicidal ideation	Have you thought about hurting yourself or wished you were dead? Is life worth living? Have you thought that others would be better off without you?

Source: Williams, J. W., Noel, P. H., Cordes, J. A., Ramirez, G., and Pigone, M. Is this patient clinically depressed? *J. Am. Med. Assoc.* 2002; **287**:1160–70.

information about precipitants and comorbidities, and assess the appropriate family, social, and prior medical history.

Most middle-aged women presenting with depression have had prior episodes as young adults. Those who have experienced two or more episodes have an 80–90% chance of repeated episodes.[6] A first episode of depressive symptoms in middle age should raise suspicion of an underlying medical condition (Table 7.3) or unrecognized bipolar disorder.

In eliciting the patient's medical history, physicians should be alert for medical and psychiatric conditions that could either exacerbate depression or complicate its treatment. All patients should be asked specifically about alcohol/substance abuse and risk of suicide. The CAGE questionnaire* is recommended to screen for alcohol abuse, although its sensitivity may be lower in women than in men.[12]

Several factors increase the risk for suicide in depressed patients (Table 7.4).[16] All patients should be asked direct questions, such as "Have you been feeling that life is not worth living or you would be better off dead?" A positive

---

* CAGE: Have you Cut down on alcohol lately? Have you gotten Annoyed by somebody telling you you should cut down on alcohol lately? Do you feel Guilty about the amount you are drinking? Do you need on Eye-opener?

Table 7.3 General medical conditions of middle-aged women associated with depression

Neurological conditions	Malignancies	Organ/systems failure	Other conditions	Medications
Stroke	CNS tumors (including secondary)	Congestive heart failure	Myocardial infarction	Clonidine
Multiple sclerosis	Pancreatic cancer	Chronic lung disease	Systemic lupus erythematosus	Opiates
Seizure disorders	Lung cancer	Renal failure	Disturbances of sodium, potassium, or calcium metabolism**	Barbiturates
Head injury	Leukemias	Hepatic failure		Benzodiazepines
Parkinson's disease		Adrenal failure (Addison's disease)*		Hypnotic agents
Normal-pressure hydrocephalus		Hypothyroid states*		Digoxin
Dementia		Hypoparathyroid states*		Antiarrhythmic medications
		Diabetes**		Antiparkinson drugs
				Indomethacin
				Corticosteroids
				Estrogen
				Progesterone
				Cimetidine

* Also associated with hyperfunctioning, e.g. Cushing's disease or Graves' disease.
** Associated with hyper- or hypoglycemia, -calcinemia, -natremia, and -kalemia.

Table 7.4 Suicide risk factors

Major depression
Hopelessness
Presence of psychosis
Substance abuse or dependence
Severe anxiety or panic disorder
Medical illness
Recent relationship loss, such as widowed or divorced
Poor social support
Prior admission to a psychiatric facility
Past suicide attempts
Family history of suicide
Active suicidal ideation
Development of suicidal plan
Access to lethal means of suicide

Source: Moscicki, E. K. Identification of suicide risk factors using epidemiologic studies *Psychiatr. Clin. North Am.* 1997; **20**:499–517.

response should be followed by questions about development of a plan. Women at high risk of suicide should be referred for psychiatric evaluation.[12] Referral for psychiatric evaluation is also necessary in severe episodes of major depression with associated psychotic features such as delusions and/or hallucinations.

Physical and laboratory assessment
Physical examination and laboratory investigations serve primarily to identify comorbid conditions that could have precipitated the episode of MDD and/or are likely to complicate its management. Investigations are targeted to the needs of the individual patient. They may include complete blood count, thyroid studies, assessment of electrolyte (sodium, potassium, calcium) and glucose levels, and evaluation of hepatic and renal function. Menopausal status may be confirmed by increased levels of follicle-stimulating hormone (FSH) (greater than 20 IU/dl) and decreased estradiol (less than 60 pg/ml) on day two or three of the menstrual cycle. Physical examination and laboratory findings are normal in many women with depression.

Management
Primary care physicians can manage successfully the vast majority of women with MDD. Therapeutic goals are to induce remission, ensure patient safety (including reducing risks of suicide and iatrogenic effects of under or over treatment), optimize function, and protect the patient from recurrent episodes of MDD.[17] For many middle-aged women, primary care physicians can build on

therapeutic alliances developed through prior experiences of health issues for the patient or family members. Trust and confidentiality are essential in assisting patients to select and adhere to the optimal treatment strategy for MDD. The many therapeutic options are divided broadly into psychotherapeutic and pharmacotherapeutic approaches (or a combination of both). Education of the patient and family about the condition, management options, anticipated course of the illness, and relapse prevention underlies all therapy.

Psychotherapy

For a mild to moderate episode of major depression, psychotherapy provides effective treatment), equivalent to antidepressant medication (American Psychiatric Association (APA) level of confidence II).[17] The most important factors in selecting psychotherapy are patient preference and her confidence in the approach. Psychotherapy may also be preferred if the patient has significant psychosocial stressors, internal conflicts, interpersonal difficulties, or a comorbid axis II disorder (APA level of confidence I).[17]

Several issues may make psychotherapy an appropriate treatment choice for a middle-aged woman. Compared with men, women are believed to be more dependent, more self-blaming, and more likely to internalize stress and pain. In addition, women may be more likely to derive self-esteem from interactions in relationships rather than mastery over their physical environment and to have low expectations or be habituated to low-prestige roles in society.[18] Psychosocial stressors for middle-aged women include aging in a youth-focused society and significant role transitions as her children mature, grandchildren are born, and her parents age. Many women become care-givers for aging, debilitated parents or dependent grandchildren. The mid-life woman is also commonly faced with chronic illness, loss of her significant other by divorce, death, or separation, and by challenges in her employment.[6] Psychotherapy must address these psychosocial features in order to improve depressive symptoms.

Problem-solving therapies such as cognitive-behavioral and interpersonal psychotherapy, may be more effective for women than less well-focused approaches[18] and have the best documented efficacy for treatment of MDD (APA level of confidence II).[17]

Cognitive-behavioral therapy focuses on changing negative thinking patterns and habits by examining thoughts and beliefs, and using problem-solving techniques and behavior modification techniques such as relaxation or meditation. It is reported to have an efficacy of around 46%,[19] but success rates specific to middle-aged women are not reported. Interpersonal therapy, which focuses on relationships, may also be suited uniquely to women because of their strong interpersonal connectedness; overall, efficacy rates of around 52% are reported.[19] Group therapy may also be more helpful for women than for men, given women's emphasis on interpersonal issues.[18] Couples therapy can be useful if relationship problems with the spouse/partner are prominent. Some primary care physicians provide cognitive therapy or interpersonal therapy, but many refer patients for these services. Care must be taken to select a therapist with appropriate expertise. The patient's response to therapy must be monitored closely (APA level of confidence I).[17] Patients may need to attend therapy sessions weekly or more frequently. All treating professionals must maintain sufficient contact with each other and with the patient to ensure exchange of relevant information and maintenance of a logical, cohesive treatment strategy (APA level of confidence I).[17] At a minimum, the primary care physician must contact the therapist and patient after four to six weeks to establish that the episode of major depression has improved or resolved.

The patient should be advised to contact the physician at any time during psychotherapy if symptoms are worsening to enable a reappraisal to be conducted and a new treatment plan to be developed. If the patient responds well to psychotherapy, some recommend continuing therapy at a lower frequency/intensity to prevent recurrence of depression.[17] *For moderate or severe major depression, an antidepressant medication combined with psychotherapy is optimal treatment*, resulting in the greatest response rate and the best relapse prevention.

Pharmacotherapy

Modern antidepressant medications are effective, safe, tolerated well, and easy to prescribe, and offer a range of effects enabling therapy to be matched more closely to the needs of each patient. These reasons may explain the increase in pharmacotherapy from 37.4% of depressed patients in 1987 to 74.5% in 1997.[20]

The agents in common use are classified as selective serotonin-reuptake inhibitors (SSRIs), tricyclic antidepressants (TCAs), and the newer antidepressants (Table 7.5). Older medications such as monoamine oxidase inhibitors (MAOIs) are used mainly in special circumstances because of the potential for adverse interactions. In general, all antidepressants appear to have similar efficacy in the outpatient treatment of MDD.[17,21] Tricyclic antidepressants are possibly more effective in severe episodes, and bupropion is probably less effective than other agents in mild to moderate depression.[22]

Approximately 60% of patients respond to the first antidepressant prescribed. More than half of chronically depressed non-responders benefit from the first change of antidepressant to one of another class,[23] and 90% eventually respond to an antidepressant medication.[22]

Selective serotonin receptor inhibitors (SSRIs) are considered first-line antidepressant treatment because of their benign adverse-effect profile, simple dosing, and safety in overdose.[17,24] The different SSRIs are equally effective in treating MDD in primary care patients. The choice of agent is made mainly on side-effect profile and cost (Table 7.5).[21,24] Any history of adverse reaction by

Table 7.5 Antidepressant medications

	Dose range (mg/day)	Average monthly cost ($)	Principal side effects*
*SSRIs**			
Citalopram	20–60	66	Drowsiness, nausea (>7.5%)
Fluoxetine	20–80 (also 90 mg/week)	153 (71 weekly)	Nausea, nervousness (>10%)
Fluvoxamine	50–300	94	Anorexia (>7.5%), Constipation (>10%) Drowsiness (>15%) Nausea (>25%)
Paroxetine	20–50	75	Dizziness, sweating (>7.5%) Fatigue (>10%) Drowsiness, nausea (>15%)
Sertraline	50–200	67	Diarrhea, insomnia (>7.5%) Nausea (>10%)
Selected tricyclics			
Amitriptyline	25–300	8	
Clomipramine	25–250	40	
Desipramine	25–300	12	
Imipramine	50–200	22	Fatigue (>7.5%) Tremors, sweating (10%) Constipation (10%), Dizziness (>20%) Dry mouth (>45%)
Nortriptyline	25–150	8	
Other antidepressants			
Bupropion	200–450	87	Dry mouth, constipation, sweating (>7.5%) Tremors, nervousness (>10%)
Venlafaxine (sustained-release)	75–375	72	Insomnia, anorexia, constipation, sweating (>7.5%) Nervousness, dizziness, dry mouth (>10%)
Mirtazapine	15–45	81	Weight gain, dry mouth (>10%) Increased appetite (>15%) Drowsiness (>35%)
Nefazodone	200–600	78	Confusion (>7.5%) Drowsiness, vision change, nausea, dry mouth (>10%)
Trazodone	100–400	14	Dizziness (>20%)

Source: Preskorn, S. *Outpatient Management of Depression: A Guide for the Primary Care Practitioner*, 2nd edition. Caddo OK: Professional Communications; 1999.
*All SSRIs can lead to sexual dysfunction (loss of libido, anorgasmia).

the patient to an antidepressant should be considered in selecting an antidepressant medication. Newer agents (venlafaxine, mirtazapine, nefazodone) are also becoming first-line treatments. All of the SSRIs and newer antidepressants are safe to prescribe for healthy women. Most can also be used safely in women with medical problems if dose adjustments are made for renal or hepatic insufficiency. Drug–drug interactions, especially those involving the cytochrome P (CYP) 450 system, must be considered. Sertraline, citalopram, venlafaxine, and mirtazapine have no to minimal effect on most CYP enzymes.[25]

SSRIs and newer agents are generally well tolerated, but sexual dysfunction can occur in up to 30% of patients. Tolerance usually develops to the gastrointestinal and other side effects (Table 7.5). For all antidepressants, starting at a low dose and gradually increasing minimizes side effects. The side-effect profile enables therapy to be targeted to the depressive symptoms of individual women. Venlafaxine, bupropion, and fluoxetine tend to be more activating and are useful for the woman who is hypersomnolent and has psychomotor retardation. Conversely, the sedating properties of mirtazapine, nefazodone, paroxetine, and fluvoxamine benefit patients who are anxious, agitated, and insomniac. If decreased appetite and weight loss are major problems, then mirtazapine is a good choice. Citalopram and sertraline are excellent choices for either the hypersomnolent/slowed-down or the activated/agitated patient. Dosing regimens may influence ease of prescribing and patient compliance. Some of the antidepressants (fluoxetine, paroxetine, sertraline, venlafaxine sustained-release, mirtazapine) allow for once-daily dosing, and an effective dose can be prescribed immediately, eliminating the need for dose titration.

Gender differences in the pharmacokinetic and pharmacodynamic properties of antidepressants mean that the drugs may have altered plasma levels, longer half-lives, more side effects and more drug toxicity in women than in men.[5] Women may need lower doses of all antidepressants, but they tend to have a more robust response to SSRIs or MAOIs than to TCAs. Women may respond less well than men to TCAs.[5]

Antidepressant medication must be taken in an adequate dose for an adequate time to achieve complete remission. If improvement is not apparent after six to eight weeks, then the situation should be reassessed (APA recommendation level I). Following any change of treatment, the patient should continue to be monitored closely and a full reappraisal made after an additional six to eight weeks (APA recommendation level I). *Once remission is achieved, the patient should be maintained on the same dose of effective medication for 16–20 weeks, with regular frequent monitoring, to prevent relapse* (APA recommendation level I). The same dose should be considered for the longer maintenance phase as there is little evidence to support the effectiveness of lower doses of medication in preventing relapse.[17] Adequate treatment time is at least six months after a good response for the first episode, and 12 months or longer after a second episode. Because women may be at increased risk for longer episodes, or more recurrence, antidepressants may need to be continued for longer durations in women than in men.

Alternative therapies

Many women with depressive symptoms use complementary and alternative therapies. Many of these therapies are controversial and not supported by reliable research evidence. Exercise (especially in groups) and stress reduction (yoga, relaxation, massage) appear to be useful adjuncts to conventional therapy, and limited evidence supports a role for acupuncture.[26] The efficacy of St John's Wort is very controversial. It may be beneficial in mild depression,[26] but it is inadequate therapy for moderate to severe depression.[27]

Although the first episode of major depression may have been inevitable, recurrences and chronicity can be improved with adequate treatment and patient education about early recognition of relapse symptoms and the necessity of promptly reinstituting treatment. Major depressive disorder should be considered a chronic condition. The risk of recurrence is dependent upon the duration of the current episode, the number of previous episodes (70% with one previous episode, 90% with two previous episodes), and family history of major depression.[22]

Hormonally related depression in mid-life women

Premenstrual dysphoric disorder

Middle-aged women who continue to menstruate are at risk for premenstrual dysphoric disorder (PMDD). The premenstrual phase is also a period of increased vulnerability to a mood disorder or to worsening symptoms of a current major depressive disorder or dysthymic disorder.[28] Suicide attempts, completed suicides, and psychiatric hospitalizations are more likely to occur during the late luteal phase. Education of women and their families about premenstrual vulnerability allows women and families to be prepared better to cope with, rather than to be "caught off guard" by, new or exacerbated symptoms.

Most menstruating women experience mild premenstrual symptoms, which remit after menses and usually do not cause significant impairment. In contrast, approximately 3–8% of women experience severe symptoms that meet criteria for PMDD. These symptoms are extremely distressing, cause significant impairment in functioning, and are a tremendous burden for the women and their families.[29] A high proportion of women with PMDD have a history of previous episodes of mood disorders, including major and minor depression, postpartum depression, and bipolar disorders.[30,31]

The diagnosis of PMDD requires documentation, usually from a daily symptom diary, of appropriate symptoms occurring consistently but only during the luteal phase of the menstrual cycle. Symptoms must interfere markedly with work, school, social activities, and relationships with others, and must be confirmed by prospective daily ratings during at least two consecutive symptomatic cycles. Symptoms must not be merely an exacerbation of another disorder, such as major depressive disorder. For diagnosis of PMDD, five or more of the cardinal symptoms (markedly depressed mood, hopelessness, self-deprecation, marked anxiety, tension, feeling "keyed up," affective lability, marked anger, irritability, increased interpersonal conflicts) must be present most of the time during the last week of the luteal phase, must begin to remit within a few days after onset of the follicular phase, and must be absent in the week postmenses in most menstrual cycles during the past year.

SSRIs are tolerated well in PMDD and rapidly reduce mood and somatic symptoms and improve functioning.[32] Conversely, TCAs are no more effective than placebo.[32] The recommended dose of SSRIs for PMDD is equal to or lower than the dose used for depression. Intermittent (luteal-phase) dosing has also been found to be effective.[33] Exercising, limiting alcohol, caffeine, sodium, and simple carbohydrates, and stress-management techniques are also recommended.

Perimenopause and menopause
Loss of ovarian follicular activity may lead to the common minor mood changes of the perimenopausal period. Minor cognitive and depressive symptoms and vasomotor instability respond well to hormone replacement therapy. Menopause is associated with an increased risk of recurrence of depressive disorders but is not a high-risk time for the new onset of depressive disorders.[18] Women who are vulnerable to depression during periods of hormonal fluctuations are likely to experience recurrent depressive episodes during perimenopause and menopause. If such a woman has a depressive episode, then hormone therapy alone is ineffective and a course of antidepressants and/or psychotherapy is required.

Other dysphoric conditions
In *adjustment disorder with depressed mood*, the patient experiences a disproportionate level of distress and/or impaired function in response to an identifiable stressor. Although distressing, this rather mild condition responds well to psychosocial support, and antidepressant medication is not indicated. The patient should be monitored for additional symptoms, such as sleep, appetite, or energy disturbance, that raise suspicion of a major or minor depressive disorder.

Dysthymia is characterized by persistent depressed mood and functioning over several years and is two to three times more likely to develop in women than in men. Dysthymic symptoms are frequently not recognized because they are perceived to be "normal" for the individual. Dysthymia usually has an insidious onset and chronic course and may be recognized only when a major depression is superimposed. Unfortunately, when dysthymia is comorbid with major depression, both conditions tend to be refractory to treatment. Management of dysthymia consists of psychosocial support, antidepressant medication, and psychotherapy.

A careful history must be taken from all women presenting with depressive symptoms to identify those who are actually in the depressive phase of a *bipolar disorder*. Inappropriate treatment of such patients can be disastrous. The patient and family members must be asked specifically about any prior episodes of mania (bipolar I disorder) or hypomania (bipolar II disorder). While a manic episode rarely goes unnoticed, hypomania may be unrecognized or considered "normal" for a high-energy, high-achieving woman. The medication management of patients in the depressive phase of bipolar disorder requires a mood stabilizer such as valproic acid, lithium, or carbamazepine plus an antidepressant if the depressive symptoms persist. Prescribing an antidepressant without a mood stabilizer to a bipolar patient can precipitate a manic episode.

Mood disorder due to a medical condition

For this diagnosis, the mood disorder must be integral to the medical condition, perhaps even sharing the pathophysiology. Depressive symptoms can be part of many medical conditions that are common in middle-aged women (Table 7.4) and sometimes are the presenting symptoms of a condition. Up to one-third of cancer survivors and their family members suffer from depression,[34] and at least half of patients with epilepsy or Parkinson's disease have depression.[35] Management consists primarily of treating the medical condition, but specific treatment of depressive symptoms may also be necessary.

Mood disorders can be induced by use of certain substances, whether prescribed, bought over the counter, or illicit (Table 7.3). In middle-aged women, exogenous hormone therapies, particularly those with high progesterone components, are important causes of depressive symptoms.

Women have lower rates of alcohol dependence than men; however, the physiological consequences of alcohol are worse for women. Estimated rates of depression in alcoholic women range from 40 to 70%.[6] For some of these women, the depression predates the alcohol abuse, perhaps indicating a tendency to self-medicate.[36] Efforts to treat the depression are ineffective until the alcohol consumption is stopped. It is not uncommon in middle-aged women for unrecognized alcoholism to explain why a depression remains refractory to treatment.

Women now in middle age were exposed to the drug culture prominent in the 1960s. Although statistics may be unreliable, 3.6% of US women older than 35 consistently report use of illicit drugs during the previous month.[6] Marijuana is the most commonly reported illicit drug (2.5% of women over

Table 7.6 Common symptoms of anxiety disorders (symptoms are severe, persistent, excessive, inappropriately triggered and are disruptive to usual or desirable functioning)

Mood symptoms	Physical symptoms	Behavioral symptoms	Cognitive symptoms
Worry	Sweating	Hand-wringing	Poor concentration
Fear	Palpitations	Pacing	Persistent/recurrent thoughts of failure
Irritability	Nausea	Nail-biting	Embarrassment
Apprehension	Diarrhea	Lip-licking	Preoccupation with impending disaster
Vigilance	Urinary frequency	Scratching	
	Muscle tension	Fidgeting	
	Trembling		
	Fatigue		

35 years), but benzodiazepine and narcotic abuse and dependence are also under-recognized in this population. Any substance abuse must be diagnosed and managed in a depressed woman, otherwise treatment of the depression will be difficult or impossible.

Bereavement

Although depressive symptoms are prominent in grief reactions or after significant loss, bereavement usually does not have prominent symptoms of worthlessness, intense or persistent suicidal ideation, marked psychomotor retardation, or significant functional impairment. By *Diagnostic and Statistical Manual*, 4th edition (DSM IV) criteria, bereavement excludes the diagnosis of major depression unless the symptoms persist for more than two months after the loss.

Anxiety

The anxiety disorders are characterized by maladaptive, abnormal response to perceived threats or stressors, with resulting mood, cognitive, or physical symptoms (Table 7.6).[37] They are the most common psychiatric disorders, with a lifetime prevalence of nearly 25% in the USA.[38] Women are twice as likely as men to develop panic disorder, simple phobia, post-traumatic stress disorder, and generalized anxiety disorder, and are at increased risk for obsessive-compulsive disorder and social phobia.[39]

Over eight million office visits per year document an anxiety-related diagnosis, and the majority of these visits are made by women aged 40–59 years.[40] Overall, anxiety accounts for about one-third of direct mental health costs in the USA,[41] but this represents only a fraction of the total burden of lost productivity, care-giver time, social services costs, decreased quality of life, and increased mortality imposed by these conditions. Patients with anxiety consult more frequently, generate more healthcare costs,[42] and are at increased risk of suicide.[40] Unfortunately, despite their disabling and distressing effects, anxiety disorders are often not recognized, possibly because patients tend to express their emotional or psychiatric distress as somatic complaints.[43] In addition, anxiety disorders are often comorbid with physical conditions, depressive disorders, substance abuse disorders, or other anxiety disorders.

Generalized anxiety disorder

The most common anxiety disorder in primary care is generalized anxiety disorder (GAD).[44] The diagnosis was made in 16.6% of women attending an inner-city practice (compared with 9.5% of men) but was rare in people younger than 30 years.[1] One-third of patients meeting criteria for GAD reported their physical health as being poor.[1] The hallmarks of GAD are chronic worrying and somatic anxiety, fatigue, muscle tension, sleep disturbances, concentration problems, restlessness, and irritability. Symptoms must be of at least six months' duration.

The lifetime prevalence is 5–6%, and GAD is twice as common in women as in men.[38] Community studies estimate prevalence rates of 2.0–4.0% for women aged 45–64 years.[45] GAD is commonly comorbid with other anxiety disorders, substance abuse, and depression.[44] Nearly 40% of GAD patients have comorbid MDD[46] or panic disorder.[47] Dysthymia may be more likely to develop in women with GAD.[48] Women with GAD are more likely than men to develop comorbid conditions, and comorbidity reduces the likelihood of remission. The spontaneous remission rate is around 20–25%.[44]

When depression and GAD are comorbid, the patient has increased disability, poor functioning, and a worse prognosis.[44] In addition, comorbidity challenges diagnostic accuracy and confounds treatment. The most common physical comorbidities appear to be gastrointestinal conditions. Half of patients with irritable bowel syndrome also meet criteria for GAD.[44]

Symptoms of GAD can be chronic or lifelong or have a fluctuating course,[44] and tend to be worse during times of stress.[49] Patients commonly have symptoms for five to ten years before the diagnosis is made. A positive response to either of two screening questions – "During the past four weeks, have you been bothered by feeling worried, tense, or anxious most of the time?" and "Are you frequently tense, irritable, and having trouble sleeping?" – should prompt further questioning for additional symptoms or use of a standardized screening instrument.[44]

Table 7.7 Common symptoms of panic attack*

Depersonalization	Palpitations, racing pulse, pounding heartbeat
Sense of unreality	Chest pain
Sense of impending death	Shortness of breath, choking
Loss of control	Dizziness, fainting, light-headedness
	Chills, hot flushes, sweating
	Trembling, shaking
	Nausea, abdominal cramps

*A panic attack is a discrete period of intense fear or discomfort, developing abruptly and peaking within ten minutes, and characterized by four (or more) of the symptoms in the table.

Phobias

Phobias are characterized by unreasonable or excessive fear of social situations (social anxiety disorder) or of specific objects or situations (specific phobia). Phobic patients strenuously attempt to avoid the trigger object or situation, and experience extreme anxiety if exposure cannot be avoided. Although sufferers relatively rarely seek medical advice, social anxiety is the most common anxiety disorder and the third most common psychiatric disorder in the USA (exceeded only by depression and alcohol dependence).[50] The overall lifetime prevalence is estimated to be 13%,[38] but the prevalence is 1.5 times greater in women than in men.[51]

The patient with social phobia has much more than excessive shyness. She experiences severe anxiety symptoms (Table 7.7), humiliation, and embarrassment in social situations and, therefore, avoids or is symptomatic in certain circumstances. Common circumstances that produce symptoms in social anxiety disorder are public speaking and performing, being the center of attention, being stared at, meeting strangers, interacting with authority figures, and writing and eating in public. *The patient develops low self-esteem and becomes impaired in social or work settings, either because of symptoms or because she avoids situations or activities that are associated with symptoms.*

Patients with specific phobias develop symptoms and/or attempt to avoid specific objects or circumstances, for example insects, storms, blood, and elevators. Although all phobias are generally mild, for a few patients they cause significant distress and restriction of activities.

Post-traumatic stress disorder

Post-traumatic stress disorder (PTSD) is an anxiety disorder that develops weeks to months after a specific or repeated life-threatening stressor or traumatic event. The patient has persistent re-experiencing of the event (intrusive recollections, flashbacks), persistent avoidance of reminders of the event, feelings of detachment, and symptoms of increased arousal (exaggerated startle response, hypervigilance, poor concentration). *Women are more likely than men to develop PTSD following a traumatic event.* The impact appears particularly significant for trauma experienced before age 15.

Sexual abuse during childhood, especially incest, is linked to potentially devastating consequences in women that may not be recognized until middle age. These women may present with comorbidities of substance abuse, eating disorders, depression and other psychiatric conditions, as well as somatic symptoms, particularly chronic pelvic pain and gynecological complaints.[39] The lifetime prevalence of PTSD is greater in women (12.5%) than in men (6.2%).[38]

The most common cause of PTSD in men is combat exposure, but women are more likely to develop PTSD after physical or sexual assault or threat or after experiencing or witnessing a life-threatening event. Women who are rape victims are almost twice as likely to have PTSD (48%) than women victimized by a non-sexual crime (25%).[52] Gender differences exist in the response to trauma: women victimized by domestic violence are more likely to develop anxiety symptoms, while men more likely to develop substance abuse.[39]

Panic disorder

Panic disorder is characterized by recurrent panic attacks with intense fear of losing control or dying during the attack. *There is such marked fear of another panic attack that certain situations or places are avoided* (Table 7.7). Approximately half of women with panic disorder also suffer from agoraphobia ("fear of the marketplace"), an intense irrational fear of being alone in places from which escape is impossible such as crowded public places or elevators.[50] The lifetime prevalence of panic disorder is 1.5–3.5% and is twice as high in women than men. The prevalence may be as high as 21% in primary care settings because women with panic disorder are likely to present with physical symptomatology and resultant excess use of medical services.[53] Panic disorder rarely begins after age 45, but it may persist or recur throughout the mid-life years.

Middle-aged women may also suffer from undiagnosed panic disorder because symptoms often mimic medical conditions or may be masked by psychiatric comorbidities, such as GAD, specific phobia, alcohol abuse and dependence, and somatization disorder.[54,55] Patients with unrecognized panic disorder commonly are heavy users of healthcare services. They frequently undergo extensive testing for cardiovascular, gastrointestinal, and other conditions in unrewarding attempts to explain their symptoms.[50] In addition to increased prevalence, women appear to have distinct features in panic disorder compared with men. Women have more individual panic-related symptoms,[56] elevated risk of agoraphobia, and more comorbidity, resulting in a more severe, refractory course and greater functional impairment.[55]

Diagnosing panic disorder can be challenging, although screening instruments are available. Common medical conditions that present as anxiety (Table 7.8) or substance abuse or withdrawal should be eliminated as causes. The family practitioner who understands the common presentations of panic disorder can avoid costly overutilization of healthcare services, save the patient exposure to unnecessary testing, and facilitate appropriate treatment.

Obsessive-compulsive disorder

At least four million Americans suffer from obsessive-compulsive disorder (OCD).[50] The condition is equally common in men and women and has a lifetime prevalence of 2–3%, although many cases are undiagnosed. Most cases begin before age 25, but OCD is a chronic, relapsing condition that may persist and be intractable in the middle-aged woman. Such women may present when they can no longer conceal the condition or a relapse is triggered by a life event. The condition may also present as a physical condition such as an intractable dermatitis of the hands due to repeated washing. Patients with OCD experience time-consuming, distressing obsessions and compulsions that impair normal functioning.

Obsessions are intrusive and recurrent thoughts, impulses or images that are intrusive and inappropriate and that cause distress and functional impairment. Common obsessions involve germs and disease, a fear of harming others or being harmed, neatness or symmetry, and disturbing images.

Compulsions are repetitive, ritualized behaviors performed to prevent or relieve anxiety. Examples of compulsions include repeated hand-washing, cleaning, checking, counting, and hoarding. Typically, women with OCD have both obsessions and compulsions and usually hide the symptoms from family and close friends for many years. Guilt, shame, and loss of self-worth occur because the patient recognizes the symptoms as senseless but is unable to change her behaviors or thoughts. Women with OCD may have a less severe clinical course than men, but the prognosis is worse for unmarried women and those with obsessional premorbid personality.[39] Comorbid depression, anxiety disorders, personality disorders, and substance abuse may complicate the diagnosis and management of OCD.

Anxiety secondary to other conditions

Clinically significant anxiety can occur during substance use or withdrawal and as part of several medical conditions (Table 7.8). A thorough history and physical assessment can help to determine whether a medical disorder or a psychiatric disorder causes the symptoms. The history should inquire

Table 7.8 Medical conditions associated with anxiety disorders

Endocrine/metabolic	Respiratory	Neurological	Cardiovascular	Medications	Other	Medication withdrawal
Hyper- or hypothyroid	COPD	Dementia	Myocardial infarction, angina pectoris	Antidepressants	Trauma	Alcohol
Hyper- or hypokalemia	Asthma	Seizure disorders	Arrhythmias	Caffeine	Anemia	Narcotic analgesics
Hyper- or hypocalcemia	Pulmonary embolism	CVA/TIA	Congestive heart failure	Alcohol	Systemic lupus erythematosus	Sedatives/hypnotics
Hyper- or hyponatremia	Pneumonia	Parkinson's disease	Cardiomyopathy	Antipsychotics		Benzodiazepines
Hypoglycemia		CNS infections	Valvular heart disease	Anticholinergics		
Cushing's syndrome		CNS tumors		Steroids		
Vitamin B deficiencies		Chronic pain		Decongestants		
				Bronchodilators		
				Calcium channel blockers		
				Digitalis		
				Antihistamines		
				Theophylline		

CNS, central nervous system; COPD, chronic obstructive pulmonary disease; CVA, cerebrovascular accident; TIA, transient ischemic attack.

Table 7.9 Pharmacotherapy of anxiety disorders

	SSRIs	Other, newer antidepressants	Tricyclics	Benzodiazepines (if no substance abuse history)	Buspirone
GAD	Usual dosing	Usual dosing	Usual dosing	If urgent symptoms	If no comorbidity
Social anxiety	Usual dosing				
PTSD	Low dosing				
OCD	Usual dosing		Clomipramine		
Panic disorder	Low dosing		Low dosing	Short-term use	

*High dose SSRI: fluoxetine 60–80 mg; fluvoxamine 300 mg; paroxetine 60 mg; sertraline 200–225 mg; citalopram 60 mg.

specifically about the use of alcohol, medications, or illicit substances, association of symptoms with social situations and emotional stressors, exposure to physical or emotional trauma, and prior or current mental illness.[57] Further assessment by examination or laboratory testing is individualized based on other potential causes of the symptoms.

If initial assessment reveals a medical disorder, then the treatment strategy should target this medical condition; the anxiety symptoms should then be reassessed after adequate treatment of the underlying medical condition. Medications can also contribute to anxiety symptoms, in which case safer medications should be substituted if possible. Regardless of the cause, anxiety associated with medical conditions can be alleviated by improved communication, since anxiety often results from inadequate, false, or insufficient information. Important aspects of communication to relieve anxiety include giving information about the condition, communicating openly, answering questions, using reassurance, and preparing the patient for unpleasant procedures.[58]

Treatment of anxiety disorders

In addition to treating underlying medical conditions and avoiding substance abuse, the specific treatment of anxiety disorders is based on medication and psychotherapies. Pharmacologic therapy is very effective, but it must be individualized to the specific anxiety disorder and take into account comorbidities, alcohol, or substance abuse history, chronicity of the disorder, and the physician's experience with the medication.[59]

The principal medications used are antidepressants, benzodiazepines, and buspirone (Table 7.9). Antidepressants have become the mainstay of treatment.

Tricyclics are effective in several of the anxiety disorders, but their side-effect profiles and toxicity in overdose have made them less desirable than some of the newer agents. *The SSRIs are used widely to treat anxiety disorders* (Tables 7.5 and 7.9), with or without comorbid depression, and have favorable side-effect profiles. As a group, the newer antidepressants have also been shown to be effective in some anxiety disorders and are generally tolerated well (see Table 7.5). Benzodiazepines, for example lorazepam and alprazolam, also play a role in the management of anxiety, especially in acute, severe, and situational anxiety symptoms. The use of benzodiazepines is limited in more chronic forms of anxiety because of the potential for abuse, dependence, and tolerance. Benzodiazepines are generally not recommended for long-term (more than four months) treatment of anxiety disorders.[59] Buspirone is effective in GAD, but it has a slower onset of action than benzodiazepines. Buspirone is unlikely to cause dependency and is usually tolerated well, although some patients complain of dizziness and nausea.

Psychotherapy is a major treatment modality for anxiety disorders. Psychoeducation aims to provide information on the anxiety disorder and can be a major building block in establishing the management of anxiety. Relaxation techniques and stress-reduction methods are useful tools for reducing and managing symptoms. Cognitive, behavioral, interpersonal, and supportive psychotherapy are beneficial.

Mixed anxiety and depression

Anxiety and depression often coexist, especially in the primary care setting. Patients with combined symptoms are the largest group with psychiatric conditions seen in the primary care office, and a substantial minority (45%) are not detected by primary care physicians.[57] Almost half of the cases of anxiety and depression occur in the same patient at the same time.[60] This comorbidity makes accurate diagnosis more difficult, treatment more complicated, and prognosis less favorable.[50] Anxiety is often the presenting symptom for depressed patients. The family physician should probe for symptoms for depression so that the depression can be identified and treated. Conversely, anxiety disorders often become comorbid with depression, and both conditions should be identified and managed. Fortunately, there is a great overlap in treatment methods, as the newer antidepressants are often indicated for the management of anxiety.

REFERENCES

1 Olfson, M., Shea, S., Feder, A., *et al.* Prevalence of anxiety, depression, and substance abuse disorders in an urban general medicine practice. *Arch. Fam. Med.* 2000; 9:876–83.

2 Williams, J. B., Spitzer, R. L., Linzer, M., *et al.* Gender differences in depression in primary care. *Am. J. Obstet. Gynecol.* 1995; **173**:654–9.

3 Kessler, R. C., McGonagle, K. A., Swartz, M., *et al.* Sex and depression in the National Comorbidity Survey. I: lifetime prevalence, chronicity, and recurrence. *J. Affect. Disord.* 1993; **29**:85–96.

4 Fava, M., Abraham, M., Alpert, J., *et al.* Gender differences in axis I comorbidity among depressed patients. *J. Affect. Disord.* 1996; **38**:129–33.

5 Kornstein, S. G. Gender differences in depression: implications for treatment. *J. Clin. Psychiatry* 1997; **58**:S12–18.

6 Choby, B. A. *Midlife Care of Women.* Monograph no. 278. Leawood, KS: American Academy of Family Physicians; 2002.

7 Sorenson, S. B. and Golding, J. M. Depressive sequelae of recent criminal victimization. *J. Trauma. Stress* 1990; **3**:337–50.

8 Tylee, A., Gastpar, M., Lepine, J. P. and Mendlewicz, J. Identification of depressed patients in the community and their treatment needs: findings from the DEPRES II (Depression Research in European Society II) survey. *Int. Clin. Psychopharmacol.* 1999; **14**:153–65.

9 Kornstein, S. G., Schatzberg, A. F., Thase, M. E., *et al.* Gender differences in chronic major and double depression. *J. Affect. Disord.* 2000; **60**:1–11.

10 Pignone, M. P., Gaynes, B. N., Rushton, J. L., *et al.* Screening for depression in adults: a summary of the evidence for the US Preventive Services Task Force. *Ann. Intern. Med.* 2002; **136**:765–76.

11 Brody, D. S., Hahn, S. R., Spitzer, R. L., *et al.* Identifying patients with depression in the primary care setting: a more efficient method. *Arch. Intern. Med.* 1998; **158**:2469–77.

12 Williams, J. W., Noel, P. H., Cordes, J. A., Ramirez, G. and Pigone, M. Is this patient clinically depressed? *J. Am. Med. Assoc.* 2002; **287**:1160–70.

13 Richter, P., Werner, J., Heerlein, A., *et al.* On the validity of the Beck Depression Inventory: a review. *Psychopathology* 1998; **31**:160–68.

14 Beck, A. T., Guth, D., Steer, R. A. and Ball, R. Screening for major depression disorders in medical inpatients with the Beck Depression Inventory for Primary care. *Behav. Res. Ther.* 1997; **35**:785–91.

15 Pignone, M. P., Gaynes, B. N., Rushten, J. L., *et al.* Screening for depression in adults: a summary of the evidence for the US Preventive Services Task Force. *Ann. Intern. Med.* 2002; **136**:765–76.

16 Moscicki, E. K. Identification of suicide risk factors using epidemiologic studies. *Psychiatr. Clin. North Am.* 1997; **20**:499–517.

17 National Guidelines Clearinghouse. Practice guideline for psychiatric evaluation of adults. http://www.guideline.gov/summary/summary.aspx?doc_id=1407. Accessed July 2002.

18 Pajer, K. New strategies in the treatment of depression in women. *J. Clin. Psychiatry* 1995; **56**:30–37.

19 Person, J. B., Thase, M. E. and Crits-Christop, P. The role of psychotherapy in the treatment of depression.; review of two practice guidelines. *Arch. Gen. Psychiatry* 1996; **53**:283–90.

20 Olfson, M., Marcus, S. C., Druss, B., Elinson, L., Tanielian, T. and Pincus, H. A. National trends in the outpatient treatment of depression. *J. Am. Med. Assoc.* 2002; **287**:203–9.

21 Simon, G. Choosing a first-line antidepressant: equal on average does not mean equal for everyone. *J. Am. Med. Assoc.* 2001; **286**:3003–3004.
22 Preskorn, S. *Outpatient Management of Depression: a Guide for the Primary Care Practitioner*, 2nd edition. Caddo, OK: Professional Communications; 1999.
23 Thase, M. E., Rush, J. and Howland, R. H. Double blind switch study of imipramine or sertraline treatment of antidepressant-resistant chronic depression. *Arch. Gen. Psychiatry.* 2002; **59**:233–9.
24 Kroenke, K., West, S. L., Swindle, R., *et al.* Similar effectiveness of paroxetine, fluoxetine, and sertraline in primary care: a randomized trial. *J. Am. Med. Assoc.* 2001; **286**:2947–55.
25 Ereshefsky, L., Riesenman, C. and Lam, Y. W. Serotonin selective reuptake inhibitor drug interactions and the cytochrome P450 system. *J. Clin. Psychiatry* 1996; **57**:17–24.
26 Manber, R., Allen, J. J. B. and Morris, M. M. Alternative treatments for depression: empirical support and relevance to women. *J. Clin. Psychiatry* 2002; **63**:628–40.
27 Hypericum Depression Trial Study Group. Effect of *Hypericum perforatum* (St. John's Wort) in major depressive disorder. *J. Am. Med. Assoc.* 2002; **287**:1807–14.
28 Endicott J. History, evolution, and diagnosis of premenstrual dysphoric disorder. *J. Clin. Psychiatry* 2000; **61**:5–8.
29 Steiner, M., Romano, S. J., Babcock, S., *et al.* The efficacy of fluoxetine in improving physical symptoms associated with premenstrual dysphoric disorder. *Br. J. Obstet. Gynaecol.* 2001; **108**:462–8.
30 Yonkers, K. A., Halbreich, U., Freeman, E., *et al.* Symptomatic improvement of premenstrual dysphoric disorder with sertraline treatment. A randomized controlled trial. *J. Am. Med. Assoc.* 1997; **278**:983–8.
31 Pearlstein, T. and Stone, A. B. Premenstrual syndrome. *Psychiatr. Clin. North Am.* 1998; **21**:577–90.
32 Freeman, E. W., Rickels, K., Sondheimer, S. J. and Polansky, M. Differential response to antidepressants in women with premenstrual syndrome/premenstrual dysphoric disorder: a randomized controlled trial. *Arch. Gen. Psychiatry* 1999; **56**:932–9.
33 Cohen, L. S., Miner, C., Brown, E., Freeman, E. W., Halbreich, U. and Sundell, K. Premenstrual daily fluoxetine for premenstrual dysphoric disorder: a placebo-controlled clinical trial using computerized diaries. *Obstet. Gynecol.* 2002; **100**:435–44.
34 Hamblin, J. E. and Schifeling, D. J. *Cancer Survivors.* Monograph no. 264. Leawood, KS: American Academy of Family Physicians; 2001.
35 Marsh, C. M. Psychiatric presentations of medical illness. *Psychiatr. Clin. North. Am.* 1997; **20**:181–204.
36 Moscato, B. S., Russell, M. and Sielezny, M. Gender differences in the relation between depressive symptoms and alcohol problems: a longitudinal perspective. *Am. J. Epidemiol.* 1997; **146**:966–74.
37 Nutt, D. J. The pharmacology of human anxiety. *Pharmacol. Ther.* 1990; **47**:233–66.
38 Kessler, R. C., McGonagle, K. A. and Shanyang, Z. Lifetime and 12-month prevalence of DSM-III-R psychiatric disorders in the United States. *Arch. Gen. Psychiatry* 1994; **51**:8–19.
39 Pigott, T. A. Gender differences in the epidemiology and treatment of anxiety disorders. *J. Clin. Psychiatry* 1999; **60**(supp 18):4–15.

40 Skaer, T. L., Robison, L. M., Sclar, D. A. and Galin, R. S. Anxiety disorders in the USA, 1990–1997 – trend in complaint, diagnosis, use of pharmacotherapy and diagnosis of comorbid depression. *Clin. Drug Invest.* 2000; **20**:237–44.

41 DuPont, R. L., Rice, D. R. and Miller, L. S. Economic costs of anxiety disorders. *Anxiety* 1996; **2**:167–72.

42 Simon, G., Ormel, J., VonKorff, M. and Barlow, W. Health care costs associated with depressive and anxiety disorders in primary care. *Am. J. Psychiatry* 1995; **152**:352–7.

43 Baughman, O. L. Rapid diagnosis and treatment of anxiety and depression in primary care: the somatizing patient. *J. Fam. Pract.* 1994; **39**:373–8.

44 Ballenger, J. C., Davidson, J. R. T. and Lecrubier, Y. Consensus statement on generalized anxiety disorder from the international consensus group on depression and anxiety. *J. Clin. Psychiatry* 2001; **62**(supp 11):53–8.

45 Blazer, D. G., Kessler, R. C., McGonagle, K. A. and Swartz, M. S. The prevalence and distribution of major depression in a community sample: the national comorbidity survey. *Am. J. Psychiatry* 1994; **151**:979–86.

46 Wittchen, H., Zhao, S., Kessler, R. C. and Eaton, W. W. DSM-III-R generalized anxiety disorder in the national comorbidity survey. *Arch. Gen. Psychiatry* 1994; **51**:355–64.

47 Yonkers, K. A., Warshaw, M. G., Massion, A. O. and Keller, M. B. Phenomenology and course of generalized anxiety disorder. *Br. J. Psychiatry* 1996; **168**:308–13.

48 Robins, L. N., Helzer, J. E. and Weissman, M. M. Lifetime prevalence of specific psychiatric disorders in three sites. *Arch. Gen. Psychiatry* 1984; **41**:949–58.

49 American Psychiatric Association. *Diagnostic and Statistical Manual of Mental Disorders*, 4th edition. Washington, DC: American Psychiatric Association; 1994.

50 Nemeroff, C. B. and Schatzberg, A. F. *Recognition and Treatment of Psychiatric Disorders*. Washington, DC: American Psychiatric Press; 1999.

51 Bisserbe, J. C., Weiller, E., Boyer, P., Lepine, J. P. and Lecrubier, Y. Social phobia in primary care: level of recognition and drug use. *Int. Clin. Psychopharmacol.* 1996; **11**(supp 3):25–8.

52 Foa, E. B. Trauma and women: course, predictors, and treatment. *J. Clin. Psychiatry* 1997; **58**(supp 9):25–8.

53 Weissman, M. M., Bland, R. C. and Canino, G. J. The cross-national epidemiology of panic disorder. *Arch. Gen. Psychiatry* 1997; **54**:305–9.

54 Marshall, J. R. Comorbidity and its effects on panic disorder. *Bull. Menninger Clin.* 1996; **60**:A39–53.

55 Yonkers, K. A., Zlotnick, C. and Allsworth, J. Is the course of panic disorder the same in women and men? *Am. J. Psychiatry* 1998; **155**:596–602.

56 Dick, C. L., Bland, R. C. and Newman, S. C. Panic disorder. *Acta Psychiatr. Scand. Suppl.* 1994; **376**:45–53.

57 Goldberg, R. J. Diagnostic dilemmas presented by patients with anxiety and depression. *Am. J. Med.* 1995; **98**:278–84.

58 House, A. and Stark, D. Anxiety in medical patients. *Br. Med. J.* 2002; **325**:207–9.

59 Rakel, R. E. Anxiety and the primary care physician. *Prim. Psychiatry* 2001; **8**:52–8.

60 Sartorius, N., Ustun, T. B., Lecrubier, Y. and Wittchen, H. U. Depression comorbid with anxiety: results from the WHO study on psychological disorders in primary health care. *Br. J. Psychiatry* 1996; **168**(supp 30):38–43.

Part II

Hormonal changes

8

Physical changes in menopause and perimenopause

Margaret Gradison, M.D.

Case: S. J. is a 47-year-old woman who presents with abnormal uterine bleeding. She had regular periods until two years ago, at which time her periods became unpredictable. Her current menses started three weeks ago; she says it alternates between needing to change pads hourly to requiring only a daily panty liner. Ms J. is obese and smokes a pack of cigarettes a day. Her only medication is thyroid supplements. Her obstetrical history is gravida three para two spontaneous abortion one (G3P2 AB 1). She uses condoms intermittently for contraception, and her first pregnancy was at age 29.

Perimenopause and menopause

Perimenopause is the time in a woman's life when she begins to experience the changes that lead to menopause. The World Health Organization (WHO) defines this as a "period immediately prior to menopause (when the endocrinological, biological, and clinical features of approaching menopause commence) and the first year after menopause."[1]

This transition is caused by a decrease in gonadotropin and ovarian hormones. The ovaries produce decreasing amounts of estrogen and the target organs become less sensitive. Some women experience significant symptomatology during this time, which leads them to seek medical assistance. Menstrual changes, hot flushes, and other signs of estrogen deficiency, such as vaginal dryness, may be the first symptoms that a woman experiences. *Perimenopause is a transition phase that usually lasts four to six years.* This is the time when women move from a state of fertility and potential childbearing to infertility and permanent amenorrhea.

Menopause is a physiologic event defined as the cessation of menses for 12 months and is, therefore, a diagnosis that can be made only retrospectively. It is not a diagnosis made based on blood tests, *because levels of follicle-stimulating hormone (FSH), luteinizing hormone (LH), and estradiol vary widely during the perimenopausal time until menses cease permanently.* Serum hormone levels do not always correlate with a woman's symptoms.

In the USA, the average age of onset of menopause is 50 years. Various factors may influence the age of menopause. Smoking and shorter menstrual cycles can cause earlier menopause, while multigravidity and use of oral contraceptive pills are associated with later menopause.[2] There may be additional factors, including cultural differences, that influence the age of menopause. There is a genetic predisposition for early menopause. Ethnic and cultural influences affect a woman's experience during this transition.[3] Women's responses to the decrease in hormones can be quite variable and individualized.

Providers can prepare women for this change in life by discussing possible symptoms as the woman becomes perimenopausal. Proactive care by the provider can help to lessen the patient's concerns and symptoms. Counseling the patient appropriately and addressing her fears and symptoms are important. As with all medicine, the communication skills of the provider will have great impact on the woman's experience through perimenopause.[4]

Symptoms

Urogenital symptoms

Estrogen-sensitive tissues in the urogenital tract atrophy, resulting in vaginal dryness, thinning, and decreased elasticity. Subsequently, women often experience dyspareunia and vaginismus. Decreased estrogen levels affect the urethra and bladder, and altered vaginal flora and acidity can cause urethral irritation, urinary tract infections, and urinary incontinence.[5,6]

The menstrual and urogenital changes associated with perimenopause can be very distressing. Seventy-five percent of postmenopausal women experience atrophic genital changes. Decreased lubrication during intercourse is often the first complaint. Some women experience vaginal trauma, resulting in pain, bleeding, and infection. Vaginal dryness is caused by the decrease in estrogen. Therefore, estrogen creams and lubricants can be of benefit. Sexual stimulation also improves vaginal symptoms. Moisturizers and lubricants can provide temporary relief.[5]

Treatment

Oral and topical hormone supplements (vaginal cream, lubricants, or rings) can improve urogenital symptoms. However, with recent data challenging the long-term use of oral estrogen and progesterone postmenopausally, topical applications may be preferred since they do not result in such elevated plasma hormone levels. More evidence is needed to confirm this.

There are a variety of forms. Estrogen cream can be prescribed for use two to four times a week initially, and then reduced to one to two times a week as the patient wishes. There is usually some systemic absorption; therefore, estrogen cream should not be used in women who have contraindications, including estrogen-sensitive cancers and thrombotic disorders. The Estring™ is a 7-cm plastic doughnut-shaped object impregnated with a form of estrogen that is not absorbed systemically. In women who cannot or do not want to have systemic absorption of estrogen, the Estring can be used to produce local vaginal lubrication and reverse atrophy. It comes in one size and is replaced every three months by the physician or the patient.

Vasomotor symptoms

Vasomotor symptoms, described as hot flushes and cold sweats, are often the most disruptive perimenopausal symptoms that a woman experiences. These symptoms can occur even before any changes in menstrual pattern. There is significant variation in an individual woman's response to these, and the symptoms can be distracting, cause insomnia, and lead to unpleasant social situations.

Although the exact cause of the hot flushes is unknown, there is an increase in skin temperature. The symptoms correlate with a decrease in estrogen; however, there is no association with the intensity and number of hot flushes and circulating hormone levels. The provider needs to make sure that these symptoms are not caused by another problem, such as anxiety, fevers, or hyperthyroidism.[7]

Pharmacological treatment

Estrogen replacement decreases vasomotor symptoms. However, the risks and benefits of this treatment must be weighed carefully. In several randomized controlled trials (RCTs), *transdermal clonidine and progestogens were found to decrease hot flushes compared with placebo.*[8] Progesterone transdermal cream has been found to decrease hot flushes by 83%.[9]

RCTs demonstrate that tibolone, a synthetic hormone not currently available in the USA, decreases hot flushes and improves vaginal symptoms at the same rate as estrogen and progesterone. Tibolone reduces vasomotor symptoms by 39% compared with placebo.[8] In other RCTs, antidepressants appear to have no effect. Methlytestosterone and estrogen used together have improved vasomotor symptoms, whereas methlytestosterone alone does not.[8] (See also Chapter 10.)

Alternative therapies

Herbal treatments have long been touted for perimenopausal symptoms. These medications are often sold in varying concentrations, so patients may receive variable doses.

Soy extracts have been found to improve vasomotor symptoms.[10,11] Increased dietary and supplemental soy products alleviate these symptoms.[12] Herbal products with potential effectiveness include soy and isoflavones, black cohosh, and St John's Wort. Other products that have been used for menopausal symptoms include evening primrose, don quai, valerian root, chasteberry, ginseng, and wild yam. However, there is no evidence that any of these are effective, and they may have detrimental side effects.[13–15] There are currently several ongoing studies, such as those at the National Institute of Health's Center for Complementary and Alternative Health, on these herbal products' effectiveness.

Menstrual changes

Menstrual patterns are altered in many ways, including menorrhagia, menometrorrhagia, oligomenorrhea, intermenstrual bleeding, polymenorrhea, postcoital bleeding, and postmenopausal bleeding. *Variety and change in menstrual pattern is the normal rather than the abnormal.* Women can normally experience one or more of these changes. In one small survey, 93% of women reported one of these changes in the five years prior to menopause.[16] The challenge for the provider is to distinguish between normal and abnormal bleeding. There is an increased incidence of endometrial cancer in this age group, so it is important to differentiate between the normal physiologic changes in menstrual flow and those that are pathological.[8]

The normal menstrual cycle ranges from 21 to 35 days in length; bleeding normally lasts one to eight days and results in a blood loss of 20–80 ml. Women describe their bleeding patterns inaccurately, even when asked specific questions,[9] so evaluating the actual amount of blood loss can be challenging. Despite this, the provider needs to assess accurately the amount of blood loss and urgency in treating the hemorrhage.[10] Menstrual periods that suddenly last more than seven to ten days, bleeding that occurs faster than a pad an hour for a day or more, periods occurring more than twice a month for more than one month, and bleeding that distresses the woman or causes problems or changes in the woman's lifestyle or work patterns can be considered beyond the range of normal. These may necessitate some investigation and evaluation. Regular or irregular bleeding that results in anemia or hypotension is definitely worthy of treatment and investigation.

The causes for abnormal bleeding are varied, and accurate diagnosis of the cause is important. Menorrhagia may be caused by anovulation or may occur with an ovulatory cycle. Etiologies of abnormal menstrual bleeding include endocrine abnormalities, pregnancy, infections (genital and systemic), neoplasms (benign and malignant) of pelvic organs, uterine abnormalities, coagulation disorders, liver disease, medication (iatrogenic) (Table 8.1), and trauma.

Table 8.1 Medications that can affect the menstrual cycle

Thyroid hormones
Steroid hormones, including prednisone
Psychotropic medications: phenothiazines, antidepressants, butyphenones
Anti-seizure medications

Evaluation

History and physical examination

A comprehensive evaluation can help to establish the cause of the bleeding abnormality. The source of the blood must be identified. Some women have difficulty distinguishing between blood from the uterus, cervix, vagina, bladder, or urethra. Systemic disease states such as liver disease, underlying bleeding disorder or coagulopathy, diabetes, and thyroid disease must be considered.

A careful medication history must be obtained, including the use of herbal medications (such as dehydroepiandrosterone, DHEA), nutritional supplements, and over-the-counter medications. Hormones such as hormone replacement therapy, contraceptives, selective estrogen receptor modulators (SERMS), and thyroid supplements can influence bleeding patterns. Anticoagulation therapy such as warfarin or excessive aspirin intake can cause bleeding.

Although fertility decreases significantly in the perimenopausal period, *pregnancy should be considered as the cause of bleeding, particularly in women not using contraception.* Women who do not want the chance of pregnancy need to use contraception until the perimenopausal period has ended.[11] Atrophic vaginitis can result in bleeding from intercourse. However, the provider should be mindful that domestic violence could cause bleeding as a result of trauma.

Endometrial lesions are frequently the source of bleeding. Benign tumors include leiomyomata uteri and endometrial or endocervical polyps. Endometrial disease or adenomyosis can be the origin of abnormal bleeding. The patient may have infections of the uterus such as pelvic inflammatory disease and endometritis. Cervical and vaginal infections should be considered.

Perimenopausal bleeding is often caused by hormonal imbalance; fluctuating levels of estrogen and progesterone are common, and thyroid levels may be decreased.

Once the provider has determined that the woman is hemodynamically stable, they must rule out endometrial neoplasia. Hyperplasia of the endometrium, with or without atypia, can advance to endometrial adenocarinoma. Perimenopausal women are at risk for endometrial hyperplasia and adenocarcinoma, caused by a decrease in progesterone. These lower levels lead to unopposed estrogen, which can result in the overstimulation of the endometrium and therefore cause hyperplasia and cancer.

Table 8.2 Risk factors for endometrial cancer

Body weight ≥ 90 kg
Age ≥45 years
History of infertility or low parity
Family history of colon carcinoma
Hypertension
Smoker
Late age at menopause
History of cholecystectomy
Polycystic ovarian syndrome
Use of exogenous estrogen (including SERMS)

Body mass index will influence a woman's perimenopausal risk and symptoms. Obese women convert adrenal androstenedione in the adipose tissue to estrone, thereby increasing estrogen levels. Obese women are therefore at higher risk for high estrogen levels, dysfunctional uterine bleeding, and endometrial carcinoma.

Risk factors for endometrial cancer are listed in Table 8.2. The use of exogenous estrogen (including SERMS), especially without progesterone, is the most significant cause of endometrial carcinoma.[13]

Laboratory testing

The laboratory and diagnostic testing for abnormal bleeding is guided by clinical presentation. Pregnancy testing is important if the patient is sexually active and using inadequate contraception. A hematocrit and hemoglobin test can evaluate anemia, and iron studies may be indicated. White blood count and differential can help to implicate an infectious etiology or hematological malignancy. Coagulation studies (platelet count, protime, prothrombin time, bleeding time) should be drawn to investigate coagulation disorders; specialized testing may be needed for von Willebrand's or other coagulopathies. Vaginal wet mount and potassium hydroxide slide may be indicated. Testing for chlamydia and gonorrhea should be considered. Liver function tests can identify hepatic abnormalities. A thyroid-stimulating hormone and prolactin test can help to rule out endocrine abnormalities. *Gonadotropin and estrogen levels have not been found to be useful in evaluating the cause of bleeding.* FSH, LH, testosterone, and DHEA-sulfate may identify polycystic ovary syndrome. A Pap smear can specify neoplastic cervical and vaginal lesions.

If the blood is from the uterus, then pathological evaluation of endometrial tissue may be necessary. In-office endometrial biopsies can be performed easily with minimal risk, cost, and discomfort. However, the yield of this procedure alone is controversial. There are several commercially available instruments for this, including Pipelle® and Gynosampler®. These have up to 90% sensitivity for endometrial cancer.[7] Many experts consider a positive test sufficient for evaluation for endometrial cancer.

A dilation and curettage (D&C) under anesthesia will result in a more complete sample for evaluation for hyperplasia or cancer. However, there are higher risks and expenses associated with this procedure. The new Tao brush may improve sampling from the endometrium without a D&C, although more data are needed for confirmation.[14]

Radiological studies

Radiological studies are being used increasingly in the initial evaluation of abnormal uterine bleeding. Ultrasonography has become the standard test in the evaluation of dysfunctional uterine and postmenopausal bleeding. Reliable differentiation between focal and diffuse endometrial and subendometrial lesions is possible. The most common anatomical findings are polyps and submucosal fibroids.[17] Transvaginal ultrasound can assess the endometrium and myometrium, including the pelvic stripe. This study has limitations if the patient is obese; unfortunately, these patients are at the highest risk for endometrial carcinoma. Transabdominal ultrasound yields less information and is, therefore, not useful in the evaluation of abnormal bleeding.

A thickened endometrial stripe or irregular endometrial surface may be indicative of hyperplasia or endometrial cancer. In a woman who is menopausal beyond doubt, an endometrial stripe of greater than 5 mm thick warrants further evaluation. A menopausal woman with an endometrial stripe of less than 5 mm has almost no chance of having endometrial cancer or hyperplasia.[18] On the other hand, if the woman is still menstruating, then greater endometrial stripe thickness is common. Some prospective studies have found that endometrial biopsy combined with vaginal sonography is sufficiently sensitive and specific to evaluate for endometrial cancer.[19]

Saline infusion sonohysterography (SIS) improves visualization of the endometrium and can increase the ability to determine the endometrial pathology, potentially decreasing the need for more expensive and invasive procedures such as D&C and hysteroscopy.[15] Hysteroscopy can be employed for both diagnostic and therapeutic treatment. The procedure that yields the most information is dependent in a large part on the operator's skill and experience. Nuclear magnetic resonance imaging (MRI) is indicated if the ultrasound or hysteroscopy results are inconclusive.[16]

Treatment of menstrual changes

For the patient with abnormal bleeding, once the etiology of the bleeding is determined, treatment should be initiated. Women with life-threatening bleeding need immediate treatment. They should be given conjugated

Table 8.3 Medical treatment for menorrhagia

Treatment	Dose
Non-steroidal agents	
Mefenamic acid	500 mg tid
Ibuprofen	400–800 mg tid
Meclofenamate	100 mg tid
Naproxen	250–500 mg tid
Hormonal therapy	
Oral contraceptive pills or patch	Various
Medroxyprogesterone acetate	5–10 mg qd, 21 days a month
Levonorgestrel-releasing intrauterine device	
Danazol	

estrogen 25 mg intravenously every four to six hours in the hospital. A D&C may be necessary for therapeutic reasons, such as severe menorrhagia. At the same time, the provider can send the tissue for pathologic evaluation. If the patient continues to have significant hemorrhaging, she should be referred to a gynecologist for surgical intervention. Pharmacological treatment for abnormal bleeding is indicated in heavy bleeding (more than 80 ml per period or more frequent than every 21 days).

Abnormal bleeding is caused by disordered prostaglandin production of the endometrium, and prostaglandins may play a role in the bleeding associated with uterine fibroids, adenomyosis, and non-hormonal intrauterine devices (IUDs) (Table 8.3). There is some evidence that non-steroidal antiinflammatory drugs (NSAIDs) decrease heavy bleeding. In addition, NSAIDs decrease dymenorrhea.[20] Mefenamic acid 500 mg three times daily, ibuprofen 400 mg three times daily, meclofenamate 100 mg three times daily, or naproxen 250 mg four times daily can be taken for the first few days of the menstrual cycle. Tranexamic acid has been found to decrease menstrual blood loss; however, it has no effect on dysmenorrhea and is indicated only for use in hemophilia. Etamsylate (ethamsylate) has also been found to decrease menstrual blood loss, but it is not currently approved by the US Food and Drug Administration (FDA). Danazol decreases blood loss, but due to its adverse effects it has not been used widely; there is not enough evidence to recommend it to most women.[21] At this time, there are no adequate trials comparing directly the above medications with each other.

Although there are few controlled studies, the oral contraceptive pill (OCP) can ameliorate dysmenorrhea, regularize cycles, decrease menstrual bleeding, and provide contraceptive protection.[22] Oral progestogens have been found to decrease blood loss if given for 21 days, but not if they are administered only in the luteal phase (ten-day regimen).

The levonorgestrel-releasing intrauterine device (LNG IUD) is as effective in decreasing blood loss as progestogen taken for 21 days.[23] Gonadotropin-releasing hormone (GnRH) does not appear to be effective and has an increased risk of adverse reactions, such as vasomotor symptoms and bone demineralization.

If contraception is needed in a patient with abnormal bleeding, then she may benefit from low-dose OCPs (assuming that she is a non-smoker and has no contraindications), oral or injectable progesterone, or LNG IUD. The use of these hormones for abnormal menstrual bleeding is not approved by the FDA. There is a variety of herbal, over-the-counter, and non-FDA-approved treatments for menorrhagia, but there are limited data on the effectiveness of most of these treatments.

If medical treatment for bleeding is not effective, then D&C may be helpful for a short period. However, the bleeding will often return to a higher level in the next cycle. If a woman has evidence of uterine malignancy, fibroids, or endometrial polyps, or if the bleeding does not respond to medical therapy, then she should be referred to a gynecologist.

Treatment for structural or neoplastic abnormalities depends on the underlying condition. Hysteroscopy is used to remove polyps, adenomyosis, and fibroids. There is debate over which procedure is best for the diagnosis and removal of uterine lesions, although currently the histopathology of the lesion cannot be determined without surgical removal of tissue.

Methods for endometrial destruction, such as resection and laser ablation, have been found to be effective in decreasing blood loss, but patient satisfaction has been low and the abnormal bleeding pattern usually returns within a few years.[24] There appears to be no evidence that myomectomy decreases blood loss.

Hysterectomy is the only way to stop menorrhagia completely. One in three women in the USA has a hysterectomy before the age of 60 years, which is approximately 600 000 yearly. At least half of these present with menorrhagia as the major symptom, although half of the women who had a hysterectomy for menorrhagia were found to have no uterine pathology. There are studies that indicate that the rate of major and minor complications after hysterectomy may be as high as one-third. The risks and benefits of this and other procedures must be explored carefully with each individual patient. The options available must be presented to help each patient make an informed decision about which is best for her medically and improves her quality of life.

Conclusion

In evaluating Ms J., you find that she is not anemic. The pathology of her endometrial biopsy reveals no hyperplasia or atypia. After counseling her about the risks and benefits, you have decided jointly that she should start on progesterone for 21 days monthly. You suggest that she follow up in three months. At that time, you find that her bleeding pattern has returned to a regular, predictable menstrual cycle.

Perimenopause is an important stage in a woman's life. In addition to the menstrual changes, she will likely have other symptoms that, although not life-threatening, can be very uncomfortable and change her quality of life. As estrogen levels decrease, she may have urogynecological and vasomotor symptoms. She may have abnormal bleeding before the complete cessation of her menses. It is important to determine the etiology of this bleeding. There are several treatments available for these symptoms, and the provider and the patient must determine jointly which is the best treatment for her. As a healthcare provider, recognizing the health risks and issues that are specific to menopause and helping the patient through this important phase in her life are important.

REFERENCES

1 World Health Organization. *World Health Report*, 1998. Geneva: World Health Organization; 1998. http://www.who.int/whr2001/2001/archives/1998/index.htm. Accessed March 13, 2003.
2 Harlow, B. L. and Signorello, L. B. Factors associated with early menopause. *Maturitas* 2002; **42** (supp 1):S87–93.
3 Obermeyer, C. M. Menopause across cultures: a review of the evidence. *Menopause* 2000; **7**:184–92.
4 La Valleur, J. Counseling the perimenopausal woman. *Obstet. Gynecol. Clin.* 2002; **29**:541–53.
5 Bachmann, G. A. and Nevadunsky, N. S. Diagnosis and treatment of atrophic vaginitis. *Am. Fam. Physician* 2000; **61**:3090–96.
6 Cutson, T. M. and Meuleman, E. Managing menopause. *Am. Fam. Physician* 2000; **61**:1391–400, 1405–6.
7 Kaunitz, A. Gynecologic problems of the perimenopause: evaluation and treatment. *Obstet. Gynecol. Clin. North Am.* 2002; **29**;455–73.
8 Rymer, J. Menopausal symptoms. In BMJ. *Clinical Evidence.* London. BMJ; 2000. pp. 1516–19.
9 Leonetti, H. B., Longo, S. and Anasti, J. N. Transdermal progesterone cream for vasomotor symptoms and post menopausal bone loss. *Obstet. Gynecol.* 1999; **94**:225–8.
10 Upmalis, D. H., Lobo, R., Bradley, L., *et al.* Vasomotor symptom relief by soy isoflavone extract tablets in postmenopausal women: a multicenter, double-blind, randomized, placebo-controlled study. *Menopause* 2000; **7**:236–42.
11 Faure, E. D., Chantre, P. and Mares, P. Effects of a standardized soy extract on hot flushes: a multicenter, double-blind, randomized, placebo-controlled study. *Menopause* 2002; **9**:329–34.
12 Ewies, A. Phytoestrogens in the management of the menopause: up-to-date. *Obstet. Gynecol. Surv.* 2002; **57**:306–13.

13 Dog, T. L., Riley, D. and Carter, T. An integrative approach to menopause. *Altern. Ther. Health Med.* 2001; **7**:45–55.

14 Rosenfeld, J. A. and Speedie, A. Patterns in the perimenopausal period. A survey. *J. Fam. Pract.*, submitted.

15 Morelli, V. and Naquin, C. Alternate therapies for traditional disease states: menopause. *Am. Fam. Physician* 2002; **66**:129–34.

16 Rosenfeld, J. A. and Speedie, A. Patterns in the perimenopausal period: a survey. *Maturitas*, submitted.

17 Davis, P. C., O'Neill, M. J., Yoder, I. C., Lee, S. I. and Mueller, P. R. Sonohystero-graphic findings of endometrial and subendometrial conditions. *Radiographics* 2002; **22**:803–16.

18 Briley, M. and Lindsell, D. R. The role of transvaginal ultrasound in the investigation of women with post-menopausal bleeding. *Clin. Radiol.* 1998; **53**:502–5.

19 O'Connell, L. P., Fries, M. H., Zeringue, E. and Brehm, W. Triage of abnormal postmenopausal bleeding: a comparison of endometrial biopsy and transvaginal sonohysterography versus fractional curettage with hysteroscopy. *Am. J. Obstet. Gynecol.* 1998; **178**:956–61.

20 Lethaby, A., Augood, C. and Duckitt, K. Nonsteroidal anti-inflammatory drugs for heavy menstrual bleeding. *Cochrane Database Syst. Rev.* 2002; issue 4.

21 Beaumont, H., Augood, C., Duckitt, K. and Lethaby, A. Danazol for heavy menstrual bleeding. *Cochrane Database Syst. Rev.* 2002; issue 4.

22 Jensen, J. T. and Speroff, L. Health benefits of oral contraceptives. *Obstet. Gynecol. Clin. North Am.* 2000; **27**:705–21.

23 Luukkainen, T. The levonorgestrel intrauterine system: therapeutic aspects. *Steroids* 2000; **65**:699–702.

24 Lethaby, A. and Hickey, M. Endometrial destruction techniques for heavy menstrual bleeding. *Cochrane Database Syst. Rev.* 2002; issue 4.

9

Spiritual and psychological aspects of menopause

Melissa H. Hunter, M.D. and Dana E. King, M.D.

Introduction

Case: Anne was 48 when she found out that she had breast cancer. She had been having frequent hot flushes, having stopped having periods one year ago, and she was still dealing with the fact that her children were no longer living at home. One child was in college and one was getting married, and now she was faced with the news that she had breast cancer. Cancer! It was almost too much to bear. She wrestled with thoughts of her changed body image, the upcoming loss of her breast, and the thought of "not being a woman any more."

Her doctor was asking her to make decisions that she did not feel ready to make, no matter how many times he explained the choices. How extensive did the surgery need to be? Should she get a complete mastectomy or a more breast-sparing procedure? Should she proceed with plastic surgery to reconstruct her breast, or was she being selfish? Where could she turn for help with these decisions? In addition to talking with her husband and reading as much as she could, she turned to spiritual resources for strength. She found great comfort in returning to religious practices that formerly she had not considered so important, like prayer and attendance at religious services. While she considered medical knowledge and skill most important in a physician, she sought a doctor who would understand her need to consult with God throughout the decision-making process.

This case illustrates some issues that can collide to bring enormous stress on the menopausal woman: physiologic change, emotional stress, medical illness and psychological health. *Menopause is a psychological and spiritual life event as well as a physical and physiologic event in women's lives.*[1] Apprehension, mood swings, feelings of grief, and family change often accompany menopause and are magnified when a woman simultaneously faces serious illness.[2] Anxiety may come from many things, including lack of knowledge about physical changes, sexual changes, loss of children in the home, mood fluctuations, and uncertainties in dealing with difficult medical decisions, as above.

Most women who go through menopause are not physically ill, but nevertheless they may have periods of self-doubt and confusion.[3] Physiologic effects of menopause are compounded by aging effects, a sense of loss that accompanies the "empty nest syndrome," and social changes.[1] Whether psychological changes are attributable directly to hormonal changes is the subject of current research and debate, but this is not the germane clinical issue. The most important issue is how to assist women facing many physiologic and psychological challenges that collide during the perimenopausal years.

Examining the spiritual facets of life and decision-making often faced in menopause, including why and how clinicians can address spiritual issues, is essential. The most common psychological features of menopause and recent research regarding anxiety, depression, and social factors will be reviewed in this chapter. The treatment options that family physicians can offer women who are having problems with coping with the changes of menopause will also be discussed.

Spiritual aspects of menopause

Spiritual aspects of menopause deal with challenges to a woman's view of herself, her world, and, often, her god. Women's religious and spiritual beliefs play an important role in their views of life and medical illness. In this chapter, "spirituality" will be defined as beliefs that give meaning to one's life and provide connection to the trascendant.[4] "Religion" will refer to a formal set of sacred beliefs, rituals, and practices. Many clinicians fail to consider the important role that spiritual and religious views play in providing women a context for interpreting life changes and illness. Failure to address spiritual and religious beliefs can frustrate the shared medical decision-making process because of lack of communication about fundamental issues. Physicians should not allow themselves to attempt to influence spiritual or religious views of their patients, but neither should they ignore patients' beliefs used to interpret the world around them.[5] Physicians must inquire about spiritual issues in order to communicate compassion and care for the whole person, and initiate referral to a minister or certified chaplain when significant issues are identified.[6]

Addressing spiritual issues

One important reason to address spiritual views in the healthcare setting is their impact on health-related decisions and behaviors. Spiritual and religious commitment is more prevalent among women than men.[7] Seventy percent of American women state that their religion is the most important influence

in their daily lives, compared with 52% of men.[8] In-patients express religious
and spiritual orientations even more strongly.[9,10] One survey of in-patients at
two hospitals revealed that 73% of patients prayed daily or more often. Ninety-
four percent of all patients and virtually all women agreed that spiritual health
is as important as physical health.

Another reason to ask about women's spiritual context is to find out about
important sources of coping.[11] Patients often use spiritual faith as a coping
resource for stress and illness. Asking about spiritual coping during discussions
of menopausal issues with women may clarify their feelings, identify sources
of strength, and give them permission to share feelings. Patients who use
religious coping have less depression and better health than those who do not
use religious coping.[12]

Clinicians can open dialog by asking female patients, "Do you have a faith
or religion that is important to you?" to express interest in spiritual or religious
needs/concerns. Another way to open dialog without a reference to religion
is to ask, "What is your source of strength when you are stressed or facing a
challenge?"[13]

Anne's situation in the earlier case demonstrates the importance of spirituality as a coping method and as an important resource in medical decision-
making.[14] It illustrates how many patients use spiritual contexts for interpreting illness. This patient sought a physician who understood her need
for spiritual support and appreciated its significance. Many patients also desire a physician who is attentive to spiritual needs in the decision-making
process.[15]

Obtaining a spiritual history

Taking a spiritual history is the process of gathering relevant information
about a patient's spiritual needs and concerns, religious beliefs and practices,
and whatever gives meaning and context to the patient's life.[5] For women
facing significant life changes, such as menopause, clinicians obtaining a routine medical history should include questions about whether the patient is
part of a religious denomination and how religious and spiritual views affect her health behavior. For patients facing hospitalization or medical crises,
history should also include coping methods, spiritual and religious concerns, and the patient's desires for availability of a minister or other spiritual
counselor.

Commonly used tools that assist in gathering spiritual and religious information from patients are the FAITH[9] (Table 9.1) and HOPE questionnaires
(Table 9.2).[13] The FAITH tool addresses issues of religious faith and may be
more useful when the clinician is aware that the patient is religious. It is also
useful in communities where religious belief is normative and accepted, making it easier to use a direct approach.

Table 9.1 FAITH spiritual history

F	Do you have a *faith* or religion that is important to you?
A	How do your beliefs *apply* to your health?
I	Are you *involved* in a church or faith community?
T	How do your spiritual beliefs affect your views about end-of-life *treatment*?
H	How can I *help* you with any spiritual concerns?

Adapted from King, D. E. Spirituality and medicine. In Mengel, M. B., Holleman, W. L. and Fields, S. (eds.). *Fundamentals of Clinical Practice: A Textbook on the Patient, Doctor, and Society.* New York: Kluwer; 2002.

Using the FAITH tool, the first question asks whether the patient has a faith or religion that is important to them. This establishes whether the patient considers herself spiritual or religious and whether such views are important in the medical context. *Determining the patient's denominational affiliation can give clinicians clues to particular health beliefs while offering a starting point for further inquiry.*

The next question focuses on how the patient's beliefs apply to their health. Are there dietary restrictions or religious customs of which the healthcare team should be aware? Are there any restrictions about the use of blood or blood products? Many religious traditions have customs or rituals about, for example, diet, prayer, religious holidays, and observances, that may affect medical care.[16]

Determining involvement in a faith community is helpful in understanding the patient's available social and spiritual support. Does the woman have someone to call for counseling or emotional support? Does the congregation offer classes or support groups for people with illness, divorce, or other life stresses?

The next question addresses whether treatment decisions may be influenced by spiritual or religious beliefs. For example, women facing decisions regarding surgery or chemotherapy may face religious and health questions, since many religious sects regard childbearing as sacred.[17] Patients who believe in an afterlife may have different outlooks from those who do not. Inquiring about spiritual and religious beliefs is particularly important when dealing with patients who are making medical decisions about life and death issues.

Finally, asking the patient about ways to help with spiritual concerns is an excellent way to open dialog about the patient's concerns. Women may share feelings or internal conflicts or may ask questions. They may also request to see the chaplain, ask for prayer, or ask the physician to pray with them. Many providers will not be comfortable praying with patients, but each provider should be prepared to respond in a compassionate and knowledgable fashion about concerns. Often, the most important thing to do is listen. In our

Table 9.2 Examples of questions for the HOPE approach to spiritual assessment

H   Sources of *hope*, meaning, comfort, strength, peace, love, and connection

We have been discussing your support systems. I was wondering, what is there in your life that gives you internal support?

What are your sources of hope, strength, comfort, and peace?

What do you hold on to during difficult times?

What sustains you and keeps you going?

For some people, their religious or spiritual beliefs act as a source of comfort and strength in dealing with life's ups and downs; is this true for you?

If the answer is "Yes," go on to O and P questions.

If the answer is "No," consider asking: Was it ever? If the answer is "Yes," ask: What changed?

O   *Organized* religion

Do you consider yourself part of an organized religion?

How important is this to you?

What aspects of your religion are helpful and not so helpful to you?

Are you part of a religious or spiritual community? Does it help you? How?

P   *Personal* spirituality/practices

Do you have personal spiritual beliefs that are independent of organized religion? What are they?

Do you believe in God? What kind of relationship do you have with God?

What aspects of your spirituality or spiritual practices do you find most helpful to your personality? (eg prayer, mediation, reading scripture, attending religious services, listening to music, hiking, communing with nature?)

E   *Effects* on medical care and end-of-life issues

Has being sick (or your current situation) affected your ability to do the things that usually help you spiritually? (Or affected your relationship with God?)

As a doctor, is there anything that I can do to help you access the resources that usually help you?

Are you worried about any conflicts between your beliefs and your medical situation/care/decisions?

Would it be helpful for you to speak to a clinical chaplain/community spiritual leader?

Are there any specific practices or restrictions I should know about in providing your medical care? (eg dietary restrictions, use of blood products)

If the patient is dying: How do your beliefs affect the kind of medical care you would like me to provide over the next few days/weeks/months?

Adapted from Anandarajah, G. and Hight, E. Spirituality and medical practice: using the HOPE questions as a practical tool for spiritual assessment. *Am. Fam. Phys.* 2000; **63**:81–8.

experience, patients are often surprised to learn that providers are interested in their spiritual concerns. Many interpret inquiry about spiritual and religious issues as a sign that the physician cares about them as a "whole person." Listening to the patient's struggles with the meaning and value of life in the midst of a health crisis can be therapeutic for the patient and also enlightening to the provider.

Integrating spiritual care into practice

Providing compassionate care to women in an emotional time of menopause means acknowledging and addressing spiritual needs of women. Most often, attending to spiritual needs entails simply listening empathetically; at other times, referral to clergy will be needed. Attentiveness to spirituality in women during the perimenopausal period will assist in identifying coping resources, in medical decision-making, and in personalizing the physician–patient interaction.

Spiritual counseling is full of ethical challenges, including issues of autonomy, authority, confidentiality, and coercion.[18,19] Physicians should refer patients to a certified chaplain or qualified minister when they identify significant spiritual needs or concerns.

Psychological aspects of menopause

Menopause as a transition

Menopause is a transition encompassing a developmental stage in the lifecycle, during which women gradually adapt to biologic, social, psychological, and spiritual changes that accompany recognized physiologic changes. While women throughout the world experience menopause, diagnosis is often difficult because it can be made only in retrospect. Along with biologic changes, significant psychological events occur during mid life, including changing relationships with children, marital instability, widowhood, and the illness or loss of parents. Menopause is a time of transition from childbearing and child-rearing to a time of growth, concentration on marital relationships, and sometimes freedom to travel. It is also a transition to "old age," increased risk of illness, disability, and grandparenting.

Contrary to medical models of menopause that characterize it as an endocrinopathy in need of hormonal treatment, women tend to view menopause as a developmental life event, or a rite of passage. One study interviewed women and found resistance to the medicalization of menopause.[20] More recently, another study evaluated middle-class, well-educated women who described menopause as a change in appearance, aging body, health, and sexuality.[21] Most women (78.7%) cited menopause as just the "cessation of periods," while just over a third of them related menopause to an end of childbearing capacity.[22] The Seattle Midlife Women's Health Study also lends further credence to women's views of menopause as a normal developmental process.

Most of the uncertainty women expressed about menopause related to their own expectations of menopause itself. Finally, the North American Menopause Society survey found that the majority of women viewed menopause and mid life as the beginning of positive life and health changes. *More than 75% of women surveyed reported making health-related lifestyle changes, such as smoking cessation, at menopause.* Hysterectomy was also a factor associated with improved spouse/partner relationships, improved sexual relationships, improved physical health, and sense of personal fulfillment.[23]

Associated demographic factors

Because life expectancy has risen considerably over the past century, women in industrialized countries expect to spend more than a third of their lives after menopause. One study found that women with poorer marital adjustment reported significantly more menopausal symptoms and perceived severity of their symptoms to be greater.[24] Significant associations occurred between women's reported menopausal symptoms and income, marital status, presence of children in the home, and perceptions of patients' mothers' experience of menopause.[25]

Women with worse symptoms were more likely to be on a low to middle income, be unmarried, have no children at home, and perceive their mothers as experiencing distress during menopause. Menopausal women who were "married with children" were physically healthier and exhibited fewer depressive symptoms. Additionally, women with only a high-school education were at a fourfold risk of developing depression, and lack of paid employment more than doubled the risk of depression, regardless of educational level.[26]

Mood and menopause

There is no agreement of the effect of menopause on psychiatric disorders, psychological symptoms, and sexual function. The important role of gonadal hormones is suggested by the prevalence of mood disorders such as depression during the reproductive years and the propensity for depressive episodes to occur during times of hormonal change. Lifetime prevalence of depression for women in the USA is consistently twice that of men, and the increased prevalence in women can also be found in other countries.[27] Lifetime prevalence depression rates of 21% in women and 13% in men were reported by the National Comorbidity Survey in 1994.[28]

Social and psychological factors also play a role in the development of depression, with happily married women having slightly lower incidence of major depression than single women. Other factors, including sexual abuse, history of domestic violence, miscarriage and abortion, death of a child or spouse, family history of depression, and mothers of children with attention deficit disorders, are all correlated with depression.[29] Cultural influences may affect the risk of depression in all women and women in the workplace who face often conflicting roles as mother, spouse, and breadwinner.[30] Sexual harassment concerns in the workplace and unequal pay with lack of advancement compared with male counterparts also place women at increased risk of depression.

Female gender is associated clearly with higher risk for affective disorders.[31] However, the effect of menopause on this risk has been controversial. Several longitudinal studies have reported no increase in moderate or severe depressive symptoms with menopause.[32,33] However, a small increase in mild symptoms peaks just before menopause.[34]

Preliminary results of the Study of Women's Health by the National Institutes on Aging indicate that African-American women have more estrogen-related symptoms at menopause, while women of Asian descent report fewer debilitating menopausal symptoms than white (2–3%) or African-American (12–14%) counterparts.[35] Other factors associated with decreased mood at menopause include prior depression, prior premenstrual syndrome (PMS), hysterectomy, psychosocial stressors, negative attitudes towards menopause, and poor health and lifestyle variables, including smoking and lack of exercise.

Much like depression, anxiety symptoms increase just before the menopause. However, several well-designed prospective studies found no increased rate of anxiety with menopause.[36,37] As with other mood disorders, women who present to menopause clinics tend to have increased rates of anxiety and other psychological symptoms.[38] Seemingly, women who present to menopausal clinics are those who are more symptomatic and more likely to request treatment, including hormone replacement therapy.

The changes in female sexuality with the menopause have been examined poorly. While sexual problems are common in women attending menopause or gynecology clinics, the picture is less clear in the general population.[39] *With increasing age, levels of sexual desire as well as frequency of sexual activity and orgasm decrease.*[39] However, the extent to which menopause contributes to these changes is unclear.

Decline in coital frequency has been associated with reductions in testosterone levels, and cross-sectional studies have found less evidence of an effect of menopausal status (including specific gonadal hormonal levels) on sexual function, the effects being some reduction in enjoyment of sexual activity and desire.[40] Overall, this suggests that reduction of libido and frequency of sexual activity and orgasm may accompany the menopause. However, satisfaction with sexual relationship remains largely unaffected in the majority of women.[41]

Social changes and context of menopause

Women have differing expectations of menopause, and cultural backgrounds may exert significant influence regarding response to menopause. This reaction is often dictated by whether a woman's status is valued or devalued by the event, with those women who define themselves in a childbearing role experiencing the most distress during menopause.[42]

Cross-cultural studies indicate that *women from different cultures cope with menopause differently*. In cultures where aging women are given elevated status or where menopause is viewed as a normal stage of the lifecycle, menopause is reported as being less problematic. Some connection between dominant values of a culture, social consequences of attitudes and values, and women's experience of menopause appear to exist.[43]

Unfortunately, women in the USA are valued in terms of youth and sexual attractiveness and are devalued as they age. This devaluation occurs with the loss of stereotypical youthful and sexual attractiveness and reproductive capacity.[44] Because of this, women often report the menopausal experience as a negative one.

Additionally, cross-cultural studies reveal considerable differences in reporting of vasomotor symptoms, such as hot flushes. Japanese women report significantly fewer hot flushes than North American and European counterparts.[45] Mayan women essentially report no menopausal symptoms, except for menstrual irregularities.[46] While cultural perceptions of menopause may modify evaluation of physical changes and symptoms, lifestyle and dietary changes may also play a part. Considerable differences in hot-flush reporting exist even within a culture, with wide variations with location intensity, and duration of flushes.[47] Positive correlation has also been found between hot-flush frequency and higher levels of perceived stress.[48]

Although menopause continues to hold potential for fear and anxiety, attitudes among women recently have become more open and accepting. Increasing attention to women's health and menopause in the media has enabled women to gain accurate information about menopause and attendant health risks and concerns. A wider variety of choices, including educational and career opportunities, delayed childbearing, and child-free or single-parenting options, have helped to reduce the emphasis on more traditional views of women's roles in the family.

Treatment

Counseling and pharmacotherapy have a role in assisting women facing challenges and symptoms of menopause. Hormone replacement has a role in alleviating some symptoms, but it has limited application for the psychological stresses of menopause. Mainstays of treatment for psychological manifestations of menopause are pharmacotherapy, exercise, and counseling.

Pharmacotherapy

Estrogen may moderate mood swings to a limited degree, but it has limited direct effects on mood in many women.[1] Estrogen may be helpful in some women with perimenopausal anxiety, irritability, and depression.[49] Because the role of estrogen is not well defined, and other proven and efficacious treatment is available, depression may be best treated with antidepressants. Treatment should also include counseling. Depression and PMS respond well to selective serotonin-reuptake inhibitors (SSRIs), including fluoxetine, sertraline, paroxetine, and citalopram. Because of gender-based pharmacokinetic differences, antidepressant plasma concentrations may be higher in women.[50] Thus, women with depression may require lower dosages of antidepressants than male counterparts. In addition, women need to be asked specifically about sexual side effects, because they generally do not report these unless asked.

Anxiety disorders should be treated with medicines indicated for that purpose, including benzodiazepines, SSRIs, and tricyclic agents. A specific diagnosis should be made to aid selection of therapy. Benzodiazepines are most useful in situational anxiety, adjustment disorder, and exacerbations of generalized anxiety disorder (GAD). Sertraline and paroxetine are indicated, approved, and effective for panic disorder, GAD, post-traumatic stress disorder, and social phobias.

Exercise

Exercise can be helpful and is highly recommended for menopausal women.[51] Running can increase bone density without increasing risk of osteoarthritis.[52] *Exercise is helpful in adjunctive medical treatment of anxiety and depression.*[53] Daily exercise should be encouraged, since activities such as daily walking and parking further from workplaces and stores ("lifestyle walking") are as effective as more structured programs.[54] Moderate walking for as little as three hours a week will bring significant health benefits and may reduce depression.[55]

Counseling

Counseling is an important therapy for a variety of psychological symptoms and conditions in menopause, and is useful for transitioning through menopause.

Familiarity with normal symptoms of menopause and common psychological concerns is paramount for the primary care provider. Brief office counseling is sufficient when reassurance and education are the main issues.[29]

Women should be counseled that menopause is a gradual process and a natural transition.[4] Reassurance and validation are important, confirming that others have similar feelings, sensations, and issues.

Counseling is also helpful in specific clinical situations. Supportive counseling is beneficial for those with marital stress or conflict caused by mood swings or other stresses.[4] Counseling is also helpful for specific anxiety disorders and depression, alone or in combination with medication. However, differentiating between adaptation difficulties and psychoses may be difficult, especially in women with pre-existing mental health disorders that occurred before menopause.[3] Referral to a psychiatrist or family therapist should be considered if psychoses or intense marital conflict are identified. Spousal/partner involvement may be needed to address the psychosocial and sexual issues often underlying emotional upheavals during menopause.[3] Referral to a certified chaplain is indicated when significant spiritual issues or conflicts are identified.[6]

Summary

Menopause is a psychological and spiritual life event as well as a physical and physiologic event. Apprehension, mood swings, feelings of grief, and family change are common. Most women who go through menopause are not physically ill, but cultural expectations about aging and appearance often affect the woman's self-esteem during this period.

In this chapter, we have discussed spiritual aspects of menopause, including how and why to address spiritual issues. We have also reviewed the most common psychological features of menopause and recent research regarding anxiety, depression, and social factors. Physicians treating patients during menopause should be alert for psychological and spiritual issues and be familiar with treatment options, including pharmacotherapy, exercise, and counseling.

REFERENCES

1 Northrup, C. Menopause. *Prim. Care* 1997; **24**:921–48.
2 Nijs, P. Counseling of the climacteric woman: diagnostic difficulties and therapeutic possibilities. *Eur. J. Obstet. Gynecol. Reprod. Biol.* 1998; **81**:273–6.
3 Cobb, J. O. Reassuring the woman facing menopause: strategies and resources. *Patient Educ. Couns.* 1998; **33**:281–8.
4 Puchalski, C. M., and Larson, D. B. Developing curricula in spirituality and medicine. *Acad. Med.* 1998; **73**:970–74.
5 King, D. E. *Faith, Spirituality, and Medicine: Toward the Making of a Healing Practitioner*. New York: Haworth Press; 2000.

6 King, D. E. Spirituality and medicine. In Mengel, M. G., Holleman, W. L. and Fields, S. (eds.). *Fundamentals of Clinical Practice: A Textbook on the Patient, Doctor, and Society*, 2nd edition. New York: Kluwer, Academic/Plenum; 2002.

7 Koenig, H. G., McCullough, M. and Larson, D. B. *Handbook of Religion and Health*. New York: Oxford University Press; 2001.

8 Gallup, G. *Religion in America 1990*. Princeton: The Princeton Religion Research Center; 1990.

9 King, D. E. and Bushwick, B. Beliefs and attitudes of hospital in-patients about faith healing and prayer. *J. Fam. Pract.* 1994; **39**:349–52.

10 Koenig, H. G., George, L. K. and Peterson, B. L. Religiosity and remission from depression in medically ill older patients. *Am. J. Psychiatry* 1998; **155**:536–42.

11 Matthews, D. A., McCullough, M. E., Larson, D. B., *et al*. Religious commitment and health status. *Arch. Fam. Med.* 1998; **7**:118–24.

12 Koenig, H. G., Cohen, H. J., Blazer, D. G., *et al*. Religious coping and depression among elderly, hospitalized, medically ill men. *Am. J. Psychiatry* 1992; **149**: 1693–700.

13 Anandarajah, G. and Hight, E. Spirituality and medical practice: using the HOPE questions as a practical tool for spiritual assessment. *Am. Fam. Phys.* 2000; **63**: 81–8.

14 Roberts, J. A., Brown, D., Elkins, T. and Larson, D. B. Factors influencing views of patients with gynecological cancer about end-of-life decisions. *Am. J. Obstet. Gynecol.* 1997; **176**:166–72.

15 Johnson, S. C. and Spilka, B. Coping with breast cancer: the roles of clergy and faith. *J. Relig. Health* 1991; **30**:21–33.

16 Rahman, F. and Marty, M. *Health and Medicine in the Islamic Tradition: Change and Identity (Health/Medicine and the Faith Traditions)*. Chicago: Kazi Publications; 1998.

17 Breuilly, E., O'Brien, J., Marty, M. E. and Palmer, M. *Religions of the World: The Illustrated Guide to Origins, Beliefs, Traditions and Festivals*. Chicago: Checkmark; 1997.

18 Sloan, R. P., Bagiella, E. and Powell, T. Religion, spirituality, and medicine. *Lancet* 1999; **353**:664–7.

19 Sloan, R. P., Bagiella, E., VandeCreek, L., Hasan, Y. and Puolos, P. Should physicians prescribe religious activities? *N. Engl. J. Med.* 2000; **342**:1913–16.

20 Martin, E. *The Woman in the Body: A Cultural Analysis of Reproduction*. Boston: Beacon Press; 1987.

21 Jones, J. Embodied meaning: menopause and the change of life. *Soc. Work Health Care* 1994; **19**:43–65.

22 Woods, F. W. and Mitchell, E. S. Anticipating menopause: observations from the Seattle Midlife Women's Health Study. *Menopause* 1999; **6**:167–73.

23 Utian, W. H. and Boggs, P. P. The North American Menopause Society 1998 Menopause Survey, part 1: postmenopausal women's perceptions about menopause and midlife. *Menopause* 1999; **6**:122–8.

24 Uphold, C. R. and Susman, E. J. Self-reported climacteric symptoms as a function of the relationships between marital adjustment and childrearing stage. *Nurs. Res.* 1981; **30**:84–8.

25 Dosey, M. F. and Dosey, M. A. The climacteric woman. *Patient Couns. Health Educ.* 1980; **2**:14–21.
26 Costello, E. J. Married with children: predictors of mental and physical health in middle-aged women. *Psychiatry* 1991; **54**:292–305.
27 Weissman, M. M., Bland, R. C. and Canino, G. J. Cross-national epidemiology of major depression and bipolar disorder. *J. Am. Med. Assoc.* 1996; **276**:293–9.
28 Kessler, R. C., McGonagle, K. A., Zhao, S., *et al.* Lifetime and 12-month prevalence of DSM-III-R psychiatric disorders in the United States. *Arch. Gen. Psychiatry* 1994; **51**:8–19.
29 McCormick, L. H. Depression in mothers of children with attention deficit hyperactivity disorder. *Fam. Med.* 1995; **27**:176–9.
30 Yonkers, K. A. and Austin, L. S. Mood disorders: women and affective disorders. *Prim. Psychiatry* 1996; **3**:27–8.
31 Leibenluft, E. Women with bipolar illness: clinical and research issues. *Am. J. Psychiatry* 1996; **153**:163–73.
32 Hallstrom, T. and Samuelson, S. Mental health in the climacteric: the longitudinal study of women in Gothenburg. *Acta Obstet. Gynecol. Scand. Suppl.* 1985; **130**: 13–18.
33 Holte, A. and Mikkelsen, A. Psychosocial determinants of climacteric complaints. *Maturitas* 1991; **13**:205–15.
34 Cawood, E. H. H. and Bancroft, J. Steroid hormones, the menopause, sexuality and well being of women. *Psychol. Med.* 1996; **26**:925–36.
35 DeAngelis, T. Menopause symptoms vary among ethnic groups. *Am. Psychiatr. Assoc. Monit.* 1997; **17**:16.
36 Garnett, T., Studd, J. W. W., Henderson, A., *et al.* Hormone implants and tachyphylaxis. *Br. J. Obstet. Gynaecol,* 1990; **97**:917–21.
37 Hay, A. G., Bancroft, J. and Johnstone, E. C. Affective symptoms in women attending a menopause clinic. *Br. J. Psychiatry* 1994; **164**:513–16.
38 Sarrel, P. M. and Whitehead, M. I. Sex and menopause: defining the issues. *Maturitas* 1985; **7**:217–24.
39 Osborn, M., Hawton, K. and Gath, D. Sexual function among middle aged women in the community. *Br. Med. J.* 1985; **296**:959–62.
40 Hawton, K., Gath, D. and Day, A. Sexual function in a community sample of middle-aged women with partners: effects of age, marital, socio-economic, psychiatric, gynaecological and menopausal factors. *Arch. Sex. Behav.* 1994; **23**: 375–95.
41 Hunter, M. S. Emotional well being, sexual behavior and hormone replacement therapy. *Maturitas* 1990; **12**:299–314.
42 Fishbein, E. G. Women at midlife: the transition to menopause. *Nurs. Clin. North. Am.* 1992; **27**:951–7.
43 Carolan, M. Beyond deficiency: broadening the view of menopause. *J. Appl. Gerontol.* 1994; **13**:193–205.
44 Berkun, C. On behalf of women over 40: understanding the importance of menopause. *Soc. Work* 1986; **31**:378–84.
45 Lock M. Ambiguities of aging: Japanese experience and perceptions of the menopause. *Cult. Med. Psychiatry* 1980; **10**:23–46.

46 Beyenne, Y. Cultural significance and physiological manifestations of menopause, a biocultural analysis. *Cult. Med. Soc.* 1986; **10**:47–71.
47 Voda, A. M. Climacteric hot flush. *Maturitas* 1981; **3**:73–90.
48 Gannon, L., Hansel, S. and Goodwin, J. Correlates of menopausal hot flushes. *J. Behav. Med.* 1987; **10**:277–85.
49 Vliet, E. L. Menopause and perimenopause: the role of ovarian hormones in common neuroendocrine syndromes in primary care. *Prim. Care* 2002; **29**:43–67.
50 Bhatia, S. Depression in women: diagnostic and treatment considerations. *Am. Fam. Physician* 1999; **60**:225–40.
51 Miszko, T. A. and Cress, M. E. A lifetime of fitness: exercise in the perimenopausal and postmenopausal woman. *Clin. Sports Med.* 2000; **19**:215–32.
52 Lane, N. A., Bloch, D. A., Hubert, H. B., *et al.* Running, osteoarthritis, and bone density: initial 2 year longitudinal study. *Am. J. Med.* 1990; **88**:452.
53 Manber, R. Alternative treatments for depression: empirical support and relevance to women. *J. Clin. Psychiatry* 2002; **63**:628–40.
54 Dunn, A. L., Marcus, B. H. and Kampert, J. B. Comparison of the lifestyle and structured intervention to increase physical activity and cardiorespiratory fitness: a randomized trial. *J. Am. Med. Assoc.* 1999; **281**:327.
55 Manson, J. E., Hu, F. B., Rich-Edwards, J. W., *et al.* A prospective study of walking as compared with vigorous exercise in the prevention of coronary heart disease in women. *N. Engl. J. Med.* 1999; **341**:651.

10

Hormone therapy

Kathy Andolsek

Case: a 51-year-old healthy woman presents to the office. She has two children, 24 and 21 years of age, both delivered by cesarean section for fetal distress. Following the second delivery, she had a bilateral tubal ligation for contraception. She has had no other medical conditions. She reports that her menses have changed over the past year, becoming shorter and lighter. She occasionally skips a period altogether. She reports hot flushes, palpitations, and some sleep disruption. She believes that the sleep disruption has led to fatigue and some mild cognitive changes, which are beginning to interfere with her work performance. She has no personal or family history of breast cancer, coronary artery disease, or thromboembolic disease. She does have a family history of osteoporosis. She is a non-smoker, drinks two beers weekly, and exercises inconsistently. Her best friend had been on hormone therapy but stopped with the recent news concerning adverse effects. She wants to know whether she should consider hormonal therapy for her hot flushes and sleeping difficulty or if there is anything "safer."

Introduction

Hormone therapy (HT) is the combined use of estrogen and progestin (EPT), or estrogen alone (ET), by postmenopausal or perimenopausal women. The US Food and Drug Administration (FDA) Office of Drug Evaluation has recently substituted the term "hormone therapy" for "hormone replacement therapy" to highlight the fact that postmenopausal hormones are *treatment* for certain conditions, not a necessary *replacement* for hormones that decrease as part of the normal menopause. In the past, EPT and ET were used both to manage the symptoms of menopause and for the primary and secondary prevention of several common chronic conditions. Clinical studies continue to inform medical decision-making.

Four thousand US women enter menopause each day, at an average age of 51.4 years. These women live, on average, nearly 30 additional years. A US woman's life expectancy in 2002 was 79.5 years.[1] In the UK, the mean age of menopause is 50.75 years. In a Scottish survey of 6096 women aged 45–54 years, 80% of women reported at least one symptom of menopause. Forty-five percent characterized one or more symptoms as "problematic."[2]

The average woman is born with over two million immature eggs but has only 300 000–600 000 eggs remaining by the time she experiences menarche at an average age of 12 years. Most women have about 400 menstrual cycles throughout their reproductive years. On average, only 25 000 eggs remain by the late thirties and no functional oocytes remain by menopause.

Estrogen and progestin production begins to decline several years before menopause and women may begin to experience symptoms during this "perimenopausal" period. *Women therefore typically spend a third to a half of their lives "post-menopause."* It was tempting to look at this "estrogen deficiency" as a medical condition that could be remedied by hormone "replacement."

In addition to natural menopause, menopause can be induced. This is usually a consequence of surgery (such as hysterectomy or bilateral oophorectomy-salpingectomy), but it may be secondary to pelvic radiation therapy as part of cancer treatment. Recommending hormone replacement for women with induced menopause has been common.

In 1995, nearly 28% of menopausal American women used HT. Forty-five per cent of menopausal women used postmenopausal hormones for at least one month; 20% of menopausal women used them for five or more years.[3] Premarin™ (a brand of conjugated estrogens), until recently, was the second most frequently prescribed medication in the USA.[4] Although stereotypically portrayed as a time of anguish and precipitous decline, in a recent survey most women reported they were happiest and most fulfilled between the ages of 50 and 65 years of age, and over three-quarters reported that they made a positive lifestyle change during this life phase.[5]

Recent studies of the safety and efficacy of EPT and ET have contradicted the conventional wisdom of the past several decades and led to confusion in women and their clinicians. Respected groups, such as the US Preventive Services Task Force (USPSTF) have reversed prior recommendations. The 1996 USPSTF recommended counseling all perimenopausal women about the potential benefits and harms of HRT (HT), acknowledging that at that point in time the evidence was insufficient to recommend for or against HRT (HT) for all women. They advised that individual decisions should be based on patient-specific risk factors, personal values, and preferences and weighed against likely benefits and harms. *Their updated 2002 recommendations now advise against the routine use of estrogen and progestin for the prevention of chronic conditions.* The USPSTF designates this conclusion a "D" recommendation (indicating that the harmful effects of HRT (HT) are likely to exceed the benefits from

Table 10.1 Recommendations for clinicians to help women decide regarding the use of HT. Clinicians should help women to:

Be actively involved in the decision-making process regarding EPT/ET
Identify her values and health beliefs
Identify her own personal, family, and medical history, especially for heart disease
   and other vascular disease, osteoporosis, certain cancers (colorectal, breast,
   ovarian), and thromboembolic disease
Identify goal(s) for HT: how does she hope to benefit?
Evaluate overall benefits or risks of HT compared with these goal(s)
Compare alternatives to HT/ET to match the goal(s) weighed against risk and benefit
   and assess their acceptability
Monitor and assess the outcome of any alternatives she tries
Compare the various choices of various preparations, routes of administration, and
   doses if she wishes HT
Develop plan to stop HT should she wish, including anticipating common side
   effects and exploring options for management of common symptoms
Interpret new studies as they become available
Reassess decision at a minimum of once a year based on newly available information
   and her own risk profile

Source: Tomic, D., Lankford, C. S. R., Whiteman, M. K. and Flaws, J. A. Postmenopausal hormone replacement therapy: where are we now? *J. Coll. Med.* 2002; 9:515–23.

prevention in most women). The USPSTF now recommends that clinicians "develop a shared decision making approach to preventing chronic disease in perimenopausal and postmenopausal women considering individual risk factors [and] preferences."[6]

Information and education by clinicians is beneficial to women in making their decision regarding HRT/ET.[7] Physicians must be able to help women differentiate what is known from what is not, to individualize this knowledge to their medical and family history and personal values, and to communicate new information as it becomes available in a timely manner (Table 10.1). Clinicians may consider establishing a database to expedite contact of women as new information becomes available and to facilitate the exchange of information. Some practices elect to do this with a newsletter, periodic group visits, or electronically through a Web page or list serve.

Hormonal changes at menopause

Estrogen levels in postmenopausal women are one-tenth of those in pre-menopausal women. Postmenopausal estrogens are produced by the adrenal glands and fat cells rather than the ovary, the primary source of premenopausal estrogen. Estrone, produced by fat, replaces estradiol as the main source of estrogen. HT approximately doubles the estrogen level of a postmenopausal woman. After menopause, progesterone is essentially absent.

Another hormone that declines around the time of menopause is testosterone, produced in men as well as in women. In women, the ovaries and the adrenal glands are the major producers of testosterone. The adrenal glands produce dihydroepiandrosterone (DHEA), which is converted to testosterone in peripheral tissues. Testosterone affects the brain, bone, muscle, skin, blood vessels, and vagina and contributes to bone density, strength, energy, hair growth, and libido in women. Levels peak when women are in their twenties and decrease to about half that level when they are in their forties. Ovaries continue producing some testosterone throughout the lifespan.

Symptoms

Because estrogen receptors are located throughout the body, menopause affects multiple organ systems (Table 10.2). HT has been used to treat these symptoms, with varying quality of evidence.

Libido is affected variably. Most women note no change. In others, libido increases, perhaps because there is no longer anxiety regarding an accidental pregnancy. For women who note a decline, a full evaluation is warranted. Etiologies may include disrupted sleep, mood changes, medical and/or environmental causes, and decreased production of testosterone.

Prevention of chronic disease

Over the past few decades, HT has been touted widely to provide both primary and secondary prevention for several major chronic conditions. More than 30 case–control and prospective observational studies have suggested that HT provided primary prevention against coronary heart disease (CHD), secondary prevention for women with prior myocardial infarction (MI), and both primary and secondary prevention against fractures from osteoporosis.

In one of the largest of these studies, the Nurses' Health Study, 70 533 postmenopausal women were followed for 20 years. HT users had a decreased risk of CHD compared with women who had never used HT.[8]

Conclusions from such observational studies can be flawed if the users are different from the non-users. *HT users are, in fact, very different from non-users.* These differences, rather than HT, are responsible for many if not all of estrogen's apparent health benefits. HT users tend to be more affluent, leaner, and more educated. They exercise more often and drink alcohol more frequently. Women who had healthier behaviors were more likely to be prescribed and to use HT.[9]

Table 10.2 Signs and symptoms from hormonal changes at menopause

Central nervous system
  Hot flushes
  Disrupted sleep
  Mood changes
  Memory difficulties
Cardiovascular system
  Increased cholesterol
  Increased risk of coronary heart disease (including myocardial infarction) and
    stroke
Breasts
  Duct and glandular tissue replaced by fat
Kidney
  Increased calcium loss
Bone
  Rapid bone loss
  Fracture and risk of deformity increases
Body shape
  Increased abdominal fat
  Increased waist circumference
Skin
  Dry, thin, easily damaged
  Decreased collagen
Urogenital
  Cessation of menses
  Vaginal dryness
  Bladder infections
  More frequent yeast infections
  Urinary frequency
  Stress incontinence
Intestines
  Less calcium absorbed from food

Rather than observational studies, the gold standard of therapeutic efficacy is the randomized controlled clinical trial (RCT). Two major studies, the Heart and Estrogen/Progestin Replacement Study (HERS) Trial and the Woman's Health Initiative (WHI), were RCTs designed prospectively to examine the benefits and harms from HT (see Chapter 12). In the HERS trial, the women who used HT experienced an increased risk of heart attack during the first year of the study. Although the risk declined in subsequent years, it was never lower than the risk of women using placebo, despite an additional three years of follow-up. In addition, HT users manifested an increased risk of blood clots in both the legs and the lungs. The HERS trial concluded that combination HT was *not* effective for the secondary prevention of coronary heart disease in

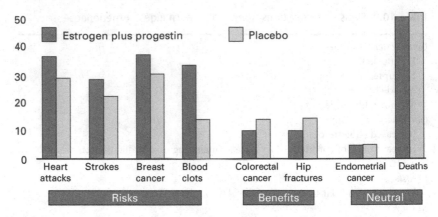

Figure 10.1 Disease rates for women on hormone replacement therapy (HRT) of estrogen plus progestin or placebo. Annual cases per 10 000 women. (From the Writing Group for the Women's Health Initiative investigators.)

women with prior MI over an average of nearly seven years of follow-up. HT users experienced more adverse outcomes than women using placebo.[10]

In the WHI, 8506 women were randomized to receive 0.625 mg conjugated equine estrogens plus 2.5 mg medroxyprogesterone acetate daily; 8102 women received placebo.[11] Compared with women who used the placebo, women who used EPT experienced:

- 26% increase in breast cancer;
- 41% increase in strokes;
- 29% increase in heart attacks;
- double the rates of blood clots of the legs and the lungs;
- 37% less colorectal cancer;
- 34% fewer hip fractures;
- no difference in mortality.

Despite the difference in disease conditions, there was no difference in overall mortality between the EPT users and the women who used placebo. Although the number of MIs was increased in HT users, there was no difference in the CHD mortality or the likelihood of coronary artery bypass graft (CABG) or angioplasty. HT users had some benefits. For every 10 000 women who use EPT for one year, five fewer will experience hip fractures and six fewer will develop colon cancer (Figure 10.1).

Despite the benefits, the WHI terminated the combined HT trial because of this increase in adverse outcomes. The WHI study arm in which 10 739 women who have had a hysterectomy were randomized to receive either ET (without progestin) or placebo is continuing as originally planned. At present, these women seem to have no excess risk. Conclusions from the estrogen-alone study are anticipated in 2005.

Table 10.3 Absolute risks of taking Prempro™ (per 1000 women per year)

Condition	Usual risk (women on placebo)	Women using HT
Breast cancer	3.0	3.8
Stroke	2.1	2.9
Heart attack	2.3	3.0
Serious blood clots	1.6	3.4

Although it is a large, well-conducted clinical trial, the WHI does not answer all clinically pertinent questions. Not all WHI participants began EPT or ET during the perimenopausal or early menopausal period, the usual time for women to initiate these drugs. Many study participants began these hormones in their seventh and eighth decades, when they had established (if unrecognized) heart disease. In addition, only one type of estrogen and one type of progestin were studied, and only one regimen (daily fixed oral administration of both estrogen and progestin) was studied. Whether the risks would be the same if different types of hormone, for example estradiol compared with conjugated estrogen, were utilized is not known. Because transdermal estradiol tends not to raise triglyceride levels, not to affect clotting, and not to cause cholelithiasis, as compared with oral conjugated estrogen, it is plausible that there would be fewer adverse outcomes with transdermal estradiol.[12]

At the heart of the WHI debate lies the concept of risk. There are two common methods for expressing risk in clinical studies. WHI data as originally published are calculated as relative risk, the percent change in the risk of HT users compared with women using placebo. After five years, 166 women were diagnosed with breast cancer among 8506 EPT users compared with 124 women among 8102 women in the placebo group. These data were extrapolated into rates per 10 000 women per year. Therefore, the rate of breast cancer in the hormone group (EPT) was 38 per 10 000 compared with 30 per 10 000 in the placebo group. The relative risk of breast cancer is calculated to be 1.26 (38/30), indicating that breast cancer risk was 0.26 greater than an equal risk of 1.0. Stated another way, there was a 26% greater chance of developing breast cancer among EPT users than non-users.

However, absolute risk may be more pertinent to guide an individual woman's decision-making. In any single year, 0.08% more HT users developed breast cancer than non-users.

Table 10.3 calculates the absolute risk for 1000 women who use EPT for one year, compared with their usual risk (determined by the risk of the women on placebo). *The absolute risk for an individual who uses HT or ET for one year is extremely small.*

Estrogen may have additional preventive benefits, including prevention of Alzheimer's disease and macular degeneration. Should these benefits be

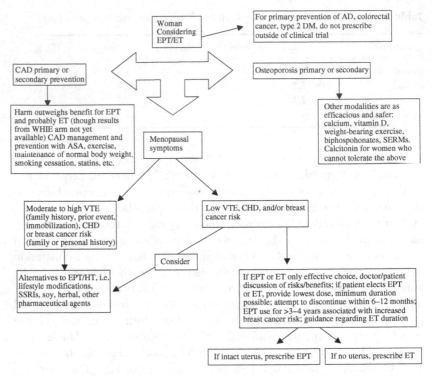

Figure 10.2 Suggested algorithm for evaluating woman for possible HT use.

proven, then the balance of risk compared with benefits for HT may shift again.

Risks of hormone therapy

Any discussion of HT risks must include the baseline risks of women not using HT or ET (Figure 10.2). Table 10.4 outlines the probability that a menopausal woman will develop chronic disease Another useful perspective may be gained by comparing these risks with risks from some common everyday activities (Table 10.5). One out of 100 women who use HT for one year will experience a net additional adverse outcome compared with non-users. Safer preventive strategies for most chronic conditions are available. Table 10.6 lists the additional adverse outcomes of 10 000 women EPT users for each year of use. There were 19 excess events in the women using EPT, or a 1% five-year risk. *Of 200 women who use HT for five years, one woman will not have an osteoporotic fracture or colorectal cancer. Four will develop invasive breast cancer, CHD, stroke, or venous thromboembolism.*[13]

Table 10.4 Estimated lifetime risk for US women of developing certain conditions or dying

Condition	% of women who will develop condition over lifetime	Lifetime probability of dying
CHD	46	1/5
Stroke	20	1/18
Hip fracture	15	
Breast cancer	10	
Endometrial cancer	2.5	
Colorectal cancer	6	
Dementia (75–84 years of age)*	>8	
Osteoporosis after 80 years of age	70	
Motor-vehicle collision		1/81
Air travel		1/5092
Dog bite		1/234 896

* 7–8% of individuals 75–84 years of age have dementia; postmenopausal women have a 1.4–3.0 higher risk of Alzheimer's disease than do men.
Source: National Safety Council, National Center for Health Statistics, US Census, Women's Health Sources, Mayo Clinic.

Table 10.5 Risks of death per 10 000 women each year by condition

Condition	Mortality rate per 10 000 women per year
Smoking	50
Motorcycling	10
Automobile driving	1.7
Continuing a pregnancy	1

Cardiovascular disease

HT is not recommended for either primary or secondary prevention of coronary heart disease. In the WHI study, seven additional women had heart attacks for every 10 000 women who used both estrogen and progesterone for one year.[13]

Stroke

HT appears to increase the risk of stroke. The Nurses' Health Study demonstrated a dose–response relationship, with the risk of stroke increasing in women who used higher hormonal dosages. In the Group Health Cooperative

Table 10.6 Outcome of 10 000 women who use EPT for one year

	Reduction in cases of the following conditions among 10 000 women who use EPT for one year		Increase in cases of the following conditions among 10 000 women who use combined EPT for one year
Hip fractures	5	Heart attacks	7
Colon cancer	6	Strokes	8
		Invasive breast cancer	8
		Pulmonary emboli/deep vein thrombosis	8

Source: Nelson, H. D., Humphrey L. L., LeBlanc, E.; *et al.* Postmenopausal Hormone Replacement Therapy for Primary Prevention of Chronic Conditions. Summary of the Evidence. http://ahrq.gov/clinic/3rduspstf/hrt/hrtsum1.htm. Accessed August 21, 2002.

Study, the risk of stroke was not associated with the current use of estrogen and progestin. *However, the risk of stroke increased two-fold during the first six months of hormone use, and the risk of ischemic stroke increased with the dose of estrogen.*[14] The stroke risk also increased in the WHI study.

Thrombotic events

Risks for thromboembolic events are highest in the first two years of use. A woman using HT has a risk approximately four-fold greater than that of a non-user. After the first year or two, the risk decreases but remains double that of non-users. The risk of thromboemoblism may also display a dose–response effect.[15]

Breast cancer

Breast cancer has been linked increasingly to the use of HT. Previous analyses have suggested a 15% increase in breast cancer for women using estrogen plus progestin for less than five years and a greater than 50% increase in risk for duration of HT for more than five years.[16] The HERS study reported a 27% increase in breast cancer after 6.8 years of use.[17]

Some studies suggest an increased risk when EPT was used compared with estrogen alone. Studies of women who had ever used HT, as opposed to studies of current HT users, did not find an increased rate of breast cancer. All six cohort studies that looked at breast cancer mortality demonstrated no effect or decreased mortality among women who had ever used HT or who had used HT for less than five years. Two studies that reported results for use longer than five years yielded conflicting results. The review concluded that benefits include fewer fractures and lower rates of colon cancer, and suggested fewer cases of dementia, which was classified as an "uncertain benefit." Harms included increased numbers of CHD events, strokes, thromboembolic events, breast cancer, and cholecystitis.[18]

The increased risk of breast cancer associated with HT decreases to that of non-users five years after HT was discontinued.[19] Risk may vary by cancer histology. HT may be associated with less aggressive and less advanced types of breast cancer.[20] In the WHI study, the risk of invasive breast cancer was increased by 26% (38 versus 30 per 10 000 woman per year). No significant difference was observed for in situ breast cancer. Increased breast cancer risk did not appear during the first four years of use.[21]

The risk of breast cancer increases with duration of use. If 100 women begin HT at 50 years of age, then the excess numbers of breast cancers diagnosed are two new cancers after five years of use, six new cancers after 10 years of use, and 12 new cancers after 15 years of use. This risk appears to dissipate five years after HT is discontinued.[22] The evidence on breast cancer mortality in longer-term users is mixed.[23,24] Although the *incidence* of breast cancer appears to be increased with HT, most studies do not demonstrate that breast cancer *mortality* is increased in ever-users or short-time users of HT.[25] One study has even demonstrated a reduced risk of death from breast cancers in HRT users.[26]

Endometrial cancer

Unopposed estrogen, the administration of estrogen alone, in women with a uterus increases the risk of endometrial cancer. Progestin given in addition to estrogen decreases this risk. Some studies suggest that the progestin must be given for more than 10 days a month.[27,28] Typical regimens give progestin in a low dose daily, as a continuous dose, or cyclically for 12–14 days per month. No definitive studies conclude that a progestin-containing intrauterine device can substitute for an oral progestin or whether the progestin dose can be given less frequently. No studies have compared the long-term safety of various progestin options.

The risk of endometrial cancer appears to be increased with duration of use and remains elevated five years following discontinuation. The risk may vary depending on the type of estrogen product used and is greater in women using conjugated versus synthetic estrogen.

In addition, women who use unopposed estrogen, an estrogen preparation without progesterone, are more likely to develop endometrial carcinoma if their uterus has not been removed. A meta-analysis of 29 observational studies demonstrated a relative risk of 2.3 for estrogen users compared with non-users, with 95% confidence interval 2.1–2.5. Increased risk was associated with increasing duration of use. Risk remained elevated five or more years following discontinuation of estrogen therapy. Conjugated estrogens were associated with a greater risk than synthetic estrogens. Endometrial cancer mortality was not elevated.[29]

Ovarian cancer

Studies linking HRT or ERT to ovarian cancer have been inconclusive.[30,31] One study followed 211 581 postmenopausal women from 1982 to 1996. Those with ten or more years of estrogen use had an increased risk of dying from ovarian cancer. The risk decreased after HT was discontinued but persisted at a higher level than in never-users.[32] Other studies seem to relate the risk of ovarian cancer to duration of use.[33]

Cognition and dementia

At the present time, *HT is not recommended as primary or secondary prevention for Alzheimer's disease* (AD).[34] Animal models have suggested biologically plausible mechanisms by which estrogen might be protective against neurodegenerative conditions such as AD.[35] The prevention of AD is particularly important for women since they are at increased risk of developing AD compared with men. Results from case–control studies and two prospective studies have been mixed. One study[36] and a meta-analysis[37] reported as much as a 30% reduced risk of AD in women who report ever using HRT compared with non-users.

Of the studies that suggest a benefit, most demonstrate a decreased risk or delay in onset of AD in postmenopausal women using HT (primary prevention) but no effect of estrogen on the clinical course of AD in women with mild to moderate established disease (secondary prevention).[38] Other studies, such as that of Seshadri and colleagues,[39] demonstrate no benefit in AD prevention with over ten years of HT use. A more recent prospective study[40] reported a decreased incidence of AD in women who used HT for ten or more years. These women did not display the anticipated increased gender risk of AD. Their adjusted risk of AD was half that of non-users. Most of the current users used unopposed estrogen (estrogen without a progestin). Nine RCTs of HT and cognition demonstrated improvement in verbal memory, vigilance, reasoning, and motor speed only among symptomatic women (with menopause-related cognitive symptoms), but not among those who were asymptomatic.[41] WHI and HERS have not reported effects of HT on cognition and dementia.

Several large RCTs on the effects of estrogen therapy on women at risk for AD are under way, including the Women's Health Initiative Memory Study (WHIMS) and the WHI Study of Cognitive Aging. These studies will examine whether ET given to women aged 65 years or older (not from the time of menopause) prevents or delays AD.

Another major study, the Women's International Study of Long Duration Oestrogen after Menopause (WISDOM), which had enrolled more than 5000 of a planned 16 000 women in England, Australia, and New Zealand and was scheduled to continue until 2016, was ended prematurely in October 2002 following the review of WHI results.[42] Raloxifene may enhance memory in women with AD,[43] but additional research is needed.[44]

Diabetes mellitus

Data from the HERS found that women who used EPT (daily treatment of 0.625 mg conjugated estrogen and 2.5 mg medroxyprogesterone acetate) had a 25% lower risk for developing type 2 diabetes mellitus over four years of follow-up in women who were predominately white.[45] This is consistent with the results from earlier studies and has been more consistent with oral as opposed to transdermal estrogens. To date, no RCT design to test this hypothesis has been conducted.

Cholelithiasis

The Nurses' Health Study reported a relative risk of 1.8 for cholecystitis for HT users compared with non-users. The risk increased with duration of use and remained elevated when HT was discontinued. HT is associated with one additional case per 250 users/year of symptomatic cholecystitis.[46]

Other adverse events

HT is far from a panacea for all women.[47] Many women never fill the initial prescription. Those who fill it initially often discontinue use because of side effects, including irregular bleeding, fluid retention, breast tenderness, headache, nausea, and dry eyes. As many as 30–40% of women experience some degree of abnormal bleeding in the first year of use. Weight is not usually affected.

The choice to use hormone/estrogen therapy

At the present time, excess adverse effects appear to outweigh benefits from the use of combination HT to prevent chronic disease.[48] HT is not protective against cardiovascular disease and may increase its risk. The American Heart Association,[49] the American College of Obstetricians and Gynecologists (ACOG),[50] and the North American Menopause Society (NAMS)[51] recommend against the use of HT for primary or secondary prevention of cardiovascular disease. Both ACOG and NAMS recommend caution if HT is used solely to prevent osteoporosis since there are equally efficacious and possibly safer strategies that deserve careful consideration.

For women at high risk of osteoporosis, combined HT should be considered only when other treatments are not tolerated, when the woman is at low cardiovascular, thrombotic, and cancer disease risk, and when the woman is fully informed of the risks and alternatives.

There are insufficient data to recommend for or against the use of ET alone for the prevention of chronic conditions in women with a hysterectomy.[52] Use of ET outside of a clinical trial is discouraged until the full WHI results become available; the initiative concludes in 2005. Clinicians should consider waiting for these results before prescribing ET for this indication for chronic disease prevention.

The principle indication for EPT and ET is the management of menopausal symptoms in women without established CHD, breast (or other hormonal-dependent) cancer, thrombosis, or risk factors for these conditions, especially if the menopausal symptoms have not responded to alternative strategies. NAMS recommends that the primary indication for EPT or ET is the treatment of menopausal symptoms.[53]

ET markedly improves menopause-related symptoms, such as hot flushes, hot disordered sleep, and vaginal dryness. Quality of life improves in the subset of women who use ET for amelioration of hot flushes and disordered sleep.[54]

Women should be counseled regarding alternative therapies for the control of menopausal symptoms. If these are not acceptable, not tolerated, or insufficient to control symptoms, women who are contemplating EPT or ET should be assessed for their individual risk profile and counseled regarding the small but possible increased risk for venous thromboembolism, CHD, and stroke within the first one to two years of therapy. For women without contraindications and who are informed of the risk, HT and ET remain reasonable for the short-term management of postmenopausal symptoms.[55] Women without a uterus should not be prescribed progestin. The only menopause-related indication for progestin is endometrial protection from unoppposed estrogen. For women with a uterus and using estrogen, clinicians should also prescribe progestin.

If, after appropriate counseling of risks and benefits, a woman still wishes EPT/ET, many experts, such as the NAMS panel, recommend the lowest dose of hormone sufficient to control symptoms for the briefest duration possible.[56]

HT is not an effective treatment for major depression in menopausal women. Clinical trials do not support the benefit of estrogen on urinary incontinence, although anecdotally some women report benefit. Although there are no data to support this recommendation, some experts suggest that women use a different estrogen/progestin formulation, a lower dosage, or another route of administration from that used in the WHI trial. However, no studies confirm that there is less risk with this approach. Table 10.7 presents the

Table 10.7 USPSTF recommendations regarding EPT and ET

Indication	EPT	ET (for women with hysterectomy)
Prevention of chronic conditions	"D" recommendation; harmful effects of HRT are likely to exceed benefit	"I" recommendation; insufficient evidence to recommend for or against the use of unopposed estrogen therapy
Menopausal symptoms, such as vasomotor symptoms (hot flushes) and urogenital symptoms	Did not evaluate	Did not evaluate

Source: US Preventive Services Task Force. Recommendations and rationale: hormone replacement therapy for primary prevention of chronic conditions. www.ahcpr.gov/clinic/3rduspstf/hrt/hrtrr.htm

recommendations regarding EPT and ET from the USPSTF. Table 10.8 summarizes the 2002 recommendations of the USPSTF regarding the use of EPT/ET and may guide clinicians in counseling women appropriately.

NAMS also believes that there is no useful distinction between long- and short-term therapy and recommends these terms be abandoned. Although some risks of HT appear related to duration of use, others seem to occur within the first year of initiating therapy. There is no clear point at which risks might outweigh benefits for one additional woman. The issue of relevance is to reassess the benefit–risk profile periodically and indications for ongoing treatment at a minimum of each visit.

How to help women make rational and individual choices

Several of the component studies of the WHI are continuing. Important additional information from these studies is expected in 2005. These studies address other forms of HT, including other estrogens, progestins, and selective estrogen receptor modulators (SERMs), hormonal effects on memory, and whether there is any prevention or delay in AD. Other studies currently in progress are examining the effects of:
• soy on CHD and osteoporosis;
• black cohosh and antidepressants on hot flushes;
• botanicals on women's health;
• plant estrogens on breast cancer;
• estrogen on cognition.
Additional information will be forthcoming.

Table 10.8 USPSTF 2002 recommendations regarding HT (EPT + ET)

EPT or ET	Good evidence of benefit	Fair to good evidence of benefit	Fair evidence of benefit	Good evidence of harm	Fair to good evidence of harm	Fair evidence of harm	Insufficient evidence of benefits or harms
EPT	↑ Bone mineral density	↓ Fracture	↓ Colorectal cancer	↑ Venous thromboembolism	↑ Breast cancer ↑ CHD	↑ Stroke ↑ Cholecystitis	Dementia Cognitive function Ovarian cancer Breast cancer mortality CHD mortality All-cause mortality
ET (unopposed)							Unable to determine whether benefits outweigh harms for women with hysterectomy

Source: US Preventive Services Task Force. Recommendations and rationale: hormone replacement therapy for primary prevention of chronic conditions. www.ahcpr.gov/clinic/3rduspstf/hrt/hrtrr.htm

In the mean time, it is important to clarify the goal(s) for the woman who is interested in HT/ET. *If she wishes to treat menopausal symptoms, then non-hormonal strategies and alternatives should be reviewed carefully.* These include behavioral therapies, herbal preparations, and other non-hormonal pharmacologic agents. She should realize, however, that there are no data to demonstrate long-term efficacy and safety for the various herbal, non-pharmacologic agents, and non-hormonal pharmacologic choices, since none of these has been subject to the rigors of an RCT such as the WHI.

Chronic disease prevention

For women interested in chronic disease prevention, safer, equally efficacious options exist. Women who desire treatment or prevention strategies for osteoporosis may benefit from calcium and vitamin D supplementation, weight-bearing exercise, strength training, SERMs, biphosphonates, and calcitonin, alone or in combination. A new product, Forteo™, was approved by the US FDA in 2002 (see Chapter 14). Women may obtain maximal protection from HT after three years of use, equal to that obtained by women using HT for more than three years. Limiting use to three years may maximize benefit and minimize adverse effects.[57] Women with increased osteoporosis risk and unable to tolerate other options may be candidates for extended use of HT.

Women who would benefit from secondary prevention for CHD can utilize weight reduction (if obese), exercise, smoking cessation (if smokers), optimal control of lipids and blood glucose, and use of beta-blockers, angiotensin-converting enzyme (ACE) inhibitors, 3-hydroxy-3-methylglutaryl coenzyme A (HMG CoA) reductase inhibitors, aspirin, and other antiplatelet agents. Folic acid may be useful if homocysteine levels are elevated.

Discontinuing hormone therapy

There are no evidence-based recommendations to guide discontinuation of HT. Women who did not have menopausal symptoms prior to starting HT appear to have few if any symptoms when it is discontinued. Similarly, there are no data on whether or how to taper use, although many clinicians will reduce a dose and maintain the woman at that dose for one to two months before decreasing again. Alternatively, some clinicians change to a different formulation of estrogen (i.e. from oral to transdermal) as part of the process.

Medications such as Prempro™ (estrogen/medroxyprogesterone acetate) can be discontinued abruptly or tapered slowly. Some clinicians taper the drug, decreasing the dose of drug by one-half each month over two to three weeks to three to six months, before discontinuing entirely. Alternatively, a form of estrogen may be prescribed to manage a predominant local symptom, such as the estrogen vaginal ring, while the systemic estrogen is being tapered and/or discontinued.

ACOG recommends that women should be counseled regarding alternatives that might reduce their risks when they discontinue HT. Women at risk for CHD should be informed regarding lifestyle modifications and the risks and benefits of statin drugs and aspirin. Women at risk for osteoporosis should explore alternative therapies, such as calcium, weight-bearing exercise, and biphosphonates.

Once HT is stopped, clinicians may want to monitor women for signs of reversal of its beneficial effects. For instance, a woman who has been on HT may have had beneficial effects on her bone mineral density regardless of whether its intent was to prevent osteoporosis. She may benefit from osteoporosis screening a year or two following cessation to determine whether osteoporosis is developing, even if prior bone mineral density (on estrogen) was within acceptable limits. This is particularly true because rapid bone loss may occur in the first year following discontinuation of estrogen, and, if identified, alternative management strategies can be instituted.[58]

Types of estrogen/progestin therapy and estrogen-alone therapy

There is a variety of available products and routes of administration for both estrogen and progestin. Most of the studies have been done on only some of these products. The WHI study, for instance, used conjugated estrogen and medroxyprogesterone (MPA). There are many different chemical kinds of estrogen and progestin as well as a variety of possible routes for administration (Table 10.9). It is not known whether different estrogen and progestin preparations carry the same risk as conjugated estrogen and MPA.

Women with a uterus are prescribed combined HT. Unopposed estrogen therapy or estrogen alone without a progestin (ET) should be used only by women who have had a hysterectomy.[59]

EPT is usually prescribed *cyclically/sequentially*, with estrogen given for 25 or 30 days per month and progestin added for 10–14 days, or *continuous combined*, with both estrogen and progestin administered daily. Progestin's role is to prevent hyperplasia of the uterine lining, which is associated with the development of uterine cancer.

All forms of estrogen are equivalent in treating menopausal symptoms such as hot flushes and vaginal dryness. Oral estrogens generally improve lipid panels favorably, particularly by increasing the high-density lipoprotein (HDL) cholesterol. In some women, however, oral estrogens may raise serum triglyceride levels.

Table 10.9 Comparisons of EPT/ET preparations

Type	Example product	Route
Estrogen only		
Conjugated equine estrogen	Premarin™	O, vaginal cream, IV
Synthetic conjugated estrogen 0.3 mg, 0.625 mg, 0.9 mg, 1.25 mg	Cenestin™	O
Esterified estrogens	Estratab™ (discontinued in USA), Menest™	O
Estropipate (piperazine estrone)	Ortho-Est™, Ogen™, generic	O
Micronized 17-beta estradiol	Estrace™, generic	O, vaginal cream
	Estring™	Vaginal ring
	Alora™, Climara™, Esclim™, Estraderm™, Vivelle™, Vivelle-Dot™, FemPatch™, generic	Transdermal (strengths range from 0.025 mg/day to 0.1 mg/day); patch sizes vary significantly, from 3.75 cm² (Vivelle Dot™ 0.0375 mg/day) to 36 cm² (Alora™ 0.1 mg/day)
Ethinyl estradiol	Estinyl™	
Dienestrol	Ortho Deinestrol™	Vaginal cream
Estradiol hemihydrate	Vagifem™	Vaginal tablet 25 µg one tablet per vagina qd × two weeks then twice weekly
Progestin		
Medroxyprogesterone acetate	Amen™, Cycrin™, Provera™	O
	Depo provera™ (not for uterine protection)	IM
Norethindrone	Micronor™, Nor-QD™	O
Norethindrone acetate	Aygestin™	O
Norgestrel	Ovrette™	O
Levonorgestrel	Mirena™	IUD
	Norplant™	Implants
Progesterone USP in peanut oil (micronized)	Prometrium™	O
Megestrol acetate	Megace™ (not for uterine protection)	O
Progesterone	Crinone™	Vaginal gel
	Progestasert™	IUD

Table 10.9 (*cont.*)

Type	Example product	Route
Combination products		
E + P		
CEE + MPA	Premphase™	O, continuous cyclic
	Prempro™	O, continuous combined
Ethinyl estradiol + norethindrone acetate	Femhrt™	O
17-beta estradiol and norethindrone acetate	Activella™	O
17-beta estradiol + norgestimate oral: 6-day cycle of estradiol × 3 days followed by combined estradiol/norgestimate × 3 days	Ortho-Prefest™	O, intermittent combined
17-beta estradiol + norethindrone acetate	Combipatch™	Transdermal (0.05 mg estrogen; 0.14 mg or 0.25 mg norethindrone) 9–16 cm^2
Estrogen–testosterone		
Estradiol cypionate + testosterone	Depo-Testadiol™	IM
Esterified estrogens/ methyltestosterone	Estratest™ Estratest HS™	O

O, oral.

Transdermal estrogen benefits HDL less than oral estrogens do, but generally it does not affect serum triglyceride levels adversely. Transdermal products have comparable benefits with oral preparations on bone density. *Transdermal preparations generally do not affect blood clotting factors or have adverse effects on the liver or gallbladder.* Patches may be slightly more expensive than pills, although a generic formulation of transdermal estradiol is available. The size of the transdermal preparations varies markedly, from 3.75 cm^2 to 30 cm^2, which may be a factor in their acceptability. Patches may cause skin irritation, but this may be managed by changing to a different patch (with a different adhesive) or a brand with a smaller patch.

Vaginal estrogens, which generally result in lower levels of circulating hormone, do not protect against bone loss, improve lipids, or impact hot flushes. At first, they are usually used nightly for one to two weeks, after which time the frequency of application is decreased to two to three times per week.[60]

Vaginal estrogens are available as creams, tablets, and an estrogen-releasing "ring." The ring, effective for up to 90 days, has been shown to be beneficial in decreasing symptoms of atrophic vaginitis and in decreasing recurrent urinary tract infections.[61]

When to start hormone therapy

In January 2003, the US FDA approved updated language for physician prescribing information and patient information leaflets for Prempro™, Premphase™, and Premarin™, building upon the revisions made by the product manufacturer in August 2002.[62] The FDA also requested all other manufacturers of estrogen and estrogen with progestin drug products for use in postmenopausal women to make similar changes to the labeling for their products.

The new warnings are posted within a box, indicating the highest level of warning. They highlight the increased risks for heart disease, heart attacks, strokes, and breast cancer, and emphasize that HT is not approved for heart disease prevention. Premarin™, Prempro™, and Premphase™ include use only when benefits clearly outweigh risks. Two of the three previously approved indications have been revised to emphasize that other therapies should be considered. Approved indications include:

- treatment of moderate to severe vasomotor symptoms (such as hot flushes) associated with the menopause (this indication has not changed);
- treatment of moderate to severe symptoms of vulvar and vaginal atrophy (dryness and irritation) associated with the menopause (the label now recommends topical vaginal products be considered when these products are being prescribed solely for the treatment of symptoms of vulvar and vaginal atrophy);
- prevention of postmenopausal osteoporosis (weak bones). The label recommends that approved non-estrogen treatments should be "carefully considered" when these products are being prescribed solely for the prevention of postmenopausal osteoporosis, and that estrogens and combined estrogen–progestin products be considered only for women with significant risk of osteoporosis that outweighs the risks of the drug.

The FDA's new labeling advises healthcare providers to prescribe estrogen and combined estrogen with progestin drug products at the lowest dose and for the shortest duration for the individual woman. Women who choose to take estrogens or combined estrogen and progestin therapies after discussion with their doctor should:

Table 10.10 Contraindications to HT

Hormone-dependent/associated neoplasia
Liver impairment
Abnormal thrombophilia screen
Venous thromboembolism
Known coronary artery disease

- have yearly breast examinations by a healthcare provider;
- perform monthly breast self-examinations;
- receive periodic mammography examinations scheduled based on their age and risk factors.

   In addition, women should consider other ways to reduce their risk factors for heart disease. Table 10.10 lists the contraindications to EPT/ET.

Pretreatment assessment

Hormone profiles are not required before the prescription of EPT/ET. A lipid panel should be considered, especially as triglycerides may sometimes increase with estrogen treatment. Blood pressure does not generally affect the decision regarding EPT/ET; however, if blood pressure is elevated, then it is an excellent time to optimize control. *Endometrial investigation need not be performed routinely before instituting EPT/ET, but it must be undertaken if there is abnormal bleeding.*

Alternatives to hormone therapy, including complementary treatments

Table 10.11 lists some of the alternatives to HT. Table 10.12 lists some ineffective and/or harmful therapies.

Hot flushes

Although over 85% of women experience hot flushes, most women find that their symptoms resolve or improve over two to five years. More than 30% of women use complementary and alternative measures, such as acupuncture, natural estrogen, herbal supplements, and plant estrogens to control symptoms. Most studies of menopausal interventions demonstrate a 20–30% improvement in the symptoms of the placebo groups regardless of whatever method is chosen for the intervention.[63] This high rate of resolution of symptoms makes it imperative that methods that purport benefit be subjected to careful scrutiny.

Chronic disease	Prevention/management	Potential adverse effect
Osteoporosis	• Weight-bearing exercise (walking, jogging, playing tennis, dancing) • Avoid smoking • Calcium and vitamin D (see table) • Strength training • SERMS, such as raloxifene	VTE, MI, stroke, hot flushes, endometrial cancer risk with tamoxifen
	• Biphosphonates (alendronate or risedronate) • Calcitonin (nasal or injection) • Phytoestrogens (have not been shown to decrease fracture, have been shown to increase BMD)	Esophageal/gastrointestinal irritation
	• Tibolone (available in Europe)	Reports of osteosarcoma in animal studies but not in human trials
	• Teriparatide (by injection) • Limit alcohol consumption • Fall prevention	No direct benefit on osteoporosis, but may decrease morbidity from a fall
CHD prevention	• Prevent and control high blood pressure • Prevent and control high blood cholesterol, including use of statins • Manage diabetes (if present) • Aspirin • Lifestyle choices (healthy diet, limiting alcohol, not smoking, maintaining healthy weight) • Physical activity • Pharmacologic options (as indicated), e.g. ACE inhibitors, beta-blockers) • Soy (the FDA believes 25 mg soy protein daily in conjunction with low-fat, low-cholesterol diet may reduce CHD risk)	

Table 10.11 (*cont.*)

Chronic disease	Prevention/management	Potential adverse effect
Cancer prevention	• Avoid or discontinue tobacco	
	• Low-fat diet may help decrease risk of colon cancer and breast cancer	
	• Limit alcohol to no more than one or two glasses a day (one glass = 4 oz wine, 12 oz beer, or 1.5 oz 80-proof spirits)	
	• Avoid unnecessary radiation exposure, such as sun exposure without sunscreen	
	• Maintain healthy weight/body mass index (BMI)	
	• Increase physical activity	
	• Eat more vegetables, fruits, and fiber	
	• Decrease intake of red meat	
	• Cancer screening (breast, colorectal cancer, cervical cancer)	
Menopausal symptom relief		
Hot flushes	• Tibolone: comparable benefit to HRT	
	• Aerobic exercise	
	• Dress in layers	
	• Sleep in a cool room; use fan; avoid warm baths near times when flushes occur; use cotton nightclothes and sheets; keep ice water at bedside; if sharing electronic blanket, use one with dual controls	
	• Avoid any food which trigger events; common culprits include spicy foods, alcohol, caffeine, and warm beverages	
	• Deep breathing and stress reduction, including meditation, t'ai chi, yoga	
	• Phytoestroegens (risks of soy are unknown, as is efficacy of pills and powders versus soy food products, such as tofu, tempeh, soy milk, soy nuts, chickpeas, lentils); one to four servings of soy-based foods per day for total of 40–60 mg soy isoflavones daily (60–90 mg possibly required for heart benefit)	
	• Red clover	

Chronic disease	Prevention/management	Potential adverse effect
	• Black cohosh; long-term studies are lacking; perhaps moderately effective, although data are inconsistent; appears to be a non-estrogenic effect, with higher doses (beyond 40 mg/day) not demonstrating additional improvement	Decrease in HDL; long-term effects unknown; in Germany combined with black cohosh; no long-term studies; use not recommended beyond six months; side effects include nausea, vomiting, dizziness, visual change, slow heartbeat
	• Chaste tree berry – mixed results	
	• Valerian root 200 mg tid + red clover	Not available in USA
	• Clonidine (clinically modest effect)	
	• Amlodipine	
	• Venlafaxine 37.5–150 mg per day (decreased hot flushes in 37–61%; higher doses worked better but also associated with greater likelihood of adverse effects)	
	• Paroxetine	
	• Sertraline 50–100 mg/day	
	• Fluoxetine 20 mg/day	
	• Megestrol acetate 20 mg bid decreased hot flushes from 5% to 21% compared with placebo	
	• Vitamin E 800 mg/day	
	• Slow, deep abdominal breathing	
	• Progestin: relatively high doses have been used when used alone without estrogen (i.e. 20 mg medroxyprogesterone qd); transdermal progesterone has been used	Constipation, dry mouth, drowsiness (xerostomia, nausea, constipation, appetite change) with higher doses); possibly helpful with disordered sleep

Table 10.11 (*cont.*)

Chronic disease	Prevention/management	Potential adverse effect
	• Testosterone: when given in combination with estrogen, a reduced dose of estrogen maintained beneficial effects	Withdrawal bleeding and appetite stimulation; adverse effects include voice change, hair growth, acne; no long-term data for safety or efficacy; foods have more evidence than supplements
	• Estradiol: the weakest of the body's own estrogens; anecdotally perhaps less breast and endometrial stimulation	
	• Gabapentin: limited studies to date	
	• Soy	
Disturbed sleep	• Physical activity (avoid later in the day)	
	• Hot shower or bath immediately before going to bed	
	• Milk products	
Vaginal dryness	• Vaginal lubricants and moisturizers: Astroglide: water-based lubricant for intercourse Replens: non-hormonal moisturizer increases the thickness of vaginal lining ProSensual: soy-based product	
	• Local estrogen	
Mood swings	• Lifestyle behaviors, including adequate sleep and physical activity	
	• Relaxation exercises/stress management techniques	
	• Antidepressant or anti-anxiety drugs if indicated	
Memory difficulties	• Mental exercises	
	• Physical activity	
	• Lifestyle behaviors (rest, avoid alcohol, relaxation)	
Libido	DHEA (one small study suggests benefit), testosterone	Multiple adverse effects
Urinary tract infections, incontinence	Topical estrogen may confer some benefit with UTIs	

Adapted from National Institutes of Health. Facts about postmenopausal hormone therapy. www.nhlbi.nih.gov/health/women/pht_facts.htm and Duke Heart Center, Management of HRT in the wake of HERS II and WHI dukemedmag.duke.edu/article.php?id.2115

Table 10.12 Ineffective therapies for menopausal symptoms

Chaste berry	
Dong quai	Adverse effects include gastrointestinal effects and photosensitization); contains coumarins and may cause bleeding if administered concurrently with warfarin
Ginseng	One study showed enhanced mood; one case of postmenopausal bleeding one case of reduction in INR in patient using warfarin
Evening primrose oil	
Wild yam cream	Contains diosgenin, which can be converted to progesterone in the laboratory but not in the human body
Vitamin E	Minimal to no benefit
Acupuncture	
Red clover	
Kava kava	May be hepatotoxic

Data from Kronenberg, F. and Gugh-Berman, A. Complementary and alternative medicine for menopausal symptoms: a review of randomized controlled trials. *Ann. Intern. Med.* 2002; **137**:805–13; Hirata, J. D., Swiersz, L. M., Zell, B., *et al.* Does dong quai have estrogenic effects in postmenopausal women? A double blinded placebo controlled trial. *Fertil. Steril.* 1999; **68**:981–6; Chenoy, R., Hussain, S., Tayob, Y., *et al.* Effects of oral gamolenic acid from evening primrose oil on menopausal flushing. *Br. Med. J.* 1994; **308**:501–3; Barton, D. L., Loprinzi, C. L., Quella, S. K., *et al.* Prospective evaluation of vitamin E for hot flushes in breast cancer survivors. *J. Clin. Oncol.* 1998; **16**:2377–81.

Behavioral therapies

Behavioral therapies have primarily anecdotal evidence to support their use. Strategies include dressing in layers, exercise, deep breathing, and stress-reduction techniques such as meditation. Many experts recommend that spicy foods and caffeine should be avoided.

Hormones

Estrogens certainly improve hot flushes.[64] Doses as low as 20 mg transdermal estrogen have been demonstrated to reduce the severity of symptoms. HT should be used only if menopausal symptoms are troublesome, alternatives are not acceptable or effective, and the woman is informed fully of the risks.

If a woman has no personal history of an estrogen-dependent cancer, coronary artery disease, clotting disorder (such as factor V Leiden or protein C or S deficiency), or thromboembolic event (such as deep vein thrombophlebitis or pulmonary embolus), then her risk from a few years of HT use is small. Nonetheless, she should be counseled regarding the risks of HT, including the increased risk of VTE, stroke, and MI, which may occur in the first year or two of use. The lowest dose of hormone for the shortest duration should be prescribed. Short-term use of HT/ET may be a reasonable option, since hot flushes, for instance, tend to decrease in most women after three to five years.

Progestin alone also improves hot flushes.[65] Testosterone may improve symptoms as well but is not approved for use in women except in combination with estrogen.

Tibolone

Tibolone is a steroid compound with estrogenic, progestogenic, and androgenic properties.[66] It is effective for reducing the frequency and severity of hot flushes and improving vaginal dryness and libido. Tibolone has been shown to increase bone mineral density, with little effect on the breast or endometrium. It should not be used in women with a history of coronary artery disease, stroke, or liver disorders. Caution is also advisable in women with kidney disease, epilepsy, migraine, diabetes, and high cholesterol. Tibolone may interact with some drugs, including anticoagulants. Its androgenic properties may cause oily skin and extra hair growth. Breast symptoms are rare. It is not available in the USA.

Phytoestrogens

Studies of phytoestrogens, naturally occurring substances found in most plants, have yielded conflicting results. Phytoestrogens are classified as *phenolic* estrogens, contrasted with *steroidal* estrogens, such as estradiol, which are manufactured by human ovaries. They are weaker than steroidal estrogens, with a potency of 1/20 000 to 1/50 that of estradiol. They mimic many estrogen effects in the body.

Isoflavones are the most estrogenically potent of the five most common types of phytoestrogens found in the human diet. They are contained primarily in legumes (chickpeas (garbanzo beans), soy, clover, lentils, and beans.) There are over 1000 isoflavones, but the most strongly estrogenic are formononetin, daidzein, biochanin, and genistein. Each acts somewhat differently. Biochanin is the most effective in blocking the effects of estradiol. If levels of steroidal estrogen are high, then isoflavones display anti-estrogenic activity, binding to estrogen receptors in place of more potent steroidal estrogens. If steroidal estrogen levels are low, then isoflavones appear to augment their estrogen effect.

Lignins are part of the cell walls of plants. They are found in the husks of seeds, especially flax seed. Coumestans have steroid-like activity. They are found in high concentrations in red clover, sunflower seeds, and bean sprouts. They have demonstrated estrogenic effects when ingested by animals.

Populations that consume high levels of dietary isoflavones report fewer hot flushes. Asian diets, for example, contain 40–80 mg active forms of isoflavones daily. However, other differences in Asian women, such as cultural factors, body mass index, and exercise patterns, may be responsible for this.

Soy is a major source of isoflavones. Most studies of the benefits of soy involve soy foods. It is not known whether dietary supplements work as well as isoflavone-containing food products. Most available dietary supplements have levels of isoflavones below the level stated on the bottle. Whether the isoflavone is present as the glycoside (sugar-bound) form or aglycone (free) form adds another source of variance. Manufacturing processes may remove the biologically active isoflavones. Two proprietary products, Rimostil™ and Promensil™, contain four isoflavones in varying proportions. Whole soy foods such as tofu, soy milk, and edamame, may be preferable to more highly processed soy, such as textured vegetable protein, for cardiovascular benefits such as lowering blood cholesterol.

Ingestion does not seem to affect the use of isoflavones for menopausal symptoms. No standard dosages have been established, but one to four servings of soy foods per day for a total of 40–50 mg soy isoflavones per day may be necessary. Several studies support the benefits of soy for menopausal symptoms.[67,68]

Women may consider substituting soy milk for use on cereals, adding cubes of tofu to soups, stews, and pasta, using tofu in casserole recipes, substituting textured vegetable protein for meat in chili, meat sauces, and meat loaf, and substituting soy flour for at least some of the wheat flour when making muffins and bread. Fermented products such as miso and tempeh are easy to digest, and the fermentation process may inactivate some of the chemicals that may impair absorption of other nutrients. Anecdotal evidence suggests that adding soy may allow a reduced dose of estrogen to control disabling menopausal symptoms.

Because soy foods can cause gas and intestinal discomfort, they should be added to the diet slowly. Soy contains chemicals that may interfere with absorption of essential nutrients such as zinc and calcium. These may be deactivated by the fermenting process. The long-term safety of soy is unknown, and it has not been tested in randomized controlled trials.[69]

Pharmaceutical-quality ipriflavone is used in Europe and Japan for the treatment of osteoporosis, but it is not available in the USA. A great deal of the available evidence on the benefits of soy is derived from observational studies, subject to the same potential bias as the early estrogen studies.

Herbal preparations: black cohosh

The German Commission E Monographs report that black cohosh has estrogen-like actions, suppresses LH, binds to estrogen receptors, and lacks contraindications to its use. Side effects include gastric discomfort, sweating, weight gain, and headache. A six-month trial funded by the manufacturer of one black cohosh product reported that women benefited from a 70% reduction in symptoms such as hot flushes, mood swings, night sweats, and insomnia. Higher doses did not improve symptoms.[70]

Overdose can result in bradycardia, nausea, vomiting, and CNS disturbance. Studies of black cohosh generally have not been blinded, enrolled more than a small number of patients, or examined duration of use beyond six months. Black cohosh is not to be confused with blue cohosh, which has nicotine properties and is potentially toxic, or with white cohosh. The American College of Obstetricians and Gynecologists (ACOG) indicates that black cohosh may be helpful for women with vasomotor symptoms but recommends that its use be limited to less than six months' duration, since little is known of its potential for adverse effects.[71]

Typical doses are 300–2000 mg orally three times daily of the dried root or 20–80 mg orally twice daily of the standardized tablet. Many experts would consider breast, ovarian, and endometrial cancer, and uterine fibroids as contraindications to its use. Potential drug interactions include red clover (enhanced estrogenic effect) and willow bark/salicylates (may potentiate salicylate effects, as the product may contain salicylates.)[72]

The National Center for Complementary and Alternative Medicine at the National Institutes of Health (NIH) is currently funding a scientific study to assess the utility of black cohosh. Remifemin® is one of the commercial preparations; it contains 20 mg root equivalent of block cohosh extract.

Other herbs and botanicals

Studies have not demonstrated efficacy for evening primrose oil, ginseng, red clover (alone), chasteberry, or dong quai compared with placebo.[73,74] Dong quai may act as a photosensitizing agent. It may contain warfarin-like compounds, resulting in a potential for many drug and herbal interactions.

St John's wort may be useful in women with mild to moderate mood disorder, but not for menopausal symptoms themselves. It is potentially photosensitizing and can interact with selective serotonin reuptake inhibitors and monamine oxidase inhibitors.

There are no good studies to support the use of valerian. Potential adverse reactions include hepatotoxicity, insomnia, sedation, and cardiac disturbance. In one case report, valerian root was associated with the onset of high-output congestive heart failure from "withdrawal."

Sellers and manufacturers of yams and yam extract have claimed that one component, diosgenin, is a precursor to progestin and DHEA. However, in humans there is no known pathway for bioconversion to these compounds; nor is there any known intrinsic biological activity. Mexican yam extract is estrogenic but would require large quantities to produce a therapeutic effect. Efficacy and safety at these higher doses is unknown. Ginseng commercial products, when tested, have frequently contained little or no ginseng and often contained caffeine, pesticide residues, and lead.

Patients should be counseled that "natural" is not equivalent to either "safe" or "effective." The adverse effects and toxicities of most of these substances, especially if used for long durations or in combination, is unknown.

Interactions with other foods substances or medications are unknown. The correct dose and even the active ingredient are frequently unknown. There is little to no standardization or quality control guaranteeing that the same dose of active ingredient is available within each pill sold. Contaminants are not uncommon. Even substances that may be efficacious when ingested as food may not be efficacious when taken in pill form.

Vaginal dryness

Approximately 40–80% of postmenopausal women have symptoms of atrophic vaginitis. These symptoms include decreased vaginal lubrication, dryness, itching, burning, dyspareunia, and urinary symptoms. Concurrent infection with *Candida trichomonas* or bacterial vaginosis exacerbates symptoms. The use of certain medications, including tricyclic antidepressants, anticholinergic agents, antipsychotics, antihistamines, cigarettes, and chemical sensitizers (such as douches and vaginal hygiene products), may contribute to the symptom of dryness.

Estrogen, regardless of the route of administration, normalizes pH and thickens and revascularizes the epithelium. Vaginal estrogen delivery systems such as creams or the vaginal ring, are effective for the control of vaginal dryness. Creams are usually used daily for three to four weeks followed by once or twice weekly. Some women require higher doses of systemic estrogen or combination systemic and vaginal estrogen for symptom amelioration. Treatment may need to be continued for 24 months. 17-Beta-estradiol tablets may be beneficial and may cause less estrogenic stimulation of the endometrium than vaginal creams.[75]

The estrogen ring allows delivery of a constant hormone concentration, infrequent application, and the avoidance of progesterone. Non-hormonal vaginal products, such as Replens™, Vagisilk™, KY Silky™, Astraglide™, and K-Y™ jelly may offer some relief from vaginal dryness.[76,77] Ginseng-containing lubricants may have estrogenic properties.

Libido

Estrogen does not increase libido, although it can increase vaginal lubrication and lead to less dyspareunia. In a few studies, testosterone has been shown to enhance libido, but it has significant adverse effects in many women.

Osteoporosis

The US Preventive Services Task Force (USPSTF) recommends that women aged 65 years and over be screened routinely for osteoporosis (B recommendation). They make no recommendation for or against routine osteoporosis screening in postmenopausal women younger than 60 or in women aged 60–64 years but not at increased risk for osteoporotic fractures

(C recommendations).[78,79] Bone mineral density measured at the femoral neck by dual-energy X-ray absorptiometry (DEXA) is the best predictor of hip fracture. A minimum of two years may be necessary to ascertain any real change or to monitor treatment.[80]

Both observational studies and RCTs demonstrate HRT has positive effects on bone density, regardless of whether the woman already has osteoporosis. The effect on fracture incidence varies: there was no reduction in hip, wrist, vertebral, or total fractures with HRT in the HERS study, but the WHI reported reductions for hip and vertebral fractures, although these were not statistically significant. The best evidence suggests that *HRT decreases the risk of vertebral fractures in the first decade after surgical menopause, the risk of non-vertebral fractures in early postmenopausal women, and the risk of vertebral fractures in women with established osteoporosis*. However, HT may confer its maximum protective effect on bones if used for only three years. A subgroup of women in the Postmenopausal Estrogen/Progestin Interventions (PEPI) trial who used HRT for three years and then discontinued it did not experience a dramatic drop in bone mineral density. Women using HT beyond three years may not acrue additional benefit.[81]

Testosterone

There are no data to suggest that women benefit from routine supplementation with testosterone.[82] A few early studies suggested that testosterone improved women's sexual function but also caused significant adverse effects, such as acne, excess facial and body hair, and abnormal lipid levels. Testosterone may improve hot flushes in women whose symptoms are resistant to estrogen or estrogen/progestin. A combination of estrogen and methyl testosterone is available for the treatment of resistant hot flushes, but it has not been approved for the treatment of sexual dysfunction.

Topical testosterone is available as a gel and two skin patches, but the doses are too high for women and currently are approved by the FDA only for use in men. Natural testosterone, not regulated by the FDA, is available from some compounding pharmacies. The correct dose is not known, and adverse effects are common. DHEA is available over the counter, but there is little evidence that it increases the body's production of testosterone. Women who use DHEA or testosterone should be monitored closely for changes in lipids or liver function and for adverse side effects.

The future

Women will continue to live an increasing proportion of their lives post-menopause, and greater numbers of women will be in this stage of life. Addressing symptomatic issues and preventing chronic disease will remain priorities for women, their healthcare providers, and public health organizations. Although the WHI trial has added a piece to the puzzle, further questions remain to be addressed.[83] The WHI is analyzing genetic and biochemical material to see whether certain subsets of women are risk. Women in the discontinued arm of the study will be followed for an additional three years or longer to determine whether their increased risk decreases following discontinuation of HT.

Additional health benefits from estrogen (e.g. effects on AD, macular degeneration, decreased risk of diabetes) remain to be established. Effective means to minimize or eliminate risk may be instigated, including, perhaps, effectively identifying women at greater risk from HT (screening for factor V Leiden or other thrombophilia markers may allow low-risk women to be offered this treatment safely). Certain routes of administration may prove safer than oral therapy, such as transdermal, vaginal, and intrauterine dosing. Some formulations of estrogen and/or progestin may have fewer adverse effects. If estrogen alone is discovered to have a reasonable cost/risk ratio, then different strategies for managing the progestin (reduced frequency, different formulation) will be identified. Safety and efficacy for commonly used herbs and botanicals will hopefully be established. Finally, alternative therapeutic agents of proven benefit and safety may become available.

FURTHER RESOURCES

National Heart, Lung, and Blood Institute, National Institutes of Health: www.nhlbi.nih.gov/health/women/pht_facts.htm

Women's Health Initiative (WHI) of the National Heart, Lung, and Blood Institute, National Institutes of Health: www.whi.org

WHI site at which publications regarding HT are linked (often full text references): http://www.whi.org/etc/pubs.asp

The Office on Women's Health, US Department of Health and Human Services: www.4women.gov/owh

North American Menopause Society: www.menopause.org

Postmenopausal women at increased risk for breast cancer can compare safety and efficacy of chemoprophylaxis (tamoxifen and raloxifene) in reducing the risk of the disease. Risk assessment tool at: www.cancer.gov/bcrisktool

Duke University site for women: www.thewomenshealthsite.org

National Osteoporosis Foundation: www.nof.org

REFERENCES

1 Maternal and Child Health Bureau. Women's Health USA 2002. www.mchb.hrsa.gov/data/women.htm. Accessed February 4, 2003.

2 Porter, M., Penney, G., Russell, D., Russell, E. and Templeton, A. A population based survey of women's experience in the menopause. Br. J. Obstet. Gynaecol. 1996; 103:1025–8.

3 Brett, K. M. and Madans, J. H. Use of postmenopausal hormone replacement therapy: estimates from a nationally representative cohort study. *Am. J. Epidemiol.* 1997; **145**:536–45.

4 Kreling, D., Mott, D., Widerholt, J., Lundy, J. and Levitt, L. *Prescription Drug Trends: A Chartbook Update.* Menlo Park, CA: Kaiser Family Foundation; 2001.

5 Utian, W. and Boggs, P. The North American Menopause Society 1998 menopause survey, part I: postmenopausal women's perceptions about menopause and midlife. *Menopause* 1998; **6**:122–8.

6 US Preventive Services Task Force. Recommendations and rationale: hormone replacement therapy for primary prevention of chronic conditions. www.ahcpr.gov/clinic/3rduspstf/hrt/hrtrr.htm. Accessed September 3, 2003.

7 McNagny, S. E. and Jacobson, T. A. Use of postmenopausal hormone replacement therapy by African American women. The importance of physician discussion. *Arch. Intern. Med.* 1997; **157**:1337–42.

8 Grodstein, F., Manson, J. E., Colditz, G. A., *et al.* A prospective observational study of postmenopausal hormone therapy and primary prevention of cardiovascular diseases. *Am. Intern. Med.* 2000; **133**:933–41.

9 Nelson, H. D., Humphrey, L. L., Nygren, P., Teutsch, S. M. and Allan, J. D. Postmenopausal hormone replacement therapy. Scientific review. *J. Am. Med. Assoc.* 2002; **288**:872–81.

10 Hulley, S., Grady, D., Bush, T., *et al.* Randomized trial of estrogen plus progestin for secondary prevention of coronary heart disease in postmenopausal women. *J. Am. Med. Assoc.* 1998; **280**:605–13.

11 Writing Group for the Women's Health Initiative Investigators. Risks and benefits of estrogen plus progestin in healthy menopausal women: principal results from the Women's Health Initiative randomized controlled trial. *J. Am. Med. Assoc.* 2002; **288**:321–33.

12 Voekler, R. Questions about hormone therapy remain puzzling. *J. Am. Med. Assoc.* 2002; **288**:2395–6.

13 Nelson, H. D., Humphrey, L. L., Le Blanc, E., *et al.* Postmenopausal Hormone Replacement Therapy for Primary Prevention of Chronic Conditions. Summary of the Evidence. http://ahrq.gov/clinic/3rduspstf/hrt/hrtusum1.htm. Accessed August 21, 2002.

14 Lemaitre, R. N., Heckbert, S. R., Psaty, B. M., Smith, N. L., Kaplan, R. C. and Longstreth, W. T. Hormone replacement therapy and associated risk of stroke in postmenopausal women. *Arch. Intern. Med.* 2002; **162**:1954–60.

15 Writing Group for the Women's Health Initiative Investigators. Risks and benefits of estrogen plus progestin in healthy menopausal women: principal results from the Women's Health Initiative randomized controlled trial. *J. Am. Med. Assoc.* 2002; **288**:321–33.

16 Collaborative Group on Hormonal Factors in Breast Cancer. Breast cancer and hormone replacement therapy: collaborative reanalysis of data from 51 epidemiological studies of 52,705 women with breast cancer and 108,411 women without breast cancer. *Lancet* 1997; **350**:1047–59.

17 Hulley, S., Furberg, C., Barrett-Connor, E., *et al.* for the HERS Research Group. Noncardiovascular disease outcomes during 6.8 years of hormone therapy: Heart

and Estrogen/progestin Replacement Study Follow up HERS II. *J. Am. Med. Assoc.* 2002; **288**:58–66.

18 Nelson, H. D., Humphrey, L. L., LeBlanc, E., *et al.* Postmenopausal Hormone Replacement Therapy for Primary Prevention of Chronic Conditions. Summary of the Evidence. http://ahrq.gov/clinic/3rdusptf/hrt/hrtsum1.htm. Accessed August 18, 2002.

19 Schairer, C., Lubin, J., Troisi, R., *et al.* Menopausal estrogen and estrogen progestin replacement therapy and breast cancer risk. *J. Am. Med. Assoc.* 2000; **283**: 485–9.

20 Schairer, C., Lubin, J., Troisi, R., *et al.* Menopausal estrogen and estrogen progestin replacement therapy and breast cancer risk. *J. Am. Med. Assoc.* 2000; **283**:485–9. [Erratum in *J. Am. Med. Assoc.* 2000; **284**:2597.]

21 Writing Group for the Women's Health Initiative Investigators. Risks and benefits of estrogen plus progestin in healthy menopausal women: principal results from the Women's Health Initiative randomized controlled trial. *J. Am. Med. Assoc.* 2002; **288**:321–33.

22 Collaborative Group on Hormonal Factors in Breast Cancer. Breast cancer and hormone replacement therapy: collaborative reanalysis of data from 51 epidemiological studies of 52,705 women with breast cancer and 108,411 women without breast cancer. *Lancet* 1997; **350**:1047–59.

23 Colditz, G., Hankinson, S., Hunter, D., *et al.* The use of estrogens and progestins and the risk of breast cancer in postmenopausal women. *N. Engl. J. Med.* 1995; **332**:1589–93.

24 Humphrey, L. L. Hormone replacement therapy and breast cancer. Systematic Evidence Review no. 14. www.ahrq.gov/clinic/serfiles.htm. Accessed January 14, 2003.

25 Ettinger, B., Friedman, G., Bush, T. and Quesenberry, C., Jr. Reduced mortality associated with long term postmenopausal estrogen therapy. *Obstet. Gynecol.* 1996; **87**:6–12.

26 Nanda, K., Bastian, L. A. and Schulz, K. Hormone replacement therapy and the risk of death from breast cancer: a systematic review. *Am. J. Obstet. Gynecol.* 2002; **186**:325–34.

27 Beresford, S., Weiss, N., Voigt, L., *et al.* Risk of endometrial cancer in relation to use of oestrogen combined with cyclic progestagen therapy in postmenopausal women. *Lancet* 1997; **349**:458–61.

28 Pike, M. C., Peters, R. K., Cozen, W., *et al.* Estrogen progestin replacement and endometrial cancer. *J. Natl Cancer Inst.* 1997; **89**:1110–16.

29 Nelson, H. D., Humphrey, L. L., LeBlanc, E., *et al.* Postmenopausal Hormone Replacement Therapy for Primary Prevention of Chronic Conditions. Summary of the Evidence. http://ahrq.gov/clinic/3rduspstf/hrt/hrtsum1.htm. Accessed August 21, 2002.

30 Lacey, J. V., Jr, Mink, P. J., Lubin, J. H., *et al.* Menopausal hormone replacement therapy and risk of ovarian cancer. *J. Am. Med. Assoc.* 2002: **288**:334–41.

31 Rodriguez, C., Patel, A. V., Calle, E. E., *et al.* Estrogen replacement therapy and ovarian cancer mortality in a large prospective study of US women. *J. Am. Med. Assoc.* 2001; **285**:14.

32 Weiss, N. S. and Rossing, M. A. Oestrogen replacement therapy and risks of ovarian cancer. *Lancet* 2001; **358**:438.

33 Riman, T., Dickman, P. W., Nilsson, S., *et al.* Hormone replacement therapy and the risk of invasive ovarian cancer in Swedish women. *J. Natl Cancer Inst.* 2002; **94**:497–504.

34 Henderson, W. V., Kelin, B. E. K. and Resnick, S. M. Menopause and disorders of neurologic function, mental health and the eye. In Wenger, N. K., Paoletti, R., Lenfant, C. I. M. and Pinn, V. W. (eds.). *International Position Paper on Women's Health and Menopause: A Comprehensive Approach*, vol 02-3284. Bethesda, MD: National Institutes of Health; 2002. pp. 251–70.

35 Novartis Foundation. Neuronal and cognitive effects of oestrogens. Monograph no. 230. Chicester, UK: John Wiley & Sons; 2002.

36 Yaffe, K., Sawaya, G., Lieberburg, I. and Gradey, D. Estrogen therapy in postmenopausal women: effects on cognitive function and dementia. *J. Am. Med. Assoc.* 1998; **279**:688–95.

37 LeBlanc, E. S., Janowsky, J., Chan, B. K. and Nelson, H. D. Hormone replacement therapy and cognition: systematic review and meta-analysis. *J. Am. Med. Assoc.* 2001; **285**:1489–99.

38 Fillit, H. M. The role of hormone replacement therapy in the prevention of Alzheimer disease. *Arch. Intern. Med.* 2002; **162**:1934–42.

39 Seshadri, S., Zornberg, F. L., Derby, L. E., *et al.* Postmenopausal estrogen replacement therapy and the risk of AD. *Arch. Neurol.* 2001; **58**:435–40.

40 Zandi, P. P., Carlson, M. C., Plassman, B. L., *et al.* Hormone replacement therapy and incidence of Alzheimer disease in older women. The Cache County Study. *J. Am. Med. Assoc.* 2002; **288**:2123–9.

41 Hlatky, M. A., Boothroyd, D., Vittinghoff, E., *et al.* Quality of life and depressive symptoms in postmenoapusal women after receiving hormone therapy. *J. Am. Med. Assoc.* 2002; **287**:591–7.

42 White, C. Second long term HRT trial stopped early. *Br. Med. J.* 2002; **325**:987.

43 Asthana, S., Baker, L. D., Craft, S., *et al.* High dose estradiol improves cognition for women with AD: results of a randomized study. *Neurology* 2001; **57**:605–12.

44 Cholerton, B., Gleason, C. E., Baker, L. D. and Asthana, S. Estrogen and Alzheimer's disease: the story so far. *Drugs Aging* 2002; **19**:405–27.

45 Kanaya, A. M., Herrington, D., Vittinghoff, E., *et al.* Glycemic effects of postmenopausal hormone therapy: the Heart and Estrogen/Progestin Replacement Study. A randomized double-blind, placebo-controlled trial. *Am. Intern. Med.* 2003; **138**:1–9.

46 Grodstein, F., Colditz, G. A. and Stampfer, M. J. Postmenopausal hormone use and cholecystectomy in a large prospective study. *Obstet. Gynecol.* 1994; **83**:5–11.

47 Barbabei, V. M., Grady, D., Stovall, D. W., *et al.* Menopausal symptoms in older women and the effects of treatment with hormone therapy. *Obstet. Gynecol.* 2002; **100**:1209–18.

48 Grady, D., Herrington, D., Bittner, V., *et al.* for the HERS Research Group. Cardiovascular disease outcomes during 6.8 years of hormone therapy. Heart and Estrogen/Progestin Replacement Study Follow-up (HERS II). *J. Am. Med. Assoc.* 2002; **288**:49–57.

49 American Heart Association. Estrogen and Cardiovascular Disease *in Women*. http://www.americanheart.org/presenter.jhtml?identifier=4536. Accessed January 12, 2003.

50 American College of Obstetricians and Gynecologists. Questions and Answers on Hormone Therapy. http://www.acog.org/from_home/publications/press_releases/ nr08-30-02.cfm.

51 North American Menopause Society. Amended report from the NAMS Advisory Panel on Postmenopausal hormone therapy. *Menopause* 2003; **10**:6–12.

52 US Preventive Services Task Force. Hormone replacement therapy for primary prevention of chronic conditions. http://www.ahcpr.gov/clinic/3rduspstf/ hrt/hrtrr.htm.

53 Voelker, R. Questions about hormone therapy remain puzzling. *J. Am. Med. Assoc.* 2000; **288**:2395–6.

54 Hlatky, M. A., Boothroyd, D., Vittinghoff, E., *et al.* Heart and Estrogen Progestin Replacement Study Research Group. Quality of life and depressive symptoms in postmenopausal women after receiving hormone therapy: results from the Heart and Estrogen Progestin Replacement Study Trial. *J. Am. Med. Assoc.* 2002; **287**: 591–6.

55 Soloman, C. G. and Dhluly, R. G. Rethinking postmenopausal hormone therapy. *N. Engl. J. Med.* 2002; **348**:579–80.

56 Voelker, R. Questions about hormone therapy remain puzzling. *J. Am. Med. Assoc.* 2000; **288**:2395–6.

57 Greendale, G. A., Espeland, M., Slone, S., Marcus, R. and Barrett-Connor, E. Bone mass response to discontinuation of long-term hormone replacement therapy: results from the Postmenopausal Estrogen/Progestin Interventions (PEPI) Safety follow-up study. *Arch. Intern. Med.* 2002; **162**:665–72.

58 Gallagher, J. C., Rapuri, P. B., Haynatzki, G. and Detter, J. R. Effect of discontinuation of estrogen, calcitrol, and the combination of both on bone density and bone markers. *J. Clin. Endocrinol. Metab.* 2002; **87**:4914–23.

59 New Zealand Guidelines Group. Best practice evidence-based guideline for the appropriate prescribing of hormone replacement therapy. www.guidelines.gov. September 2002.

60 Ansbacker, R. The pharmacokinetics and efficacy of different estrogens are not equivalent. *Am. J. Obstet. Gynecol.* 2001; **184**:255–63.

61 Eriksen, B. A randomized open parallel-group study on the preventive effects of an estradiol-releasing vaginal ring on current urinary tract infections in postmenopausal women. *Am. J. Obstet. Gynecol.* 1999; **180**:1072–9.

62 US Food and Drug Administration. FDA approves new labels for estrogen and estrogen with progestin therapies for postmenopausal women following review of women's health initiative data. http://www.fda.gov/bbs/topics/NEWS/ 2003/NEW00863.html. Accessed January 9, 2003.

63 American College of Obstetricians and Gynecologists. Use of botanicals for management of menopausal symptoms. Clinical Management Guidelines for Obstetrician-Gynecologists. ACOG Practice Bulletin No. 28, June 2001. www.acog.org/from_home/publications/misc/pb028.htm.

64 Nelson, H. D. Assessing benefits and harms of hormone replacement therapy clinical applications. *J. Am. Med. Assoc.* 2002; **288**:882–4.

65 Leonetti, H. B., Longo, S. and Anasti, J. N. Transdermal progesterone cream for vasomotor symptoms and postmenopausal bone loss. *Obstet. Gynecol.* 1999; **94**: 225–8.

66 Moore, R. A. Livial: a review of clinical studies. *Br. J. Obstet. Gynaecol.* 1999; **106**(supp 19):1–21.

67 Faure, E. D., Chantre, P. and Mares, P. Effects of a standardized soy extract on hot flushes: a multicenter, double blind randomized placebo controlled study. *Menopause* 2002; **9**:329–34.

68 Han, K. K., Soares, J. M., Haidar, M. A., de Lima, G. R. and Baracat, E. C. Benefits of soy isoflavones therapeutic regimen on menopausal symptoms. *Obstet. Gynecol.* 2002; **99**:389–94.

69 Hughes, C. Easing menopausal symptoms with soy. http://dukehealth.org/news/healthtip_october02.asp. Accessed November 4, 2002.

70 Liske, E., Hanggi, W., Henneicke-von Zepelin, H. H., Boblitz, N., Wustenberg, P. and Rahlfs, V. W. Physiological investigation of a unique extract of black cohosh (Cimicifugae racemosae rhizoma): a 6-month clinical study demonstrates no systemic estrogenic effect. *J. Womens Health Gend Based Med.* 2002; **11**:163–74.

71 American College of Obstetricians and Gynecologists. Use of botanicals for management of menopausal symptoms. Clinical Management Guidelines for Obstetrician–Gynecologists. ACOG Practice Bulletin No. 28, June 2001. www.acog.org/from_home/publications/misc/pb028.htm. Accessed December 14, 2002.

72 Office of Dietary Supplements, National Institutes of Health. Questions and answers about black cohosh and the symptoms of menopause. http://ods.od.nih.gov/factsheets/blackcohosh.html.

73 Office of Dietary Supplements NIH/The National Center for Complementary and Alternative Medicine at the NIH. Dietary supplements, complementary or alternative medicines. www.nlm.nih.gov/services/dietsup.html.

74 American College of Obstetricians and Gynecologists. Use of botanicals for management of menopausal symptoms. Clinical Management Guidelines for Obstetrician–Gynecologists. ACOG Practice Bulletin No. 28, June 2001. www.acog.org/from_home/publications/misc/pb028.htm. Accessed January 7, 2003.

75 Rious, J. E., Devlin, C., Gelfant, M. M., *et al.* 17 beta estradiol vaginal tablet versus conjugated equine estrogen vaginal cream to relieve menopausal atrophic vaginitis. *Menopause* 2000; **7**:140–42.

76 Grady, D. A 60 year old woman trying to discontinue hormone replacement therapy. *J. Am. Med. Assoc.* 2002; **287**:2130–37.

77 Nelson, H. D. Assessing benefits and harms of HRT: clinical applications. *J. Am. Med. Assoc.* 2002; **288**:882–4.

78 US Preventive Services Task Force. Screening for osteoporosis in postmenopausal women: recommendations and rationale. *Am. Fam. Physician* 2002; **66**:1430–32.

79 US Preventive Services Task Force. Screening for osteoporosis in postmenopausal women: recommendations and rationale. *Am. Intern. Med.* 2002; **137**:526–8.

80 Greendale, G. A., Espeland, M., Slone, S., Marcus, R. and Barrett-Connor, E. Bone mass response to discontinuation of long-term hormone replacement therapy. *Arch. Intern. Med.* 2002; **162**:665–72.

81 Davis, S. R. Androgens and female sexuality. *J. Gend. Specif. Med.* 2000; **3**:36–40.
82 Solomon, C. G. and Dluhy, R. G. Rethinking postmenopausal hormone therapy. *N. Engl. J. Med.* 2003; **348**:579–81.
83 Grodstein, F., Clarkson, T. B. and Manson, J. E. Understanding the divergent data on postmenopausal hormone therapy. *N. Engl. J. Med.* 2003; **348**:645–50.

11

Contraception and fertility

Tracey D. Conti

Case: S.J. is a 42-year-old woman who has recently remarried four years after her divorce. She used condoms as a teenager, oral contraception in her twenties and mid thirties, and abstinence over the past four years. She is unsure whether she wants to restart hormonal contraception. In her latest job, she works at night, this makes it hard to remember regular contraception. She is menstruating regularly and so assumes she is still fertile; she does not want to become pregnant.

Introduction

The need for reliable, safe, and reversible contraception has become more evident, and the duration of their use has increased as many women opt to delay childbearing into the late third and fourth decades. Though the decision to delay childbearing results in greater satisfaction, reproductive health discussions must now include a frank and evidence-based presentation of the potential health risks, complications, and decreased fertility rates associated with delayed childbearing and advanced maternal age.

Contraception

Contraceptive methods can be classified into types – physical barriers and hormonal methods – or as folk methods, traditional methods, and contemporary methods (Table 11.1).

Individual decisions regarding contraceptive methods vary widely among women. Factors that may influence decision-making include age, attitudes and beliefs regarding family planning, and concerns over the use of exogenous hormones, most notably regarding cancer and thromboembolic disease.[1] Failure rates vary by the method (Table 11.2).

Table 11.1 Classification of contraceptive methods

	Folk	Traditional	Contemporary
Physical barriers		Condom	IUD
		Diaphragm	Tubal sterilization
		Sponge	Vasectomy
		Rhythm	
		Spermicides	
Hormonal devices			Oral contraceptives
			Injections
			Topical devices
Other methods	Coitus interruptus		
	Postcoital douche		
	Prolonged lactation		

Barrier devices

Tubal ligation

Since the advent of tubal sterilization in 1823, many techniques have been described. Rates of tubal sterilization have risen steadily among all age groups since 1970. Fifty percent of women aged 40–44 years using any contraception have been sterilized, and 20% have a partner who has had a vasectomy.[2]

Presently, sterilization procedures (tubal sterilization and vasectomy) are some of the most common forms of contraception worldwide and in the USA, along with oral contraceptives and condoms.

Many psychosocial and economic factors will continue to affect women's contraceptive decision-making and undoubtedly will continue to influence rates of tubal sterilization.

Tubal sterilization is generally considered an irreversible form of contraception. Approximately 80% of women are satisfied with tubal ligation. Reasons for dissatisfaction include heavier menses and irreversibility. However, the percentage of women requesting tubal ligation reversal remains at 1–2%. Rates of successful reversal are related directly to the amount of viable fallopian tube preserved, which is related largely to surgical technique. Relatively low rates of successful reversal of tubal sterilization should prompt the clinician to engage the patient in comprehensive pre-procedure counseling. Many US states have developed policies that guide practitioners in the timing of this counseling, even prohibiting immediately postpartum consent for tubal sterilization.

Practitioners should be mindful of specific and indirect cues that might suggest indecision on the part of the patient or their partner. It is important to note, however, that US Federal law does not require spousal written consent with regard to women's fertility decisions.

Table 11.2 Failure rates of contraceptives

Contraceptive	Failure rate (per 100 woman-years)
Male condom	11
Diaphragm	17
Sponge	14–28
Spermicide	25–50
Oral contraceptives	
Combined	1
Progestin-only	2
Patch	1
Vaginal ring	1
Postcoital contraceptives	Prevents 80%
Injection (Depo-Provera^{TM})	<1
Monthly (Lunelle^{TM})	<1
Implant	<1
IUD	<1
Periodic abstinence	20
Surgical sterilization of women	<1
Surgical sterilization of men	<1

Data from Food and Drug Administration. Birth control guide. (www.fda.gov/fdac/features/1997/babytabl.html. Accessed March 14, 2003.

Morbidity and failure rates for tubal sterilization remain low. The pregnancy rate after tubal ligation is approximately one in 250 postpartum tubal ligations and one in 400 tubal ligations done at other times. Intraoperative and postoperative complications include bowel perforation, dehiscence, and postoperative infection.

More common complications include postoperative pain and menstrual irregularity. There is considerable debate as to whether these rates are any higher than in women who have not undergone the procedure. Menstrual irregularities and pain in all women are influenced more by contraceptive selection rather than a history of tubal sterilization.

Tubal sterilization, however, is associated with increased rates of ectopic pregnancy and hysterectomy. The risks of ectopic pregnancy and failure rates are lower in older women.[3] There is no evidence that women who have undergone tubal sterilization experience higher rates of psychological disturbance such as anxiety, depression, psychosis, or adjustment disorder. This procedure is an excellent option for women who have completed their families.

Vasectomy
Vasectomy, like tubal sterilization, should be considered an irreversible sterilization procedure. However, reversal rates are considerably higher when

compared with tubal sterilization.[4] Usually performed as an office procedure, under local anesthesia, it involves excision of small segments of the right and left vas deferens after a small scrotal incision. Failure rates have been reported consistently as less than 0.1%. A three-month post-procedure ejaculate that is sperm-free denotes definitive sterilization.

Vasectomy reversal (vasovasostomy) rates are considerably higher than for tubal sterilization, approaching 70–75%. Though reversal rates are relatively high, post-reversal pregnancy rates may be as low as 20%. Risks and benefits should be explained carefully and followed by written, informed consent.

Complication rates for vasectomy and vasovasostomy are low, but include bleeding, secondary skin infection, and drug allergy due to the use of local anesthesia. The vasectomy offers a relatively safe outpatient procedure that may prove attractive, particularly in the partners of older women in whom the complication rate for tubal procedures may be markedly higher.

Condoms

Condom use is the most common form of contraception worldwide. The advantages of condoms are that they are inexpensive and highly effective barrier devices against both pregnancy and the transmission of sexually transmitted diseases. Many condoms now incorporate a spermicide as an added failsafe method against unanticipated sperm deposition.

Condom failure rates are reported at less than 0.1% and are most commonly the result of improper condom application, failure to withdraw the penis before detumescence, thus allowing escape of semen, and physical imperfections with the condom itself. Failure rates are decreased when condom and spermicide use is coupled with a contraceptive vaginal foam or jelly.

Intrauterine devices

Intrauterine devices (IUDs) continue to be used, although their exact mechanism of action remains unclear. Constructed of plastic, metal, or combinations, IUDs offer long-term contraception at a relatively low cost. Furthermore, devices require a single procedure for insertion, may be inserted by properly trained non-physicians, and allow for restored fertility soon after removal. No compelling evidence exists to suggest that infertility rates are significantly higher than in non-IUD wearers after removal.

IUD insertion may be performed at any time. However, insertion just after menstruation is generally considered most desirable because of the relatively low likelihood of pregnancy and the increased patency of the cervix, allowing for easier access to the endometrial cavity. IUD insertion requires formal training, but the learning curve is not particularly steep.

The most common complications of IUD insertion include pelvic pain or discomfort, often reported as non-specific pain or intense menstrual cramps.[5]

Wider IUDs produce comparatively more discomfort, and nulliparous women have more subjective pain complaints. Far less common complications include traumatic uterine perforation. Uterine perforation rates are related directly to technique. Other negative events include post-IUD insertion pregnancy and IUD expulsion.

Pregnancy rates among women with IUDs are variable but relatively low and are related to age and parity. The pregnancy rate is very low – less than three per 1000 woman-years. However, the tubal pregnancy rate is not decreased. If a woman with an IUD becomes pregnant, then the risk of a tubal pregnancy is higher. If pregnancy does occur, then an immediate ultrasound will show placement of the IUD and the pregnancy. If the IUD is still intrauterine, it should be removed, which will reduce the spontaneous abortion rate. The rate of spontaneous abortion associated with forceful IUD removal outweighs the risk of pregnancy with an in situ IUD. Other indications for IUD removal include severe or persistent menorrhagia or menometrorrhagia, high clinical suspicion or clinical evidence of partial or complete uterine perforation, and evidence of improper placement.

Considerable debate remains regarding IUD removal because of the risk of the development of endometritis or salpingitis. Contraindications for IUD placement include pregnancy, genitourinary malignancy, cervicitis, recent abnormal Pap smear, dysfunctional uterine bleeding of unknown etiology, salpingitis, and history of previous ectopic pregnancy.

Women should inspect themselves and locate the strings of the IUD. Though expulsion rates are relatively low (less than 0.01%), suspected expulsion should prompt physician examination to confirm expulsion and to be certain that all components of the device have been removed.

An IUD may be considered in any non-pregnant woman of childbearing age and who has no underlying gynecologic pre-existing pathology, in post-abortion and postpartum women with no evidence of pelvic infection, and in monogamous women with a relatively high degree of certainty regarding the reciprocal monogamy of their partner. Hormone-containing IUDs may reduce perimenopausal metrorrhagia and dyspareunia.[6] IUDs typically require replacement every ten years, making them particularly appealing to older women, who may require only one IUD for the remainder of their fertile period.

Diaphragms
Like the IUD, these devices require pelvic examination before insertion. However, properly trained non-physicians may insert them. Failure rates remain consistently between 2% and 5% and are related to improper fitting and/or placement resulting in dislodgement during intercourse. Failure rates may be increased in older women because of relaxation of the pelvic muscles. Frequent checks may be necessary to ensure proper fitting.

Sponges

The rates of conception associated with this barrier device are similar to those reported with the diaphragm. Constructed of polyurethane, sponges are easy to insert and remove. Properly lubricated before coitus and augmented by the act of intercourse, the spermicide nonoxynol-9 provides up to 24 hours of spermicidal effectiveness.

Hormonal methods

Oral contraceptives

The oral contraceptive pill (OCP) remains one of the most common forms of contraception in the USA, followed by condoms. The OCP is extremely effective when taken regularly.

Advantages to OCP use include apparent protection against benign breast disease, pelvic inflammatory disease (PID), and some forms of cancer. OCPs have the lowest rates of ectopic pregnancy compared with other methods of contraception. *Combination OCPs provide significant reduction in endometrial cancer risk, which peaks at a reduced risk of nearly 30% at five years and persisting for up to ten years after discontinuing the pill.*[7] Additional observed advantages include decreased incidence of dysmenorrhea and decreased incidence of ascending bacterial pelvic infections.

The major concern regarding OCP use centers around malignancy risk and the development of thromboembolic disease – deep venous thrombosis, pulmonary embolism, cerebral thrombosis, and coronary artery thrombosis (Table 11.3). Despite the apparent protective effects of OCP use with respect to endometrial malignancy, there is increased relative risk of both breast and cervical cancer, which may remain for up to ten years after discontinuing the OCP. Cancer risk is not related to OCP preparation or duration of use.

Thromboembolic events are three to six times greater among OCP users compared with non-users. This risk is even greater among OCP users who smoke cigarettes, regardless of age or parity. OCP users also have significantly increased risk of postpartum development of DVT when compared with postpartum women who have not used OCPs. Use of OCPs in women over age 35 and who smoke is contraindicated because of increased thromboembolic risk.

Other potential adverse effects of OCP use include metabolic changes similar to pregnancy, including elevations in thyroid binding proteins and thyroxin, elevations in total cholesterol and triglycerides (in combination pills), decreased glucose tolerance, and the development of biliary diseases, including cholelithiasis, cholecystitis, and cholestatic jaundice.

There is a variety of OCPs, many of which now vary or reduce the amount of progesterone and estrogen throughout the cycle. Those with lower estrogen doses and/or lower progestin doses may be tolerated better by older menstruating women.

Table 11.3 Contraindications to hormonal contraception

Absolute
  History of thromboembolic disease – Pulmonary embolism, stroke, or CVA
  Structural heart disease
  Estrogen-dependent cancers – Breast, uterine
  Pregnancy
  Major surgery and/or prolonged immobilization
  Unexplained or continuing liver or gallbladder disease
  Age over 35 years and smoker
  Uncontrolled hypertension

Relatively contraindicated
  Undiagnosed vaginal bleeding
  Pregnancy, postpartum, lactation
  Interacting drugs
  Gallstones
  Severe headaches
  Uncontrolled diabetes
  Sickle cell disease
  Lipid disorder

Women may use hormonal therapy into their fifties and menopause, if they have no contraindications and are not smokers.[8] However, menopause will then need to be diagnosed, because the woman will continue to cycle, even when menopausal, if she is still taking OCPs. After age 50, a follicle stimulating hormone (FSH) level should be obtained on the fifth to seventh afternoon of her week on placebos (withdrawal bleeding week). If her FSH level is 25 IU/dl or more, she is menopausal and should stop her OCP. She may still have a withdrawal bleed.[8]

One variation of OCP use includes non-stop progestin or the "mini-pill," which provides the daily medication without a special or preset schedule, and with a significant reduction in anovulatory bleeding and reduced side effects compared with OCPs containing estrogen. The precise mechanism of action of the mini-pill remains unknown. Failure rates of progestin-only pills are lower with older women (less than 0.3 per 100 women-years) than younger women.[9]

Progesterone-only OCPs may be a good choice for some women in this age group, especially those who smoke or who are on multiple medications or drugs that are metabolized by the liver, especially the P450 system, such as anti-seizure drugs, antidepressants, and phenothiazines. They cause more breakthrough bleeding and increased incidence of bloating and nausea than combination estrogen–progesterone pills, but taking them at the same time every day reduces the amount of breakthrough bleeding.

Table 11.4 Some proprietary methods of emergency contraception

Preven®	Two tablets; repeat in 12 hours
Plan B®	One tablet; repeat in 12 hours
Lo-Ovral®	Four tablets; repeat in 12 hours
Levlen®, Triphasil, TriLevlen, Nordette	Four tablets; repeat in 12 hours
Ovral®	Two tablets; repeat in 12 hours
Ovrette	Twelve tablets; repeat in 12 hours

Data from Andolsek, K. Contraception. In J. A. Rosenfeld (ed.). *Handbook of Women's Health*. Cambridge: Cambridge University Press; 2001. p. 159.

Emergency contraception

Emergency contraception may occasionally still be needed by women in this age range, especially in those using condoms or diaphragms. Used for breaks or failure to use contraception, emergency contraception hinders ovulation and may impede implantation. It does not interrupt an already established pregnancy. Emergency contraception can prevent approximately 75–80% of pregnancies if taken within 72 hours. It is more effective the earlier it is used. Physicians can provide women with emergency prescriptions on hand or easy methods of obtaining them, when needed. Consider using a prophylactic antiemetic. Table 11.4 lists some methods of emergency contraception.

Injectable contraceptives

Intramuscular injections of synthetic sex hormones provide varying durations of contraception, depending upon the specific agent and dose. In most cases, the mechanism of contraception occurs through suppression along the pituitary axis. Injection of a depot of higher-dose sex hormones leads to endometrial atrophy, resulting in irregular or absent uterine bleeding that may persist for months after discontinuing the regimen. Women contemplating this method must be counseled regarding the possibility that restoration of regular menses and fertility make take one year or more following discontinuing the agent.

There are two types of injectable hormones – a progestin-only (Depo-Provera) drug and a combination (Lunelle). The combination hormonal injection acts similarly to oral agents and carries the same risks with regards to estrogen. The progestin-only injection does not carry the risks associated with estrogen but commonly produces irregular bleeding, as discussed previously; such bleeding may be problematic. Further evidence suggests a possible link to decreased bone density with long-term use. However, none of these studies have targeted older women.

Transdermal and other hormonal contraception

Transdermal agents are the newest forms of hormonal contraception. Clinical investigations have been limited to their use in younger women of reproductive age.

The hormones used in these devices are similar to the hormones in combination OCPs, with the same risks and benefits. Perhaps the most attractive benefit is ease of use; patches are placed weekly with a free week after the third patch to allow menstruation to occur. The risk of missed daily doses is essentially eliminated, because women have to medicate themselves only three times monthly.

Another contraceptive option is the vaginal ring. This combination hormone device is inserted into the vagina, where it remains in place for three weeks. The fourth week is a hormone-free week. Considered an appealing contraceptive method due to its ease of use, it is an in-dwelling rather than a transdermal device. The vaginal ring provides women with a once-monthly contraceptive option. As with a diaphragm, dislodgement is an uncommon but legitimate concern; it is particularly possible in older women, whose changing pelvic musculature can increase the risk of dislodgement. Women need a back-up contraceptive method during the first seven consecutive days following insertion and in the event that the ring has been out of place for more than three hours.

Rhythm methods

Also known as periodic abstinence or natural family planning, this method is based on the knowledge of the relatively small window of fertility during the menstrual cycle. The premise is simple – timed coitus to minimize the likelihood of a released ovum and sperm meeting in the oviduct. The period of fertility extends for two to three days following ovulation.

Women must attempt to predict ovulation accurately. Generally, the three established methods in increasing reliability and cost are the calendar method, measurement and recording basal body temperature, and serum peak luteinizing hormone (LH) levels. This mechanism can be more challenging in the perimenopausal woman, due to changes in the timing and frequency of the menstrual cycle.

Spermicidal devices

These devices come in various preparations, including jellies, suppositories, creams, and foams. They provide a direct killing effect on sperm while also forming a physical barrier between the vagina and the cervix. The effectiveness

of a properly applied, non-defective condom with a properly applied spermicidal device has a failure rate of virtually zero. Though not optimally effective
as a prevention strategy for sexually transmitted disease (STDs), evidence
suggests that spermicidal preparations afford women significant protection
against most common STDs, including gonorrhea, trichomonas, syphilis, and
human papilloma virus (HPV).

Less reliable methods

Common folk methods that have varying degrees of reliability include coitus
interruptus (withdrawal of the penis before ejaculation), postcoital douching,
and prolongation of lactation following pregnancy.

Abortion

Abortion is a less frequent although still practiced method of contraception
in this age group. Although only 1.4% of births occur in women over age
40 years, 39% of pregnancies in women of this age end in abortion, compared
with only 20% of pregnancies in women aged 25–34 years.

Summary

Ultimately, reproductive health decisions and contraceptive choices must be
left to women, hopefully in conjunction with their partners. Practitioners
provide an important role, often as facilitators of the discussion of the advantages, disadvantages, risks, and benefits of the various contraceptive methods.
Numerous societal, biological, psychological, and legal factors must be considered when counseling women about their reproductive health. As with any
physician–patient encounter, careful documentation must accompany any discussion regarding reproduction and contraceptive choices.

Discussions regarding reproductive health, contraception, and sterilization
must make the clear distinction between contraception and protection from
STDs.

Choice of method

Many women in this age group are in a long-term relationship in which they
are comfortable using one form of contraception. Some long-term couples
use withdrawal or abstinence with good success over many years.

For women aged 45–65, the choice of contraception may be different from
that of younger menstruating women. Reversibility may be less important
than permanence. Younger women may tolerate some side effects for some

Table 11.5 Chronic conditions, disability, and hormonal contraception

Condition	Use of combination OCPs	Use of progestin-only OCPs, depot, injectable
Blindness	Not if caused by diabetes, glaucoma, or vascular disease	Not if caused by diabetes, glaucoma, or vascular disease
Cancer of breast or reproductive system	Contraindicated	Contraindicated
Cerebrovascular accident or TIA	Contraindicated	Contraindicated
Coronary artery disease, MI	Not contraindicated, but other methods should be used instead	Possibly
Coumidin use	Contraindicated	Possibly
Diabetes	Yes, if under control; may worsen control	Yes, if under control
Epilepsy	Relatively contraindicated because medications interact	Possibly – watch antiepileptic drug levels
Hypertension	Yes, if under control; watch types of antihypertensive medications, especially if they are metabolized in the liver	Yes, if under control
Migraine headaches	Contraindicated if OCP worsens headaches; should be used only very carefully	Possibly
Muscular diseases, multiple sclerosis	May increase the risk of thromboembolism, relatively contraindicated	Possibly
Rheumatoid arthritis	May worsen disease; use cautiously	May worsen disease; use cautiously
Ulcerative colitis (Crohn's disease)	Not contraindicated	Not contraindicated

gains that will not interest older women, such as the use of OCPs, which may give breakthrough bleeding but will allow for the advantages of decreased breast tenderness and improvement of acne. Some methods have lower failure rates in older women, such as progestin-only pills. Some methods become relatively contraindicated as older women develop chronic diseases and disability (see Table 11.5).

Sterilization by tubal ligation is one of the more common choices because of its permanence and relatively low incidence of side effects. Women may continue to use hormonal contraception, especially if they are non-smokers. OCPs may be more risky than pregnancy for women over age 35 and who smoke.[10]

For women using hormonal methods, long-term injectable hormones may be less used because of concerns with osteoporosis. *Low-estrogen and/or progestin-only OCPs may be more advisable because of the age-associated increasing risk of hypertension and thromboembolic disease.* Progestin-only OCPs may be advisable for women with migraines, hypertension, seizures, or depression and those on antidepressants.

Infertility and assisted fertilization

If women continue to opt to delay childbearing, many will require assistance with fertilization. Methods have become increasingly more effective over the past several decades, making assisted fertilization a somewhat commonplace, though still expensive, method of childbearing assistance. Broad categories of assisted fertilization include hormonal assistance designed to induce ovulation and in vitro fertilization.[11]

Infertility

Infertility is the inability of a couple to become pregnant after one year. Infertility, affecting approximately 10–15% of the total population, is increased with chronic disease, age, certain medications, smoking, alcohol abuse, and obesity.[12] The duration of infertility and age of the patient are the most important factors determining the prognosis.[13]

Evaluation

A woman who is in this age group and is having difficulty becoming pregnant needs specialist attention because of the limited time involved.[14] Medications that may affect cycles, including hormones, steroids, and psychotropic drugs, should be changed or stopped (Table 11.6).

The woman should be evaluated for thyroid and other hormonal diseases. FSH and LH levels may be elevated if the woman has ovarian failure or menopause.

In vitro fertilization

The first live birth resulting from in vitro fertilization (IVF) occurred in the late 1970s.[15] The resulting wave of scientific discovery has led to countless successes and new techniques. Consequently, the improved techniques have ushered in an era of debate regarding scientific intervention into the physiology, biochemistry, and genetics of conception.

Table 11.6 Drugs that may affect
fertility adversely

Alcohol
Antibiotics – tetracycline, nitrofurantoin
Calcium channel blockers
Cancer therapeutic agents
Cigarette smoking
Colchicine
Steroids
Sulfasalazine

Indications for IVF include severe tubal dysfunction, endometriosis, antisperm antibodies, oligospermia, and infertility of unexplained origin.[16] Assisted fertilization is indicated if the probability of conception by IVF exceeds the likelihood of successful conception using conventional means.

IVF begins with hormone-induced superovulation followed by egg aspiration. Superovulation employs numerous therapies utilizing one or more medications, including clomiphene citrate, human menopausal gonadotropins (hMG), FSH, and luteinizing hormone releasing hormone (LHRH). Egg aspiration requires direct laparoscopy or ultrasound-guided percutaneous technique, the latter being performed easily as an outpatient or same-day procedure. The process proceeds with fertilization with capacitated sperm, followed by culture of fertilized eggs and fertilized egg replacement into the uterus.

IVF has relatively few complications, apart from those associated with laparoscopy, general anesthesia, and conscious sedation. There is no evidence of increased rates of congenital birth defects or ectopic pregnancy.

Rates of spontaneous conception at 24 months are comparable between natural conception, hormone-induced ovulation, and IVF. Compared with the relatively low rates of conception at 24 months for women with even mild tubal disease (less than 80%), IVF provides a viable reproductive option for those with the patience and financial means.

The psychological effects of infertility are varied. Many women cope with the stresses of not achieving pregnancy and the demands of IVF, including the side effects of medication and timing intercourse. Some, however, may have ambivalent feelings about their body, concerns about body image, sexuality, place in the marital relationship, and guilt and shame about being unable to conceive. There may be sexual difficulties, reduced sexual desire, and anorgasmia. The woman may avoid family and friends with children, becoming socially isolated. Psychological counseling may be needed.

Summary

Contraception and conception may continue to be concerns of women of this age. Although choices may be different, both are achievable.

FURTHER RESOURCES

National Library of Medicine – birth control/contraception: www.nlm.nih.gov/medlineplus/birthcontrolcontraception.html

Food and Drug Administration birth control guide: www.fda.gov/fdac/ features/1997/babytabl.html

Contraception Online: www.contraceptiononline.org/

Alan Guttmacher Institute. www.agi-usa.org

www.ivf-infertility.co.uk. Designed by infertility specialists primarily for couples who are experiencing difficulty in having a child and who think that they might need medical help.

REFERENCES

1 Riphagen, F. E., Fortney J. A. and Koelb, S. Contraception in women over forty. *J. Biosoc. Sci.* 1988; **20**:127–42.

2 The Alan Guttmacher Institute. Facts in brief: contraceptive use. www.agi-usa.org/pubs/fb_contr_use.html. Accessed March 17, 2003.

3 Bouyer, J., Coste, J., Fernandez, H., Pouly, J. L. and Job-Spira, N. Sites of ectopic pregnancy: a 10-year population-based study of 1800 cases. *Hum. Reprod.* 2002; **17**:3224–30.

4 Anderson, R. A. and Baird, D. T. Male contraception. *Endocr. Rev.* 2002; **23**:735–62.

5 Stanford, J. B. and Mikolojczyk, R. T. Mechanisms of action of intrauterine devices: update and estimation of postfertilization effects. *Am. J. Obstet. Gynecol.* 2002; **187**:1699–708.

6 Wildemeersch, D., Schacht, E. and Wildemeersch, P. Performance and acceptability of intrauterine release of levonorgestrel with a miniature delivery system for hormonal substitution therapy, contraception and treatment in peri and post-menopausal women. *Maturitas* 2003; **44**:237–45.

7 Schneider, H. P. Hazards. I: perimenopausal contraception. *Eur. J. Contracept. Reprod. Health Care* 1997; **2**:95–100.

8 Creinin, M. D. Laboratory criteria for menopause in women using oral contraceptives. *Fertil. Steril.* 1996; **66**:101–4.

9 Speroff, L. and Darney, P. *A Clinical Guide for Contraception.* Philadelphia: Williams and Wilkins; 1996. p. 120.

10 Andolsek, K. Contraception. In J. A. Rosenfeld (ed.) *Handbook of Women's Health.* Cambridge: Cambridge University Press; 2001. p. 155.

11 Aboulghar, M. A., Mansour, R. T., Serour, G. I. and Al-Inany HG. Diagnosis and management of unexplained fertility: an update. *Arch. Gynecol. Obstet.* 2003; **267**:177–88.

12 Jones, H. The infertile couple. *N. Engl. J. Med.* 1993; **329**:1710–15.
13 Hargreave, T. B. and Mills, A. Investigating and managing infertility in the general practice. *Br. Med. J.* 1998; **316**:1438–41.
14 Cohen, M. and Sauer, M. Fertility in perimenopausal women. *Clin. Obstet. Gynecol.* 1998; **41**:958–65.
15 Burrage, J. infertility treatment in women aged over 40 years. *Nurs. Stand.* 1998; **13**:43–5.
16 Hesla, J. S. Current concepts in assisted reproductive technology. In J. A. Rock, S. Faro and N. F. Gant, Jr, *et al. Advances in Obstetrics and Gynecology*, vol. 1. St Louis, MO: Mosby; 1994. pp. 231–58.

Part III

Disease prevention

12

Prevention of coronary heart disease in women

Valerie K. Ulstad, M.D., M.P.H., M.P.A., F.A.C.C.

Case 1: a 62-year-old woman comes to you as a new patient. She has no complaints but needs preventive care. She smokes one pack of cigarettes per day and is on no medications. She does no regular physical exercise and has a desk job. She has no chronic medical problems. Her blood pressure is 150/90 mmHg, and she has a body mass index (BMI) of 38 kg/m² and a waist-to-hip ratio of 1.2. There are no other physical exam abnormalities. You order fasting screening labs, which show total cholesterol of 265 mg/dl (6.9 mmol/l), low-density lipoprotein (LDL) 180 mg/dl (4.7 mmol/l), high-density lipoprotein (HDL) 25 mg/dl (0.65 mmol/l), triglycerides 300 mg/dl (3.4 mmol/l), and glucose 180 mg/dl.

Case 2: a 65-year-old woman presents for new patient evaluation after a recent hospitalization for an inferior myocardial infarction (MI). She was treated acutely with angioplasty and stent placement in the right coronary artery. She also has a 30% left anterior descending coronary artery lesion and a 20% circumflex lesion. Her ejection fraction is 40%. She has had no further angina and denies symptoms of congestive heart failure. She smokes half a pack of cigarettes per day and proudly tells you this is much less than she used to smoke. She has no other chronic medical problems.

She is taking atenolol, aspirin, and atorvastatin. Her blood pressure is 160/100 mmHg, pulse is 90 bpm, BMI is 35 kg/m², and the reminder of her examination is unremarkable. In hospital, her cholesterol was 330 mg/dl (8.5 mmol/l), LDL 190 mg/dl (4.9 mmol/l), HDL 40 mg/dl (1.0 mmol/l), triglycerides 500 mg/dl (5.6 mmol/l), and hemoglobin A1C 6.0%.

What can be offered in each of these cases to reduce the patients' coronary heart disease (CHD) risk/risk of CHD reoccurrence?

Introduction

Cardiovascular disease (CVD) is the major cause of death in women in the USA and in the UK[1,2] Coronary heart disease (CHD) presents as myocardial infarction (MI), unstable angina, and chronic stable angina pectoris. CVD also includes cerebrovascular disease, primarily in the form of stroke, and peripheral vascular disease. CHD is the leading cause of premature death, death, and disability in women (and men) in both countries.[1,2]

CHD is a disease of the endothelium or lining of the blood vessel wall. In the healthy endothelium, a balance between vasodilation and vasoconstriction and between prothrombotic and anti-thrombotic factors exists.[3] Atherosclerosis begins after injury to the endothelium perturbs this balance. There are many sources of endothelial injury, including (but not limited to) passive and active smoking, hyperlipidemia, systolic and diastolic hypertension, and diabetes. These are among the major risk factors for clinical vascular disease identified by the Framingham Heart Study[4] and the Nurse's Health Study.[5] These and other factors injure directly or indirectly the vascular endothelium and promote the development of clinical vascular disease.

Risk factors for atherosclerosis

There are three classes of risk factor for atherosclerosis. *Causal risk factors are those where evidence supports a direct cause-and-effect role. These risk factors include nicotine use, high blood pressure, elevated serum cholesterol or LDL, low HDL, and high plasma glucose.*

Conditional risk factors are those where the existence of a cause-and-effect relationship and the magnitude of the relationship are less clear. These risk factors include elevated triglycerides, lipoprotein (a), small LDL particles, homocysteine, fibrinogen, plasminogen activator inhibitor, and C reactive protein.

Predisposing risk factors are those that most likely intensify the causal risk factors. They include obesity (BMI >30), abdominal obesity (waist >88 cm in women), physical inactivity, family history of premature coronary artery disease (CAD), behavioral factors (depression, anger, hostility), and ethnic characteristics.[6]

The Framingham coronary heart disease prediction equation: a new tool to improve coronary heart disease risk stratification in primary prevention

Risk factors for CHD are graded. One does not simply go from having risk to not having risk by crossing some numerical threshold. The magnitude of the risk factor is important. The actual value of the risk factors can be used to predict CHD risk more accurately.[7] Readily available calculators that are easily downloaded from the Internet into handheld devices should now be used routinely to assess the patient's CHD risk. These calculators work by incorporating multiple patient data, including age, sex, level of LDL cholesterol, systolic and diastolic blood pressure, smoking status, and presence or absence of diabetes.[8] The tool allows calculation of the ten-year absolute CHD risk and, thus, allows targeting of high-risk primary-prevention patients for more aggressive intervention. Application of this tool is readily becoming the standard of care in individualizing risk assessment. It should be applied in the care of patients to help identify people who have a constellation of risk factors that put them at very high risk, thereby triggering clinical decisions regarding the aggressiveness for the application of preventive measures.

Primary prevention

Efforts to prevent the development of vascular disease in otherwise healthy women are called primary prevention. Primary prevention should focus on the major risk factors of passive and active smoking, systolic and diastolic hypertension, elevated serum total and LDL cholesterol, low HDL cholesterol, diabetes, physical inactivity, and obesity. Advancing age is also a potent risk factor for CHD in women.

Smoking

Approximately 22% of US women and 26% of UK women are currently cigarette smokers.[1,2] In general, *a woman who smokes has two to six times the risk of a heart attack of a non-smoking woman.*[9] Absolute smoking cessation (as opposed to decreased cigarette use) should be the goal, because a woman who smokes one to four cigarettes a day is at twice the risk of an acute MI as a non-smoker, while a woman who smokes more than 45 cigarettes a day has a risk that is 11 times higher than that of a non-smoker.[10]

Smoking by women causes 1.5 times as many deaths from CHD as from lung cancer.[9] Active or passive exposure to nicotine and its by-products impairs endothelial function. Exposure to nicotine increases clotting proteins (fibrinogen), enhances the reactivity of platelets (making thrombosis more likely), and increases the viscosity of the blood. Smoking also decreases the advantageous HDL cholesterol.[11] Nicotine exposure injures the endothelium and destabilizes previously established atherosclerotic plaques by promoting plaque rupture and the development of superimposed coronary thrombosis. The process of plaque ruptures and superimposed thrombosis is the sequence of events now accepted to be at the root of most MIs.

Complete cessation of nicotine use and avoidance of passive nicotine inhalation should be the goals. Women should be offered access to formal smoking-cessation programs, which can provide counseling, temporary nicotine replacement therapy, and behavioral therapy.

Hypertension

Approximately half of women over age 45 years have an elevated blood pressure.[12] Systolic and/or diastolic hypertension, defined as a blood pressure of more than 140/90 mmHg or the use of antihypertensive medication, increases independently and powerfully the risk of CHD in women.[13,14] Optimal blood pressure is <120/<80 mmHg and high normal blood pressure is 130–139/85–89 mmHg (see Chapter 13 for more details).

In a patient with no established vascular disease or diabetes, then drug therapy should be used when a non-pharmacological approach fails to bring blood pressure below 140/90 mmHg or when blood pressure is very high (>160/>100 mmHg).[13] The thresholds for patients with established vascular disease or diabetes are discussed below.

Non-pharmacological treatment of hypertension can be extremely effective. Regular physical activity, weight loss, smoking cessation, avoidance of alcohol, a well-balanced diet that is low in saturated fat and high in fiber, with moderate sodium restriction, and stress-management techniques (yoga, meditation) are important elements in a non-pharmacological approach.[12,15]

Diabetes

The prevalence of diabetes is increasing in the USA and in Europe. In the UK, approximately 3% of adults have diabetes; in the USA, the prevalence is 7%.[1,2] Approximately 20% of middle-aged American adults and 35% of older Americans have some degree of glucose intolerance.[16]

Diabetes is a powerful risk factor for CHD in women. In diabetic women, the risk of CHD is three- to seven-fold higher compared with non-diabetic women. With diabetes, the CHD risk increases two to three times in men.[12] In addition to controlling blood glucose, controlling other CHD risk factors such as elevated LDL cholesterol, hypertension, cigarette smoking, obesity, and physical inactivity will reduce the onset of CHD and its complications in women with diabetes.[16]

Diabetes is now considered a "CHD equivalent" because it confers a high risk of new CHD within ten years. The term "CHD equivalent" is used to describe conditions that are associated with a risk for major coronary events equal to that of established CHD, i.e. >20% per ten years. CHD risk equivalents include diabetes, other clinical forms of atherosclerotic disease (peripheral arterial

Table 12.1 Normal lipoprotein levels

Lipoprotein	Suggested maintenance level
LDL cholesterol normal	<100 mg/dl (2.6 mmol/l)
Low HDL cholesterol normal	<40 mg/dl (1.0 mmol/l)
Triglycerides – normal	<150 mg/dl (1.7 mmol/l)
Borderline high	150–199 mg/dl (1.7–2.3 mmol/l)
High	200–499 mg/dl (2.3–5.6 mmol/l)
Very high	>500 mg/dl (5.6 mmol/l)

Data from Executive Summary of the Third Report of the National Cholesterol Education Program (NCEP) Expert Panel on Detection, Evaluation, and Treatment of High Blood Cholesterol in Adults (Adult Treatment Panel III). *J. Am. Med. Assoc.* 2001; **285**:2486–97.

disease, abdominal aortic aneurysm, symptomatic carotid artery disease), and multiple risk factors that confer a ten-year risk for CHD >20%.[17]

The goal in diabetic patients is maintenance of preprandial blood glucose at 80–100 mg/dl (4.4–5.6 mmol/l) and bedtime glucose at 100–140 mg/dl (5.6–7.8 mmol/l). The hemoglobin A1C should be less than 7%, LDL cholesterol less than 100 mg/dl (2.6 mmol/l), and triglycerides less than 150 mg/dl (1.7 mmol/l), and blood pressure should be maintained at less than 130/85 mmHg.[12,16,17] Glucose and hemoglobin A1C should be monitored routinely in diabetic women, and a fasting glucose test should be part of a screening evaluation in obese, non-diabetic women.[12] Regular physical activity should also be encouraged.

Serum lipids

The desirable total cholesterol level is below 200 mg/dl (5.2 mmol/l).[2,17] In the USA, 40% of women older than 55 have an elevated serum cholesterol.[12] In Europe, 91% of women age 65–74 have an elevated cholesterol.[2] *Serum cholesterol rises with age.*[1,2] The higher the blood cholesterol level, the higher the CHD risk.[4]

The new National Cholesterol Education Program – Adult Treatment Panel (NCEP-ATP) III guidelines have made several changes to the recommendations for cholesterol screening and optimal levels for the components.[17] A complete fasting lipoprotein profile with assessment of total cholesterol, LDL, HDL, and triglycerides is recommended as the initial test. The optimal levels are shown in Table 12.1.

LDL cholesterol remains the primary target for lipid intervention to prevent CHD. The recommended levels of LDL cholesterol continue to depend on the number of risk factors present. Risk factors considered in determining the

Table 12.2 Use of risk factors to determine target LDL levels

Age (male >45, female >55)
Family history of premature CHD
Current cigarette smoking
Hypertension
Treatment with antihypertensive medications
Low HDL cholesterol
Diabetes mellitus

target LDL levels for primary prevention include age (men over 45, or women over 55), family history of premature CHD, current cigarette smoking, hypertension or treatment with antihypertensive medications, low HDL cholesterol, and diabetes mellitus.

An HDL level greater than 60 mg/dl or 1.6 mmol/l is considered protective against CHD. When zero or one risk factor is present, then the target LDL is less than 160 mg/dl or 4.1 mmol/l. When there are more than two risk factors, then the target LDL cholesterol is less than 130 mg/dl or 3.4 mmol/l. When CHD is present, or when diabetes, other vascular disease, or multiple risk factors are present, then the target LDL level is less than 100 mg/dl or 2.6 mmol/l.

The new guidelines focus on the importance of diabetes and/or multiple risk factors in CHD risk. People with diabetes mellitus are now considered to have CHD for the purposes of determining their ideal LDL level (CHD equivalent). The Framingham ten-year absolute risk projections should now be used to determine which patients are high risk with a ten-year CHD risk above 20%.[6–8] The target LDL level in these patients and in diabetics should be less than 100 mg/dl or 2.6 mmol/l (Table 12.2).[17]

Lipid management is also critically important in patients with the metabolic syndrome, because it may be involved in most premature CHD in women.[17] The metabolic syndrome exists in women when more than three of the following are present: abdominal obesity (waist circumference >88 cm), triglycerides above 150 mg/dl or 17 mmol/l, HDL cholesterol below 50 mg/dl or 1.3 mmol/l, blood pressure above 130/>85 mmHg, and fasting glucose above 110 mg/dl or 1.0 mmol/l. Approximately 24% of American adults and 43% over the age of 60 have the metabolic syndrome.[18] Women with the metabolic syndrome should be treated promptly with a diet of less than 7% saturated fat and dietary cholesterol less than 200 mg/dl. They should be encouraged to change their diet to lower LDL by eating 5–10 g/day of soluble fiber and 2 g/day of plant stanols/sterols, found in commercial margarines, in fruits and vegetables, or in the form of soy protein (25–40 g/day) to replace animal food products. These patients should also be advised to increase their physical activity and reduce their weight.[17]

In the Cardiovascular Health Study, *the use of statins is associated with a decreased risk of cardiovascular events in older women and men aged 65 or older and with no known previous CHD.*[19] In another large primary prevention study, therapy with lovastatin reduced the risk of first major coronary event by 54% in women and by 34% in men.[20] The major benefit of statin therapy is probably due to its LDL-lowering and HDL-elevating effects. Statin-treated individuals have less CHD than patients with the same cholesterol levels not being treated with statins.[21-23] Statins also inhibit smooth-muscle proliferation and platelet aggregation (important steps in the atherogenic process), enhance endothelial function, and provide anti-inflammatory actions.[24]

Statin therapy is very effective and quite safe. However, there are side effects with the use of these agents. They are absolutely contraindicated in patients with active or chronic liver disease. They are relatively contraindicated in women who concomitantly use ciclosporin, fibrates, niacin, macrolide antibiotics, various antifungal agents, and cytochrome P450 inhibitors.[25] Fibrates are often used in combination with statins in patients with high triglycerides, but these patients should be monitored carefully.

Statins are usually tolerated well. Elevated liver enzymes occur in 0.5–2.0% of treated patients; these elevations are dose-dependent.[25] Approximately 5% of patients complain of muscle aches and joint pains without an elevation of their creatinine phosphokinase (CPK) levels. Severe myositis is rare (approximately 0.08%), and rates of development do not differ between the agents used in the USA, which include atorvastatin, fluvastatin, lovastatin, pravastatin, and impastatin. Cervistatin was observed to have a markedly higher rate of serious side effects and was removed from the market.

Before starting statin therapy, baseline measurements should include a lipid profile, and creatine kinase (CK), alanine transferase (ALT), and aspartate transferase (AST) levels. Elevations of less than three times normal are not contraindications to starting, continuing, or increasing doses of these drugs, but these patients should be monitored carefully.[17,25] Statins should be discontinued if CK levels are more than ten times normal in a patient with muscle tenderness or pain.[25] If a patient has symptoms and a modest or no CK elevation (three to ten times normal), then the patient's symptoms and CK levels should be followed weekly until the trajectory of the problem is clear. If symptoms progress and CK levels rise, it is best to stop the agent. For routine use, ALT and AST should be rechecked after the patient has been on treatment for 12 weeks and then checked annually thereafter, unless symptoms arise.[25]

Obesity

Overweight women are more likely to develop CHD, even if they have no other risk factors. The more overweight the person is, the higher the risk.[26] Body mass index (BMI) is now the common measure of obesity. The risk of CHD is over three times higher among women with a BMI greater than 29 kg/m^2 compared with lean women. Even women who are mildly to moderately overweight (BMI 25–28.9 kg/m^2) have twice the risk of CHD.[27]

BMI is not a perfect measure, however, because it does not consider body fat distribution. In women, a BMI less than 21 kg/m^2 is associated with the greatest protection from CHD. However, for some women, a BMI near 30 kg/m^2 may not be of serious concern if the increased body fat is in the pelvis and not in the abdomen.[28] An increased waist circumference or an increased waist-to-hip ratio predicts morbidity and mortality from CHD.[28] The risk of CHD rises steeply among women whose waist-to-hip ratio is higher than 0.8.[29] In general, the target BMI should be less than 25 kg/m^2 and the waist circumference should be less than 88 cm in women.[12] Gradual and sustained weight loss is the goal.

Physical inactivity

Over 70% of USA and UK women do not get adequate physical exercise.[1,2] Active women have a graded reduction in CHD risk compared with sedentary women.[30,31] *Regular physical activity can also help to lower blood pressure, prevent diabetes, decrease total and LDL cholesterol, raise HDL cholesterol, and help to treat or prevent obesity.*[32] Every woman should accumulate 30 minutes or more of moderate-intensity physical activity on most days of the week.[33,34] Strength training and flexibility are two other additional components of physical fitness.[12,32]

Aspirin for primary prevention

Aspirin has a role in preventing CHD in women. A study of more than 87 000 women showed that those who took a low dose of aspirin regularly were less likely to have a first MI than women who took no aspirin.[35] However, regular aspirin ingestion is associated with side effects such as gastrointestinal bleeding and hemorrhagic stroke.

The risk/benefit ratio for aspirin to decrease the incidence of CHD is favorable if the woman's risk of CHD is greater than 1.5% per year.[36,37] The risk of CHD can be calculated using the Framingham equation and readily available calculators.[6–8] The recommended dose of aspirin is 80–100 mg/day.[37]

Secondary prevention

In secondary prevention, atherosclerosis is the therapeutic target. The pillars of secondary prevention are antiplatelet therapy (usually with aspirin), beta-blockers (regardless of blood pressure), angiotensin-converting enzyme inhibitors (ACEIs) (regardless of blood pressure or ejection fraction), statins (regardless of LDL cholesterol level), cardiac rehabilitation, a Mediterranean diet, and folic acid.

Aspirin

Aspirin has been shown to significantly reduce reinfarction, non-fatal stroke, the need for revisualization, and death in patients with established vascular disease.[38,39] Low-dose aspirin (75–325 mg) is as effective as high-dose aspirin (1200 mg), but with fewer side effects.[39] Aspirin should be continued indefinitely. Patients who are intolerant to aspirin should receive clopidogrel 75 mg/day.[39,40]

Beta-blockers

Beta-blockers reduce the incidence of recurrent MI, sudden cardiac death, and all-cause mortality in the post-infarction patient.[41] Beta-blockers reduce myocardial workload by reducing heart rate, blood pressure, and myocardial contractility. They also increase the threshold for ventricular fibrillation. The highest-risk patients benefit the most; such patients include those with large anterior MI, left ventricular systolic dysfunction, and ventricular arrhythmias, and elderly patients.[40]

Contraindications for the use of beta-blockers include a pulse less than 50, significant hypotension, decompensated heart failure, asthma or reactive airways disease requiring bronchodilators and/or steroids, and second- or third-degree atrioventricular block.[42] Diabetes, peripheral vascular disease, mild/moderate asthma or chronic obstructive pulmonary disease (COPD), asymptomatic bradycardia, and compensated congestive heart failure are not contraindications to the use of beta-blockers.[42]

Beta-blockers should be administered to all post-MI patients without contraindications and should be continued indefinitely. They should be the preferential agent for angina, arrhythmias, and hypertension in the patient with established vascular disease.[40] Beta-blockers should also be considered in all patients with atherosclerosis, since they reduce the risk of MI and make it more likely that the patient will survive an MI.[41] The most common agents in use are atenolol and metoprolol.

Statins

Statins yield a significant decrease in mortality, recurrent MI, recurrent episodes of unstable angina, stroke, the need for revascularization, and hospitalization in patients with established atherosclerosis.[43–45] Statins reduce inflammation and stabilize vulnerable plaques and have been shown to benefit patients with total cholesterol and LDL cholesterol in low, normal, and high ranges.[43–45]

The Medical Research Council (MRC)/British Heart Foundation (BHF) Heart Protection Study examined statin use in 20 536 high-risk individuals (women and men) aged 40–80 years in the UK.[46] These patients either had established vascular disease or diabetes or they were men with hypertension and aged over 60 years. They were randomized to 40 mg/day of simvastatin or placebo and followed for five years. The study found that statin drugs protect a great variety of individuals who were at risk for CVD events. Statins cut the risk of events in patients with CHD and with CHD equivalents, including those with normal or low cholesterol. In the study, 33% had LDL below 116 mg/dl or 3.0 mmol/l, 25% had LDL levels of 116–135 mg/dl or 3.0–3.5 mmol/l, and 42% had LDL above 135 mg/dl or 3.5 mmol/l; simvastatin provided the same significant benefit, irrespective of blood cholesterol. Statins were equally effective in the elderly and in women. Diabetics without prior CVD had a 28% reduction in the incidence of MI.[46] This study will likely cause a rethinking of the recent cholesterol guidelines that now recommend statins to be used to keep LDL cholesterol below 100 mg/dl or 2.6 mmol/l in patients with established vascular disease or CHD equivalents. Given these recent data, all patients with established vascular disease or CHD equivalents should be on a statin.

Angiotensin-converting enzyme inhibitors

ACEIs are powerful secondary prevention agents with very potent cardioprotective and vascular effects. The Heart Outcomes Prevention Evaluation (HOPE) trial was a landmark study carried out in 9297 high-risk patients with either vascular disease or diabetes and one other risk factor. This study included women and men who were at least 55 years of age. The subjects were randomized to ramipril (Altace®) 10 mg/day or placebo for five years. The study was stopped early because of a greater than anticipated protective effect of ramipril in preventing MI, stroke, and cardiovascular death. This study showed a 16% reduction in mortality with ACEIs and a 32% reduction in stroke and a 20% decrease in MI. ACEI use was also associated with fewer diabetic complications, less congestive heart failure, a marked reduction in the development of new diabetes, the need for fewer revascularization procedures, and fewer cardiac arrests.[47]

ACEIs should be used in all patients with atherosclerosis and in all diabetics with or without vascular disease. These agents should be used even if the blood pressure and ejection fraction are normal.[47] These should be started early (12–24 hours) post-MI, and adequate doses should be used (Table 12.3). ACEIs are contraindicated in pregnant women and in women with a history of angioedema or current hyperkalemia. Angiotensin receptor antagonists should be used in ACEI-intolerant patients.[40]

Table 12.3 Adequate doses of ACEIs
for secondary prevention

Drug	Dose (mg/day)
Captopril	150
Enalapril	20
Lisinopril	40
Ramipril	10
Quinapril	40
Trandolapril	4

Synergy of medications

The potential cumulative impact of the use of aspirin, beta-blockers, statins, and ACEIs is dramatic. Since each agent alone produces a relative risk reduction of 25%, together they can potentially reduce the relative risk by more than 75%.[48] Thus, systematic pharmacologic secondary prevention can bring CHD patients great benefit.

Cardiac rehabilitation

Cardiac rehabilitation offers many benefits to post-MI patients, including improved functional capacity and quality of life, improved medication compliance, reduced risk of subsequent events, and cardiovascular mortality.[49] Only 15% of qualifying patients participate in rehab programs, and evidence suggests that women are less likely to be referred than men.[50]

Mediterranean diet

The best data on a diet that prevents recurrent CHD events are from the Lyon Diet Heart Study.[51] This study found that the Mediterranean diet, rich in linolenic acid, reduced cardiovascular events in patients who had survived their first heart attack.[51] In the study, the treatment group was advised to eat more bread, more vegetables, more fruit, more fish, and less meat, and to replace butter and cream with canola (rapeseed) oil margarine. The treatment group also ate 50% more fruit than the usual care group. The trial was stopped after 27 months because of a 70% relative risk reduction in death in the intervention group. The effect remained significant at 46 months of follow-up.[51]

The components of the Mediterranean diet include cold-water fish (salmon and halibut), olive oil, low glycemic carbohydrates, plenty of fruits, vegetables (onion and garlic), and nuts, and small amounts of red wine (quercetin), which amounts to a diet composed of 20–25% protein, 30–35% healthy fats, and 45–50% carbohydrates.[52]

Folic acid and other B vitamins

Homocysteine is an amino acid that is produced in the body and that requires adequate amounts of certain B vitamins for its breakdown. Homocysteine levels in the blood correlate independently with the risk and severity of coronary artery disease and predict mortality in patients with established vascular disease.[53,54] *A homocysteine level greater than 10.0 μmol/l is considered high risk for heart disease.*[55,56]

A recent study in patients post-percutaneous coronary intervention showed that treatment with folic acid and vitamins B12 and B6 decreased significantly the need for revascularization and the overall rate of adverse events compared with placebo.[57] Until additional large clinical trials showing that treatment actually makes a difference are completed, an emphasis should be on achieving adequate amounts of B vitamins through the consumption of vegetables, fruits, legumes, meats, fish, and fortified grains and cereals. In patients with established vascular disease, if dietary changes fail to lower the homocysteine level below 10.0 μmol/l, then supplementation with folic acid 1–2 mg/day, vitamin B12 0.5–1.0 mg/day, and vitamin B6 25–100 mg/day should be offered, but only after underlying B12 deficiency is ruled out.[55]

Hormone replacement therapy: a preventive therapy that has fallen from favor

Physicians have had to rethink the use of hormone replacement therapy (HRT) for primary and secondary prevention of CHD, given the results of recent studies. The first surprise came with the results of the Hormone Replacement Study (HERS) in postmenopausal women with established vascular disease. This large, randomized clinical trial of combined estrogen and progesterone versus placebo showed that at 6.8 years of follow-up, combined HRT did not reduce the risk of subsequent cardiovascular events in women who already had CHD.[58] The HERS trial did not have an estrogen-only arm.

The next major and even more significant blow to the use of combined HRT for CHD prevention came when the Women's Health Initiative (WHI) was stopped early, at just over five years rather than after the planned 8.5 years. The WHI showed that in healthy women without vascular disease, treatment with combined HRT actually increased the risk of heart disease and breast cancer.[59] Even though the increased risk was small, women on HRT had more MIs, strokes, and blood clots. The WHI is continuing to investigate the effects of estrogen alone used for women who have had a hysterectomy. Experts now feel that *there is no basis for the use of combined estrogen and progesterone to prevent CHD in either primary or secondary prevention.*

Conclusions

Future heart attacks are prevented by the prevention of atherosclerosis or plaque formation in the coronary arteries and by the stabilization and regression of existing plaque through lifestyle modification and medication. *Coronary bypass surgery and angioplasty with stent placement do not prevent future heart attacks in patients with chronic CHD.* These procedures only relieve ischemia in the distribution of established stenoses. All women must take personal preventive action to prevent CHD death and disability by working to prevent plaque formation and promote stabilization of existing atherosclerotic disease. This is the basis of CHD prevention in women.

REFERENCES

1 American Heart Association. *2002 Heart and Stroke Statistical Update.* Dallas: American Heart Association; 2001.

2 European Heart Network. www.ehnheart.org/statistics/summary. Accessed September 23, 2002.

3 Verma, S. and Anderson, T. J. Fundamentals of endothelial function for the clinical cardiologist. *Circulation* 2002; **105**:546–9.

4 Lerner, D. J. and Kannel, W. B. Patterns of coronary heart disease morbidity and mortality in the sexes: a 26-year follow-up of the Framingham population. *Am. Heart J.* 1986; **111**:383–90.

5 Rich-Edwards, J. W., Manson, J. E., Hennekens, C. H and Buring, J. E. The primary prevention of coronary heart disease in women. *N. Engl. J. Med.* 1995; **332**: 1758–66.

6 Grundy, S. M., Pasternak, R., Greenland, P., *et al.* Assessment of cardiovascular risk by use of multiple risk factor equations: a statement for healthcare professionals from the American Heart Association and the American College of Cardiology. *J. Am. Coll. Cardiol.* 1999; **34**:1348–59.

7 Wilson, P. W. F., D'Agostino, R. B., Levy, D., *et al.* Prediction of coronary risks using risk factor categories. *Circulation* 1998; **97**:1837–47.

8 www.statcoder.com. Accessed September 23, 2002.

9 www.nhlbi.nih.gov/health/public/heart/other/hhw/index.htm. Accessed September 23, 2002.

10 Willett, W. C., Green, A., Stampfer, M. J., *et al.* Relative and absolute excess risk of coronary heart disease among women who smoke cigarettes. *N. Engl. J. Med.* 1987; **317**:1303–9.

11 Ockene, I. S. and Miller, N. H. Cigarette smoking, cardiovascular disease, and stroke: a statement for healthcare professionals from the American Heart Association. *Circulation* 1997; **96**:3243–7.

12 Mosca, L., Grundy, S., Judelson, D., *et al.* Guide to preventive cardiology for women. AHA/ACC Scientific statement: consensus panel statement. *J. Am. Coll. Cardiol.* 1999; **33**:1751–5.

13 The sixth report of the Joint National Committee on prevention, detection, evaluation, and treatment of high blood pressure. *Arch. Intern. Med.* 1997; **157**:2413–46.

14 Moser, M., Hebert, P. and Hennekens, C. H. An overview of the meta-analyses of the hypertension treatment trials. *Arch. Intern. Med.* 1991; **151**:1277–9.

15 Labarthe, D. and Ayala, C. Non-drug interventions in hypertension prevention and control. *Cardiol. Clin.* 2002; **20**:249–63.

16 Grundy, S. M., Howard, B., Smith, S., *et al.* Prevention conference VI: diabetes and cardiovascular disease. Executive summary. Conference proceeding for healthcare professionals from a special writing group of the American Heart Association. *Circulation* 2002; **105**:2231–9.

17 Expert Panel on Detection, Evaluation, and Treatment of High Blood Cholesterol. Executive Summary of the Third Report of the National Cholesterol Education Program (NCEP) Expert Panel on Detection, Evaluation, and Treatment of High Blood Cholesterol in Adults (Adult Treatment Panel III). *J. Am. Med. Assoc.* 2001; **285**:2486–97.

18 Ford, E. S., Giles, W. H. and Dietz, W. H. Prevalence of the metabolic syndrome among U.S. adults: findings from the third National Health and Nutrition Survey. *J. Am. Med. Assoc.* 2002; **287**:356–9.

19 Lemaitre, R. N., Psaty, B. M., Heckbert, S. R., *et al.* Therapy with hydroxymethylglutaryl coenzyme A reductase inhibitors (statins) and associated risk of incident cardiovascular events in older adults – evidence from the cardiovascular health study. *Arch. Intern. Med.* 2002; **162**:1395–400.

20 Downs, J. R., Clearfield, M., Weis, S., *et al.* Primary prevention of acute coronary events with lovastatin in men and women with average cholesterol levels: results of AFCAPS/TexCAPS. *J. Am. Med. Assoc.* 1998; **279**:1615–22.

21 Sacks, F. M., Pfeffer, M. A., Moye, L. A., *et al.* The effect of pravastatin on coronary events after myocardial infarction in patients with average cholesterol levels: cholesterol and recurrent events trial investigators. *N. Engl. J. Med.* 1996; **335**:1001–9.

22 Packard, C. J. Influence of pravastatin and plasma lipids on clinical events in the West of Scotland Coronary Prevention Study (WOSCOPS). *Circulation* 1998; **87**: 1440–45.

23 LaRosa, J. C., He, J. and Vupputuri, S. Effect of statins on the risk of coronary disease: a meta-analysis of randomized controlled trials. *J. Am. Med. Assoc.* 1999; **282**:2340–46.

24 Yeung, A. C. and Tsao, P. Statin therapy: beyond cholesterol lowering and antiinflammatory effects. *Circulation* 2002; **105**:2937–38.

25 Pasternak, R. C., Smith, S. C., Jr, Bairey-Merz, C. N., *et al.* ACC/AHA/NHLBI advisory on the use and safety of statins. *J. Am. Coll. Cardiol.* 2002; **40**:567–72.

26 Field, A. E., Coakley, E. H., Must, A., *et al.* Impact of overweight on the risk of developing common chronic diseases during a 10-year period. *Arch. Intern. Med.* 2001; **161**:1581–6.

27 Manson, J. E., Stampfer, M. J., Colditz, G. A., *et al.* A prospective study of obesity and the risk of coronary heart disease in women. *N. Engl. J. Med.* 1990; **322**:882–9.

28 Eckel, R. H. Obesity and heart disease: a statement for healthcare professionals from the Nutrition Committee, American Heart Association. *Circulation* 1997; **96**:3248–50.

29 Bjorntorp, P. Regional patterns of fat distribution. *Ann. Intern. Med.* 1985; **103**: 994–5.

30 Lemaitre, R. N., Heckbert, S. R., Psaty, B. M. and Siscovick, D. S. Leisure-time physical activity and the risk of nonfatal myocardial infarction in postmenopausal women. *Arch. Intern. Med.* 1995; **155**:2302–8.

31 Kushi, L. H., Fee, R. M., Folsom, A. R., *et al.* Physical activity and mortality in postmenopausal women. *J. Am. Med. Assoc.* 1997; **277**:1287–92.

32 Fletcher, G. F., Balady, G., Blair, S. N., *et al.* Statement on exercise: benefits and recommendations for physical activity programs for all Americans. A statement for healthcare professionals by the Committee on Exercise and Cardiac Rehabilitation of the Council on Clinical Cardiology, American Heart Association. *Circulation* 1996; **94**:857–62.

33 Physical activity and cardiovascular health. NIH Consensus Development Panel on Physical Activity and Cardiovascular Health. *J. Am. Med. Assoc.* 1996; **276**:241–6.

34 US Department of Health and Human Services. *Physical Activity and Health: A Report of the Surgeon General.* Atlanta, GA: US Department of Health and Human Services, Public Health Service, CDC, National Center for Chronic Disease Prevention and Health Promotion; 1996.

35 Manson, J. E., Stampfer, M. J., Colditz, G. A., *et al.* A prospective study of aspirin use and primary prevention of cardiovascular disease in women. *J. Am. Med. Assoc.* 1991; **266**:521–7.

36 US Preventive Services Task Force. Aspirin for the primary prevention of cardiovascular events: recommendation and rationale. *Ann. Intern. Med.* 2002; **136**:157–60.

37 Lauer, M. Aspirin for the primary prevention of coronary events. *N. Engl. J. Med.* 2002; **346**:1468–74.

38 Antiplatelet Trialists' Collaboration. Collaborative overview of randomised trials of antiplatelet therapy – I: prevention of death, myocardial infarction, and stroke by prolonged antiplatelet therapy in various categories of patients. *Br. Med. J.* 1994; **308**:81–106.

39 Hennekens, C. H., Dyken, M. L. and Fuster, V. Aspirin as a therapeutic agent in cardiovascular disease. A statement for health care professionals from the American Heart Association. *Circulation* 1997; **96**:2751–3.

40 Smith, S. C., Blair, S. N., Bonow, R. O., *et al.* AHA/ACC Guidelines for preventing heart attack and death in patients with atherosclerotic cardiovascular disease: 2001 update. *Circulation* 2001; **104**:1577–9.

41 Frishman, W. H. and Cheng, A. Secondary prevention of myocardial infarction: role of beta-adrenergic blockers and angiotensin-converting enzyme inhibitors. *Am. Heart J.* 1999; **137**:S25–34.

42 Gheorghiade, M. and Golstein, S. Beta blockers in the post-myocardial infarction patient. *Circulation* 2002; **106**: 394–8.

43 Scandinavian Simvastatin Survival Study Group. Randomised trial of cholesterol lowering in 4444 patients with coronary heart disease: the Scandinavian simvastatin survival study (4S). *Lancet* 1994; **344**:1383–9.

44 Lewis, S. J., Sacks, F. M., Mitchell, J. S., *et al.* Effect of pravastatin on cardiovascular events in women after myocardial infarction: the Cholesterol and Recurrent Events (CARE) Trial. *J. Am. Coll. Cardiol.* 1998; **32**:140–46.

45 The Long-Term Intervention with Pravastatin in Ischaemic Disease (LIPID) Study Group. Prevention of cardiovascular events and deaths with pravastatin in patients with coronary heart disease and a broad range of initial cholesterol levels. *N. Engl. J. Med.* 1998; **339**:1349–57.

46 Heart Protection Study Collaborative Group. MRC/BHF Heart Protection Study of cholesterol lowering with simvastatin in 20,536 high risk individuals: a randomized placebo-controlled trial. *Lancet* 2002; **360**:7–22.

47 The Heart Outcomes Prevention Evaluation Study Investigators. Effects of an angiotensin-converting enzyme inhibitor, ramipril, on cardiovascular events in high-risk patients. *N. Engl. J. Med.* 2000; **342**:145–53.

48 Yusuf, S. Two decades of progress in preventing vascular disease. *Lancet* 2002; **360**:2–3.

49 American College of Cardiology and American Heart Association Task Force on Practice Guidelines. ACC/AHA guidelines for the management of patients with acute myocardial infarction. www.acc.org/clinical/guidelines/nov96/1999/index.htm. Accessed September 23, 2002.

50 Mosca, L., Manson, J. E., Sutherland, S. E., *et al.* Cardiovascular disease in women. A statement for healthcare professionals from the American Heart Association. *Circulation* 1997; **96**:2468–82.

51 DeLorgeril, M., Salen, P., Martin, J. L., *et al.* Mediterranean diet, traditional risk factors, and the rate of cardiovascular complications after myocardial infarction: final report of the Lyon Diet Heart Study. *Circulation* 1999; **99**:779–85.

52 American Heart Association. www.americanheart.org. Accessed September 23, 2002.

53 Boushey, C. J., Beresford, S. A. A., Omenn, G. S. and Motulsky, A. G. A quantitative assessment of plasma homocysteine as a risk factor for vascular disease; probable benefits of increasing folic acid intakes. *J. Am. Med. Assoc.* 1995; **274**:1049–57.

54 Nygard, O., Nordrehaug, J. E., Refsum, H., *et al.* Plasma homocysteine levels and mortality in patients with coronary artery disease. *N. Engl. J. Med.* 1997; **337**:230–36.

55 Malinow, M. R., Bostom, A. G., Krauss, R. M. Homocysteine, diet and cardiovascular diseases: a statement for health care professionals from the nutrition committee, American Heart Association. *Circulation* 1999; **99**:178–82.

56 Homocysteine Lowering Trialists' Collaboration. Lowering blood homocysteine with folic acid based supplements: meta-analysis of randomised trials. *Br. Med. J.* 1998; **316**:894–8.

57 Schnyder, G., Roffi, M., Flammer, Y., Pin, R. and Hess, O. M. Effect of homocysteine-lowering therapy with folic acid, vitamin B 12, and vitamin B 6 on clinical outcomes after percutaneous coronary intervention: the Swiss Heart Study: a randomized controlled trial. *J. Am. Med. Assoc.* 2002; **288**:973–9.

58 Grady, D., Herrington, D., Bittner, V., *et al.* Cardiovascular disease outcomes during 6.8 years of hormone replacement therapy: Heart and Estrogen/Progestin Replacement Study follow-up (HERS II). *J. Am. Med. Assoc.* 2002; **288**:49–57.

59 Writing Group for the Women's Health Initiative Investigators. Risks and benefits of estrogen plus progestin in healthy postmenopausal women: principal results form the Women's Health Initiative randomized controlled trial. *J. Am. Med. Assoc.* 2002; **288**:321–33.

13

Hypertension and stroke

Jo Ann Rosenfeld

Case: M.M. is a 54-year-old obese woman who has not seen a physician in two years. She has a history of hypertension and high cholesterol. She works full time as an accountant for a medium-sized firm and has spent all her spare time for the past two years caring for her mother, who died two years after being incapacitated by a stroke. She has two married daughters who live across the country. She wants to control her hypertension so she doesn't end up like her mother and as a burden to her children.

Introduction

Hypertension has been termed the "silent killer." Working with women to control their hypertension can positively affect their future health. Treating and controlling hypertension can decrease the risks of heart disease, death, myocardial infarction (MI), kidney disease, and stroke. Yet, fewer than half of individuals with hypertension receive treatment, and of those who are under treatment fewer than half are controlled well.[1,2] Strokes may be prevented primarily or secondarily in individuals with certain risk factors, but the treatment is not completely effective.

Hypertension

Impact

Approximately one-fifth of adults over the age of 40 have high blood pressure. Hypertension is the most common cause of stroke in the UK and the most common cause of renal failure in the USA.[1] Women are more likely than men to have hypertension, and the risk of hypertension increases with age.

Uncontrolled hypertension affects health profoundly negatively, and improving hypertension improves health. Hypertensive women have four times the rate of stroke as non-hypertensive women.[3] The noteworthy truth about hypertension is that treating it reduces risks of other diseases. *Small reductions in blood pressures will decrease many other risks, including the increased risk of stroke.*[1] For women over age 50, one-half of the reduction of stroke mortality in white women and two-thirds the reduction in African-American women is linked to the reduction of high blood pressure.[4]

The etiology of high blood pressure is known in only 5% of individuals.[1] The remaining 95%, who have what is termed "essential hypertension," show a variety of genetic patterns, including no patterns, suggesting that there is a variety of types of essential hypertension. Secondary causes of hypertension include alcohol abuse, renal vascular and parenchymal disease, and certain endocrine states, including pheochromocytoma, Cushing's syndrome, and primary aldosteronism.

Diagnosis

Blood pressure measurement is a specific science, and the relevance of any one blood pressure reading is questionable. Blood pressure should be measured with the woman sitting, after resting for 15 minutes, and at least 15 minutes since smoking a cigarette and/or drinking coffee. The cuff should be the correct size, approximately two-thirds the length of the upper arm. Readings of greater than 140/90 mmHg at more than one visit are considered indicative of hypertension, while readings of greater than 135/80–85 mmHg are considered borderline. Borderline blood pressure readings are becoming more important because recent evidence suggests that treating even borderline high blood pressure may reduce morbidity and mortality.

Whether "white-coat hypertension" exists and its relevance are disputed. Some experts believe that if a woman has high blood pressure readings, even only at the physician's office, then she will or can have them elsewhere, even if her readings at home or elsewhere are often normal. However, a recent study suggested that the pressure reading in the physician's office is the least specific (only 43%) in predicting hypertension, although it is fairly sensitive (85%). Blood pressure readings taken at home by the patient, ambulatory blood pressure evaluations, or home nurse-taken blood pressures are more specific.[5] At any rate, if the woman takes a series of blood pressure readings at home and discusses these with her physician, then a more accurate picture of the trend will be obtained.

The initial evaluation of the woman with hypertension is minimal, because most women have essential hypertension. If these preliminary tests are normal and the woman responds to medication, then no further testing is needed. Serum electrolytes, blood urea nitrogen, thyroid-stimulating hormone and creatinine levels, and a urine analysis are the minimum tests needed. Fasting serum lipid, glucose, and glycosolated hemoglobin levels may be obtained to examine for other risk factors of heart disease.

A history of sudden emergent severely high blood pressure, alcohol abuse or kidney disease, and/or a physical examination that showed signs of end-stage damage or Cushing's syndrome, including striae, truncal obesity, a hump, and bruising, would suggest that a more extensive evaluation is needed. Similarly, abnormal electrolytes, especially potassium levels, might indicate the need to evaluate for endocrinopathies. An elevated blood urea nitrogen or creatinine level or an abnormal urine analysis would indicate the need to examine renal functions with 24-hour urine tests, serum levels of metanephrines, urine culture, morning and/or afternoon cortisol levels, and intravenous pyleograms and renal ultrasounds.

Treatment

Most studies of treatment have primarily enrolled men. Many studies have not separated women from men in the results. However, a meta-analysis of more than seven drug studies with more than 20 000 women and men found that treatment significantly improved the risk of fatal coronary events, stroke, and fatal stroke in women as well as men.[6]

"Control" or goal levels for hypertension are a systolic blood pressure (SBP) below 140 mmHg and a diastolic blood pressure (DBP) below 85 mmHg.

Lifestyle changes and non-pharmacological therapy

The primary treatment of hypertension definitely starts with lifestyle changes, especially in individuals with borderline hypertension.

Diet and weight reduction, if needed, are the primary treatments. A low-fat, low-salt diet is important. Weight loss of 10–20% may obviate or reduce the need for pharmacological therapy. *Patients who lose weight may be able to stop medication.* A weight loss of 10 kg may reduced a woman's risk of hypertension by 26%. Alternatively, an increase in weight of 1 kg is associated with a 12% risk of developing hypertension.[7] Reducing alcohol consumption is also important.

Sodium reduction does not have to be excessive to impact blood pressure levels. Reducing intake from the normal 12–15 g daily of salt to 5–7 g daily can reduce systolic blood pressure by an average of 7.6 mm in women.[8]

Exercise is another important part of therapy. At a minimum, 20–30 minutes of concentrated activity three times a week is necessary and may aid in weight loss. Walking, swimming, aqua therapy including walking in pools, and low-impact aerobics can be a good first start, especially in elderly women, obese women, and those who have had little exercise recently.

Pharmacological therapy

Pharmacological therapy is initiated in individuals in whom lifestyle changes are not accomplished or are inadequate to control hypertension and in those individuals who have sustained blood pressure readings greater than 160 mmHg systolic and/or 100 mmHg diastolic.[9] In individuals with diabetes or who have evidence of end-stage target organ damage, treatment should be started if blood pressure is higher than 140/90 mmHg.[3]

Recent studies have found that *the most important factor is getting the blood pressure controlled, and "this is more important than the means."*[10] Similarly, most patients will need more than one medication. Several commissions have suggested that the first-line drugs should be low-dose thiazide diuretics or beta-blockers, in the absence of other factors. Beta-blockers, especially the cardioselective types, are good medications for many individuals. Data suggest that use of beta-blockers may reduce the incidence of strokes but not total mortality.[11] They are especially good choices in patients with tachycardia, anxiety, migraine headaches, and angina. They should be avoided in asthmatics, patients with bradycardia or atrioventricular blocks, and diabetic patients using insulin who may become hypoglycemic. Beta-blockers can make the individual feel slow, tired, or depressed. Their effects on women's sexual function are not known.

Diuretics are effective antihypertensive medications, but they may worsen incontinence and glycemic and lipid control, and they may cause hypokalemia.

Angiotensin-converting enzyme inhibitors (ACEIs) are effective treatment and have many other effects, some of which are not understood. They protect renal function in diabetics, and one study found recently that ramipril decreased the risk of stroke, even in diabetic individuals who were not overtly hypertensive.[12] However, up to 49% of women on, ACEIs may develop a cough. The angiotensin II inhibitors are another good choice and have been found to be as effective in reducing blood pressure and microalbuminuria in diabetic hypertensive patients.[13]

The short-acting calcium-channel blocker nifedipine has been implicated in increasing heart failure and in increasing the risk of breast cancer. However, sustained-release forms are effective and a good choice in treating hypertension, especially in individuals with angina, atrial tachycardias, or migraines.

Comparison of different classes of drugs has produced a variety of results. One study of more than 6000 patients aged 70–84 found no difference in control of blood pressure or morbidity or mortality between use of diuretics, beta-blockers, calcium-channel blockers, and ACEIs.[14] A meta-analysis found that ACEIs and calcium-channel blockers reduced cardiovascular mortality and morbidity as well as beta-blockers and thiazide diuretics.[15] The Antihypertensive and Lipid-Lowering Treatment to Prevent Heart Attack Trial (ALLHAT) study, a randomized, double-blind, controlled clinical trial examining 42 418 patients with mild to moderate hypertension and aged 55 years

Table 13.1 Medications that can interfere with blood pressure medications or worsen hypertension

Dietary: alcohol, caffeine, licorice
Appetite suppressants
Anesthetics
Analgesics: non-steroidal anti-inflammatory drugs
Medications containing sodium: antacids, antibiotics
Hormones: adrenal steroids, chronic steroid use, erythropoietin; oral contraceptives
Illegal substances: cocaine, amphetamines, androgen steroids

or older, examined the results of one of four antihypertensive treatments: the diuretic chlortalidone (12.5–25 mg daily), the ACEI lisinopril (10–40 mg daily), the calcium-channel blocker amlodipine (2.5–10 mg daily), and the alpha-blocker doxazosin (1–8 mg daily). More than 15 000 participants were women, and more than 10 000 were African-American. The effects of all drugs except doxazosin were similar in reduction of mortality and heart disease. However, lisinopril was significantly less effective than the diuretic at reducing stroke and combined cardiovascular disease, and chlortalidone use reduced the incidence of heart failure.[16] A recent editorial from the *British Medical Journal* states: "What matters most is getting blood pressure controlled, and this is overwhelmingly more important than the means."[17]

Concomitant illnesses may indicate the need for different first-line drugs. Diabetics should be given ACEIs, whereas patients with cardiac disease may need medications that are also anti-anginal, such as calcium-channel blockers.

Difficult-to-treat hypertension

Hypertension may be difficult to control because the blood pressure levels have been measured inaccurately, because the disease has progressed with time, because it is caused by another disease or medication, and/or because the medication used is suboptimal.

The patient may be taking too much sodium and/or inadequate diuretics. Certain medications or diets may interfere with blood pressure medicines (Table 13.1)[2]. One in ten individuals uses non-steroidal anti-inflammatory drugs (NSAIDs), and two meta-analyses have found that NSAIDs raise the blood pressure by an average of 3.3–5 mmHg in individuals with hypertension.[18,19]

Concomitant diseases can make high blood pressure difficult to control. *Alcohol or cigarette abuse can worsen hypertensive control.* Individuals with panic attacks or generalized anxiety disorder, pain disorders, or delirium, because of autonomic excess, may have difficult-to-control blood pressure levels. Approximately 40% of those with hypertension are obese.[2]

Table 13.2 Risk factors for stroke

Hypertension
Atrial fibrillation
Diabetes
History of recent MI
Cigarette smoking
Alcohol abuse
High-fat, high-salt diet
Obesity
Low exercise
Hyperlipidemia

Stroke

Strokes are one of the most important causes of disability and the second most common cause of death worldwide.[20] Although there have been recent advances in treatment, few patients receive thrombolysis and its importance is disputed. Treatment may include immediate thrombolysis, long-term rehabilitation, and avoidance of complications and prevention of repeat strokes. Prevention, both primary and secondary, has thus become more important.

Diagnosis

An individual with stroke presents with the sudden onset of a focal neurological deficit. Clinical history and physical examination cannot distinguish a thrombotic from a hemorrhagic stroke, although the symptoms of a thrombotic stroke may resolve within an hour while those of a hemorrhagic stroke seldom do. Radiological examination is imperative. A computed tomography (CT) scan done within two weeks should distinguish between the types of stroke. Magnetic resonance imaging (MRI) may show a smaller hemorrhage or area of thrombosis and is more accurate in the brainstem.

Examination for the causes of stroke is important. An electrocardiogram (EKG) may show atrial fibrillation. An echocardiogram may show valvular disease, left atrial enlargement, or thrombus, and/or left ventricular dysfunction. Any of these may indicate the need for long-term anticoagulation.

Primary and secondary prevention

Primary prevention focuses on reducing risk factors for stroke. *The six most important factors are hypertension, atrial fibrillation, history of recent MI, diabetes, cigarette smoking, and alcohol abuse.* Weight reduction in obese people and control of hyperlipidemia can reduce the risk of stroke (Table 13.2).

Table 13.3 Individuals in whom warfarin use is recommended to reduce the risk of stroke

---

Patients with atrial fibrillation and one or more of the following: previous TIA, previous
 stroke, previous embolism, hypertension or left ventricular function, age >75 years
Patients with atrial fibrillation, aged 65–75, and with no risk factors
Patients with MI and who have other risk factors, including non-valvular atrial fibrillation,
 decreased left ventricular ejection fraction, and left ventricular thrombus

---

Data from Gubitz, G. and Sandercock, P. Prevention of ischaemic stroke. *Br. Med. J.*
2000; **321**:1455–9.

Secondary prevention may be implemented in individuals who have had transient ischemic attacks (TIAs), a history of vascular disease with occlusion, or those who have survived a previous stroke. Eighty per cent of individuals survive a stroke; of these, 10% will have another one within one year and the risk of another stroke continues at 5% per year.[12]

Control of hypertension is the single most important way to reduce the risk of stroke; for every 7.5-mm increase in diastolic blood pressure, the risk of stroke doubles.[21] The greatest reduction in risk is in the elderly.

Dietary and lifestyle changes have been shown to reduce risk of stroke. A low-salt, low-fat diet, control of hyperlipidemia, reduction of obesity, and exercise may reduce the risk of a first stroke. Reducing or quitting cigarette smoking is important. Once a woman stops smoking, her risk of stroke returns to that of a non-smoker within three to five years.[22]

Reduction of cholesterol levels by use of statin drugs, especially in patients with coexisting coronary heart disease, has been recommended to reduce the risk of fatal and non-fatal stroke.[23]

Anticoagulation

Anticoagulation in patients with atrial fibrillation will definitely reduce the risk of primary stroke by 48–72%.[24] Warfarin was significantly more effective than aspirin as prevention for both primary and second strokes. Guidelines suggest warfarin use in patients of any age with atrial fibrillation and any of the risk factors for stroke listed in Table 13.3.

Anticoagulation for patients in normal sinus rhythm is not indicated and even increases the risk of hemorrhagic stroke.

Primary prevention by use of therapeutic agents

Recently, use of ACEIs, particularly ramipril (10 mg daily), in diabetic non-hypertensive patients has been shown to reduce the risk of stroke by 32%.[15] Use of aspirin also reduces the risk of ischemic stroke. Although various daily doses (82–600 mg) are effective, the risk of bleeding increases with the dose. Thus, the lowest possible daily dose is suggested.

Secondary prevention

Once a patient has had a TIA or stroke, then risk factor reduction is even more important. Risk of recurrence of another stroke after the first stroke is 8% per year; after a TIA, the risk of a stroke is 8% in the first month, then 5% after a year.[24]

As with primary prevention, there are several modifiable risk factors. Changing to a low-fat, low-salt diet, reducing or eliminating alcohol and tobacco use, controlling diabetes and cholesterol levels, reducing weight, and increasing exercise are important. Although evidence as to whether hypertensive control is as important in reducing the risk of a second stroke is disputed,[25] anticoagulation of individuals with atrial fibrillation will also reduce the risk of a second stroke.[16]

Anticoagulation

Use of antiplatelet drugs, specifically aspirin and anticoagulants, reduces the risk of stroke in individuals with atrial fibrillation and who have had a previous ischemic stroke.[26] Anticoagulation of individuals in normal sinus rhythm with warfarin to levels of international normalized ratio (INR) 2.0–3.0 does not decrease the risk of thrombotic stroke but *increases* the risk of hemorrhagic stroke.[27] Use of clopidogrel shows a modest reduction in stroke risk greater than aspirin. *Anticoagulation with warfarin is indicated in all individuals who have atrial fibrillation and who have had a TIA or stroke and who have no contraindications.* The range of anticoagulation should be 2.0–3.0 INR. For those individuals in whom warfarin is contraindicated or problematic (history of gastrointestinal bleeding, peptic ulcer disease, frequent falls or seizures, alcohol abuse, unreliable social history, etc.), use of aspirin is an acceptable alternative, because it does reduce the risk of stroke by as much as 2.5% per year for secondary prevention.[28]

Surgical treatment of carotid artery stenosis

Although it is disputed as to whether treatment of carotid artery stenosis by endarectomy in asymptomatic individuals reduces the risk of stroke, its use in symptomatic patients (patients with a stroke or a CVA) is clearer. For symptomatic individuals with severe stenosis (defined as greater than 70% but less than 100% by angiography), surgery nearly eliminates the risk of ipsilateral stroke. Individuals with moderate (40–60%) occlusion also benefit.[29]

Summary

Treatment of hypertension is one of the best, and best-proven, methods of reducing morbidity and mortality. Accurate diagnosis, close concordance and relationship between physician and patient, and adequate therapy with lifestyle changes, exercise, and pharmocotherapy are essential. Primary and secondary prevention of stroke by lifestyle changes, control of hypertension and diabetes, and therapeutic use of aspirin, warfarin, or ACEIs will prevent further morbidity and mortality.

REFERENCES

1 Brown, M. J. Science, medicine and the future. Hypertension. *Br. Med. J.* 1997; **314**:1258.

2 O'Rorke, J. E. and Richardson, W. S. Evidence based management of hypertension: what to do when blood pressure is difficult to control. *Br. Med. J.* 2001; **322**:1229–32.

3 Mercuro, G., Sonco, S., Pilia I., *et al.* Effects of acute administration of transdermal estrogen on postmenopausal women with systemic hypertension. *Am. J. Cardiol.* 1997; **80**:652–7.

4 Joint National Committee on Prevention, Detection, Evaluation, and Treatment of High Blood Pressure. The Sixth Report of the Joint National Committee on Prevention, Detection, Evaluation, and Treatment of High Blood Pressure. NIH publication no. 98-4080. Bethesda, MD: National Institutes of Health; 1997.

5 Little, P., Barnett, J., Barnsley, L., *et al.* Comparison of agreement between different measures of blood pressure in primary care and daytime ambulatory blood pressure. *Br. Med. J.* 200; **325**:254–7.

6 Gueyffier, F., Boutitie, F., Boissel, J. P., *et al.* Effect of antihypertensive drug treatment on cardiovascular outcomes in women and men. *Ann. Intern. Med.* 1997; **126**:761–7.

7 Huang, Z., Willett, W. C., Mason, J. E., *et al.* Body weight, weight change and the risk for hypertension in women. *Ann. Intern. Med.* 1998; **128**:81–8.

8 Geleijnse, J. M., Wetteman, J. C., Back, A. A., Breijen, J. H. and Grobee D. E. Reduction in blood pressure with a low sodium, high potassium, high magnesium salt in older subjects with mild to moderate hypertension. *Br. Med. J.* 1994; **309**:436–40.

9 Ramsay, L., Williams, B., Johnston, G., *et al.* Guidelines for management of hypertension: report of the third working party of the British Hypertension Society. *J. Hum. Hypertens.* 1999; **13**:569–92.

10 Williams, B. Drug treatment of hypertension. *Br. Med. J. USA* 2003; **3**:127–9.

11 Mulrow, C. D. and Pignone, M. Evidence based management of hypertension: what are the elements of good treatment for hypertension? *Br. Med. J.* 2001; **322**:1107–9.

12 Bosch, J., Yusuf, S., Pogue, J., *et al.* Use of ramipril in preventing stroke: double blind randomised trial. *Br. Med. J.* 2002; **324**:699–702.

13 Mogensen, C. E., Neldam, S., Tikkanen, I., *et al.* Randomised controlled trial of dual blockade of renin–angiotensin system in patients with hypertension, microalbuminuria, and non-insulin dependent diabetes: the candesartan and lisinopril microalbuminuria (CALM) study. *Br. Med. J.* 2000; **321**:1440–44.

14 Hansson, L., Lindholm, L. H., Ekbom, T., *et al.* Randomised trial of old and new antihypertensive drugs in elderly patients: cardiovascular mortality and morbidity. The Swedish Trial in Old Patients with Hypertension-2 study. *Lancet* 1999; **354**: 1751–6.

15 Collaboration Blood Pressure Lowering Treatment Trialists. Effects of angiotensin converting enzyme inhibitors, calcium antagonists and other blood pressure lowering drugs on mortality and major cardiovascular morbidity. *Lancet* 2000; **356**: 1955–64.

16 The ALLHAT Officers and Co-ordinators for the ALLHAT Collaborative Research
    Group. Major cardiovascular events in hypertensive patients randomly assigned to
    doxazosin vs chlorthalidone: the antihypertensive and lipid lowering treatment to
    prevent heart attack trial (ALLHAT). *J. Am. Med. Assoc.* 2002; **283**:1967–75.
17 Williams, B. Drug treatment of hypertension. *Br. Med. J.* 2003; **326**:61–2.
18 Pope, J. E., Anderson, J. J. and Felson, D. T. A metaanalysis of the effects of non-
    steroidal anti-inflammatory drugs on blood pressure. *Arch Intern. Med.* 1992;
    153:477–84.
19 Johnson, A. G., Nguyen, T. V. and Day, R. O. Do nonsteroidal anti-inflammatory
    drugs affect blood pressure? A meta-analysis. *Ann. Intern. Med.* 1994; **121**:289–90.
20 Gubitz, G. and Sandercock, P. Prevention of ischaemic stroke. *Br. Med. J.* 2000;
    321:1455–9.
21 Alberts, M. tPA in acute ischemic stroke. United States experience and issues for
    the future. *Neurology* 1988; **51** (supp 3):53–5S.
22 Lees, K. R., Bath, P. M. W. and Naylor, A. R. ABC of arterial and venous disease:
    secondary prevention of transient ischaemic attack and stroke. *Br. Med. J.* 2000;
    320:991–4.
23 Gorelick, P. B., Sacco, R. L., Smith, D. B. *et al.* Prevention of a first stroke. A review
    of guidelines and a multidisciplinary consensus statement from the National Stroke
    Association. *J. Am. Med. Assoc.* 1999; **281**:1112–20.
24 Hart, R. G., Benavente, O., McBride, R. and Pearce, L. A. Antithrombotic therapy
    to prevent stroke in patients with atrial fibrillation: a meta-analysis. *Ann. Intern.
    Med.* 1999; **131**:492–501.
25 PROGRESS Management Committee. Blood pressure lowering for the secondary
    prevention of stroke: rationale and design of PROGRESS. *J. Hypertens.* 1996; **14**
    (supp 2):41–6S.
26 Antiplatelet Trialists' Collaboration. Collaborative overview of randomised trials
    of antiplatelet therapy. I: prevention of death, myocardial infarction, and stroke by
    prolonged antiplatelet therapy in various categories of patients. *Br. Med. J.* 1994;
    308:81–106.
27 The Stroke Prevention in Reversible Ischaemia Trial (SPIRIT) Study Group. A
    randomised trial of anticoagulant versus aspirin after cerebral ischemia of presumed
    arterial origin. *Ann. Neurol.* 1997; **42**:857–65.
28 Hart, R. G., Benavente, O., McBride, R. and Pearce, L. A. Antithrombotic therapy
    to prevent stroke in patients with atrial fibrillation: a meta analysis. *Ann. Intern.
    Med.* 1999; **131**:492–501.
29 Cina, C., Clase, C. and Haynes, R. Carotid endarterectomy for symptomatic stenosis.
    In: *Cochrane Library*, Issue 3. Oxford: Update Software; 1999.

14

Diagnosis and treatment of osteoporosis

Jeannette E. South-Paul, M.D.

Introduction

Osteoporosis is a major public health problem, affecting more than 40 million people, one-third of postmenopausal women, and a substantial portion of the elderly in the USA, Europe, and Japan. An additional 54% of postmenopausal women have low bone density measured at the hip, spine, or wrist. *Osteoporosis results in more than 1 500 000 fractures annually in the USA.*

The direct expenditures for osteoporotic fractures have increased during the past decade from $5 billion to approximately $15 billion annually. Of the 25 million women in the USA who have osteoporosis, eight million have a documented fracture.[1] The female-to-male fracture ratios are 7 : 1 for vertebral fractures, 1.5 : 1 for distal forearm fractures, and 2 : 1 for hip fractures.[2,3] Approximately 70% of hip fractures in individuals older than 65 years of age occur in women. Osteoporosis-related fracture in older men is associated with lower femoral neck bone mineral density (BMD), quadriceps weakness, higher body sway, lower body weight, and decreased stature.[4]

Osteoporotic fractures are more common in white people and Asian people than in African-Americans and Hispanics, and more common in women than in men. Little is known regarding the influence of ethnicity on bone turnover.[5] Factors such as differences in bone accretion are likely to be responsible for much of the ethnic variation in adult BMD.

Prevention

Nutritional prevention

Bone mineralization depends on adequate nutritional status in childhood and adolescence. Therefore, measures to prevent osteoporosis should begin with improving the nutritional status of adolescents to increase bone mineralization, including increasing milk intake.[6] Because other nutrients

Table 14.1 Risk factors for osteoporosis

Female gender
Petite body frame
Caucasian or Asian race
Sedentary lifestyle/immobilization
Nulliparity
Increasing age
High caffeine intake
Renal disease
Lifelong low calcium intake
Smoking
Excessive alcohol use
Long-term use of certain drugs
Postmenopausal status
Low body weight
Impaired calcium absorption

besides calcium are essential for bone health, adolescents must maintain a balance between the intake of calcium, protein, phosphorus, and other calorie sources. Substituting phosphorus-laden soft drinks for calcium-rich dairy products and juices compromises calcium uptake by bone and thereby promotes decreased bone mass.

Although the fetus utilizes much of the maternal calcium during pregnancy and lactation, this bone mineral loss appears to be restored completely 6–12 months after weaning.[7]

A summary of risk factors for osteoporosis is shown in Table 14.1. *Sedentary lifestyle and/or immobility (those confined to bed or wheelchair), low body weight, cigarette smoking, and excessive alcohol consumption all influence bone mass negatively.*

Eating disorders affect BMD because the inability to maintain normal body mass promotes bone loss. The body-weight history of women with anorexia nervosa has been found to be the most important predictor of the presence of osteoporosis as well as the likelihood of recovery.[8] The BMD of these patients does not increase to the normal range, even several years after recovery from the disorder. All individuals with a history of an eating disorder remain at high risk for osteoporosis in the future.

Behavioral measures that decrease the risk of bone loss include eliminating both tobacco use and excessive consumption of alcohol and caffeine.[4] Maintaining estrogen levels in women is important. Measurement of bone density should be considered in patients who present with risk factors. Whether risk factors alone should be the reason to institute preventive measures is not well proven.

Regular physical exercise can reduce the risk of osteoporosis and delay the physiological decrease of BMD.[9] Exercise training (walking, jogging, stair-climbing) in healthy, sedentary, postmenopausal women results in improved bone mineral content.[10] Weight-bearing exercise results in increased bone mineral content, but the bone mass reverts to baseline levels when weight-bearing exercise is discontinued.[11–13] In the elderly, progressive strength training is a safe and effective form of exercise that reduces risk factors for falling and may enhance BMD.[14]

Estrogen deficiency results in diminished bone density in younger and older women. Athletes who exercise much more intensely and consistently than the average person usually have above-average bone mass. However, the positive effect of exercise on the bones of young women is dependent upon normal levels of endogenous estrogen. The low estrogen state of exercise-induced amenorrhea outweighs the positive effects of exercise and results in diminished bone density.[15] When mechanical stress or gravitational force on the skeleton is removed, as in bedrest, space flight, immobilization of the limbs, or paralysis, bone loss is rapid and extensive.[15] Furthermore, *weight-bearing exercise and estrogen replacement therapy (ERT) have independent and additive effects on the BMD of the limb, spine and Ward's triangle (hip).*[12]

No randomized prospective studies have systematically compared the effects of various activities on bone mass. Recommended activities include walking and jogging, weight-training, aerobics, stair-climbing, field sports, racquet sports, court sports, and dancing. Swimming is of questionable value to bone density because it is not a weight-bearing activity. There are no data on cycling, skating, or skiing. Any increase in physical activity may have a positive effect on bone mass for women who have been very sedentary. To be beneficial, the duration of exercise should be at least 30–60 minutes and should occur at least three times per week.

Evaluation

Symptoms and signs

The history and physical examination are important in screening for secondary forms of osteoporosis and directing the evaluation, although they are neither sensitive enough nor sufficient for diagnosing primary osteoporosis. A medical history provides valuable clues to the presence of chronic conditions, behaviors, physical fitness, and/or the use of long-term medications that could influence bone density. *Patients already affected by complications of osteoporosis may complain of upper or mid-thoracic back pain associated with activity, aggravated by long periods of sitting or standing, and easily relieved by rest in the recumbent position.* Low bone density, a propensity to fall, greater height, and presence of previous fractures confer increased fracture risk.

Table 14.2 Indications for measuring bone density

Concerned perimenopausal woman willing to start therapy

Radiographic evidence of bone loss

Patient on long-term glucocorticoid therapy (more than one month at ≥ 7.5 mg prednisone/day)

Asymptomatic hyperparathyroidism, where osteoporosis would suggest parathyroidectomy

Monitoring therapeutic response in woman undergoing treatment for osteoporosis if the result of the test would affect the clinical decision

A thorough physical examination is important for the same reasons. Lid lag and/or enlargement or nodularity of the thyroid suggests hyperthyroidism. Moon facies, thin skin, and a buffalo hump suggest hypercortisolism. Cachexia mandates screening for an eating disorder or malignancy. A pelvic examination is one aspect of the total evaluation of hormonal status and a necessary part of the physical examination in women. Osteoporotic fractures are late physical manifestations. Common fracture sites are the vertebrae, forearm, femoral neck, and proximal humerus. The presence of a dowager's hump in elderly patients indicates multiple vertebral fractures and decreased bone volume.

Laboratory findings

Basic chemical analysis of serum is indicated when history suggests other clinical conditions influencing the bone density. These tests provide clues to serious illnesses that may otherwise have gone undetected and that, if treated, could result in resolution or modification of the bone loss. Specific biochemical markers, such as human osteocalcin, bone alkaline phosphatase, immunoassays for pyridinoline cross-links, and type 1 collagen-related peptides in urine, which reflect the overall rate of bone formation and bone resorption, are now available. However, these markers are primarily of research interest and are not recommended as part of the basic work-up for osteoporosis.[16] They suffer from a high degree of biologic variability and diurnal variation and do not differentiate between causes of altered bone metabolism.[16–18]

Imaging tests

Plain radiographs are not sensitive enough to diagnose osteoporosis until total bone density has decreased by 50%, but bone densitometry is useful for measuring bone density and monitoring the course of therapy (Table 14.2).[19] Single-photon absorptiometry (SPA) and dual-photon absorptiometry (DPA) have been used in the past, but these provide poorer resolution, less accurate analysis, and more radiation exposure than X-ray absorptiometry. The most widely used techniques of assessing bone mineral density are dual-energy X-ray

Table 14.3 Classification of DEXA scan results

Normal: no further therapy
Osteopenic: counseled, treated, and followed so that no further bone loss develops
Osteoporotic: active therapy aimed at increasing bone density and decreasing fracture
   risk

absorptiometry (DEXA) and quantitative computerized tomography (CT).[20] These methods have errors in precision of 0.5–2%. Quantitative CT is the most sensitive method, but it results in substantially greater radiation exposure than DEXA.

Special tests

Of these methods, DEXA is the most precise and the diagnostic measure of choice. Smaller, less expensive systems for assessing the peripheral skeleton are now available. These include DEXA scans of the distal forearm and the middle phalanx of the non-dominant hand and a variety of devices for performing quantitative ultrasound (QUS) measurements on bone. *The predictive value of these peripheral measures to assess fracture risk at the hip or vertebra is not clear.* Ideally, therefore, measurements should be taken at both a central and a peripheral site for baseline. Follow-up BMD measures must be done using the same instruments to ensure reliability of data.

Bone densitometry reports provide a T-score (the number of standard deviations above or below the mean BMD for sex and race matched to young controls) or Z- score (comparing the patient with a population adjusted for age, sex, and race). The BMD result allows the classification of patients into three categories: normal, osteopenic and osteoporotic (Table 14.3). Osteoporosis is a T-score of more than 2.5 standard deviations below the sex-adjusted mean for normal young adults at peak bone mass.[21] Z-scores are of little value to the practicing clinician.

Women who receive bone density screening have better outcomes (improved bone density or fewer falls) than women who are not screened. The US Preventive Services Task Force suggests that the primary argument for screening is that postmenopausal women with low bone density are at increased risk for subsequent fractures of the hip, vertebrae, and wrist, and that interventions can slow the decline in bone density after menopause.[22] The presence of multiple risk factors (age >80 years, poor health, limited physical activity, poor vision, prior postmenopausal fracture, psychotropic drug use, and others) is a stronger predictor of hip fracture than low bone density.[22] The patient who is asymptomatic and has only one or two risk factors can benefit from BMD screening. Indications for BMD screening are outlined in Table 14.2.

Differential diagnosis and screening

The greatest challenge for clinicians is to know which asymptomatic patients would benefit from screening for osteoporosis, rather than determining a treatment regimen for those with known disease. All women and girls should be counseled regarding appropriate calcium intake and physical activity. Assessment of osteoporosis risk is also important when following a patient for a chronic disease known to cause secondary osteoporosis. Preventive measures are always the first step in therapy.

Recognizing the variety of conditions conferring risk of osteoporosis, the National Osteoporosis Foundation makes the following recommendations to physicians:
- Counsel all women on the risk factors for osteoporosis. Osteoporosis is a "silent" risk factor for fracture, just as hypertension is for stroke; one out of two white women will experience an osteoporotic fracture at some point in her lifetime.
- Perform evaluation for osteoporosis on all postmenopausal women who present with fractures, using BMD testing to confirm the diagnosis and determine the disease severity.
- *Recommend BMD testing to postmenopausal women under age 65 years and who have one or more additional risk factors for osteoporosis besides menopause.*
- Recommend BMD testing to all women aged 65 years and older, regardless of additional risk factors.
- Advise all patients to obtain an adequate intake of dietary calcium (at least 1140 mg/day, including supplements if necessary).
- Recommend regular weight-bearing and muscle-strengthening exercise to reduce the risk of falls and fractures.
- Advise patients to avoid tobacco smoking and to keep alcohol intake moderate.
- Consider all postmenopausal women who present with vertebral or hip fractures candidates for osteoporosis treatment.
- Initiate therapy to reduce fracture risk in women with BMD T-scores below -2 in the absence of risk factors and in women with T-scores below -1.5 if other risk factors are present.
- Pharmacologic options for osteoporosis prevention and/or treatment are hormone replacement therapy, alendronate, raloxifene (prevention), and calcitonin (treatment).[2]

Treatment

Treatment for osteoporosis is instituted to prevent early or continuing bone loss, with the belief that there can be an immediate impact on the patient's wellbeing and a willingness to comply with the patient's desires. Bone

Table 14.4 Conditions qualifying for Medicare coverage of densitometry

---

Estrogen-deficient woman at clinical risk for osteoporosis
Individual with vertebral abnormalities (e.g. osteopenia, vertebral fractures, osteoporosis)
Individual receiving long-term (more than three months) glucocorticoid therapy
Primary hyperparathyroidism
Individual being monitored to assess response to osteoporosis drug therapy

---

densitometry can assist in the decision-making process if the patient's age confers risk. However, because there are seldom early manifestations of disease, the decision is usually centered on prevention rather than treatment. BMD measurements can also assist in therapy when there are relative contraindications to a specific agent, and demonstrating efficacy could encourage continuation of therapy.

In the USA, Medicare currently reimburses costs of bone densitometry according to the guidelines outlined in Table 14.4. The decision to intervene with pharmacologic therapy involves clinical judgment based upon a global assessment rather than BMD measurement alone.

Estrogen

Adequate estrogen levels remain the single most important therapy for maintaining adequate bone density in women.[23,24]

Before 2002, estrogen replacement therapy was considered for all women with decreased bone density and who did not have contraindications. However, in July 2002, the Women's Health Initiative (WHI) randomized, controlled, primary prevention trial was stopped at a mean 5.2 years of follow-up by the data and safety monitoring board, because the test statistic for invasive breast cancer exceeded the stopping boundary for the adverse effect of estrogen and progesterone versus placebo. Estimated hazard ratios were excessive for coronary heart disease, breast cancer, and strokes, but were less than 1.0 for colorectal cancer, endometrial cancer, and hip fracture.[25] The arm of the study involving estrogen replacement only is continuing. Results are expected by 2006.

These results are consistent with two earlier reports, the Hormone Replacement Study (HERS) trial and a follow-up survey of postmenopausal women in the Nurses' Health Study in 1992.[26] In the Nurses' Health Study, the risk of breast cancer was increased significantly among women who were currently using estrogen alone or estrogen plus progestin, as compared with postmenopausal women who had never used hormones. Women currently taking hormones who had used such therapy for five to nine years had an adjusted relative risk of breast cancer of 1.46, as did those currently using hormones

Table 14.5 Overall treatment strategies

Calcium-rich diet plus/minus vitamin D supplements
Weight-bearing exercise
Avoidance of alcohol, tobacco products, excess caffeine, and drugs
Estrogen replacement within five years of menopause, and used for at least ten years
Alendronate
Raloxifene
Calcitonin

---

and who had done so for ten or more years (relative risk 1.46). The addition of progestins to estrogen therapy does not reduce the risk of breast cancer among postmenopausal women. Therefore, careful risk assessment is needed for each patient to determine whether the improvement of risk for hip fracture balances the risk for cardiovascular and breast disease.

Calcium and vitamin D

Calcium supplementation produces small beneficial effects on bone mass throughout postmenopausal life and may reduce fracture rates by more than the change in BMD would predict – possibly as much as 50%.[27] Postmenopausal women receiving supplemental calcium over a three-year period in a placebo-controlled, randomized clinical trial had stable total body calcium and bone density in the lumbar spine, femoral neck, and trochanter compared with the placebo group.[28]

Vitamin D increases calcium absorption in the gastrointestinal tract, with the result that more calcium is available in the circulation and subsequently reabsorbed in the renal proximal tubules. Significant reductions in non-vertebral fracture rates occur from physiologic replacement of vitamin D in the elderly.[29] Vitamin D supplementation is important in people of all ages with limited exposure to sunlight.

Dietary calcium augmentation should be recommended to maintain lifetime calcium levels and to help to prevent early postmenopausal bone loss (Table 14.5). Adults should ingest 1000 mg of elemental calcium per day for optimal bone health.[21,30] Teenagers, pregnant/lactating women, women over 50 years of age and taking ERT, and all people over 65 years of age should ingest 1500 mg of elemental calcium per day for optimal bone health. If this cannot be achieved by diet alone, then calcium supplementation is recommended.

Calcitonin

Calcitonin, a hormone directly inhibiting osteoclastic bone resorption, is an alternative for patients with established osteoporosis and in whom estrogen replacement therapy is not recommended.[30] Calcitonin produces an analgesic effect with respect to bone pain. Thus, it is often prescribed for patients who have suffered an acute osteoporotic fracture.

Treatment should be continued until pain is controlled, followed by tapering of medication over four to six weeks. Calcitonin decreases further bone loss at vertebral and femoral sites in patients with documented osteoporosis, but it has a questionable effect on fracture frequency.[31] Calcitonin prevents trabecular bone loss during the first few years of menopause, but it is unclear whether it has any impact on cortical bone.[29]

The Prevent Recurrence of Osteoporotic Fractures (PROOF) study – a five-year double-blind study that randomized 1255 postmenopausal women with osteoporosis to receive placebo or one of three dosages of intranasal calcitonin (100, 140, or 400 IU/day) – demonstrated a 36% reduction in the relative risk of new vertebral fractures compared with placebo.[32] There was no effect with 100 IU/day and no significant change in the reduction seen with 400 IU/day. For reasons that are poorly understood, the increase in BMD associated with calcitonin administration may be transient, or there may be the development of resistance.

Calcitonin can be provided in two forms. Nasal congestion and rhinitis are the most significant side effects of the nasal form. The injectable formulation has gastrointestinal side effects and is less convenient than the nasal preparation. The increase in bone density observed by this therapy is significantly less than that achieved by bisphosphonates or estrogen and may be limited to the spine. Nonetheless, it still has recognized value in reducing risk of fracture.

Bisphosphonates

Bisphosphonates are effective for preventing bone loss associated with estrogen deficiency, glucocorticoid treatment, and immobilization.[33] All bisphosphonates act similarly on bone in binding permanently to mineralized bone surfaces and inhibiting osteoclastic activity. Thus, less bone is degraded during the remodeling cycle.[33,34]

First-, second-, and third-generation bisphosphonates are now available (etidronate, alendronate, and residronate, respectively). The Fracture Intervention Trial investigated the effect of alendronate on the risk of fractures (both inapparent and clinically evident) in postmenopausal women with low bone mass.[35] The risk of any clinical fracture was half that of the placebo group in those taking alendronate. Because food and liquids can reduce the absorption of alendronate, it should be given with a glass of plain water 30 minutes before the first meal or beverage of the day. Patients should not lie down for at least 30 minutes to lessen the chance of esophageal irritation.

Bisphosphonates are of comparable efficacy to HRT in preventing bone loss and have a demonstrated positive effect on symptomatic and asymptomatic vertebral fracture rate as well as on non-vertebral fracture rate (forearm and hip).[35] More than four years of treatment would be needed in women with low bone density (T-score > −2.0) but without pre-existing fractures to show a significant effect in reducing the risk of clinical fracture.

In clinical trials, alendronate was generally tolerated well and no significant clinical or biological adverse experiences were observed. Alendronate is effective at doses of 5 mg daily in preventing osteoporosis induced by long-term glucocorticoid therapy. In placebo-controlled studies of men and women (aged 17–83) who were receiving glucocorticoid therapy, femoral neck bone density and the bone density of the trochanter and total body increased significantly in patients treated with alendronate.[36]

Risedronate is a pyridinyl bisphosphonate approved as treatment for several metabolic bone diseases. In doses of 5 mg daily, risedronate reduces the incidence of vertebral fractures in women with two or more fractures by rapidly increasing BMD at sites of cortical and trabecular bone.[37] A randomized trial of more than 1400 postmenopausal women with diagnosed osteoporosis showed a 40% reduction in risk of new vertebral fractures and reduction in incidence of non-vertebral fractures.[38] Risedronate significantly reduces the risk of hip fracture in women with osteoporosis.[39] Bisphosphonates should be prescribed for three to four years in women with osteoporosis and low bone density. Intravenous pamidronate is being studied for quarterly use to treat osteoporosis.[40]

Selective estrogen receptor modulators

Raloxifene, the first of a new class of drugs, termed selective estrogen receptor modulators (SERMs), has estrogen agonist effects on bone and antagonist effects on breast and endometrium. It blocks estrogen in a similar manner to tamoxifen, while also binding and stimulating other tissue receptors to act like estrogen. *Raloxifene inhibits trabecular and vertebral bone loss in a manner similar, but not identical, to estrogen* – i.e. by blocking the activity of cytokines that stimulate bone resorption.

Raloxifene therapy results in decreased serum total and low-density lipoprotein (LDL) *cholesterol* without any beneficial effects on serum total high-density lipoprotein (HDL) cholesterol or triglycerides.[41,42] The side effects of raloxifene are vaginitis and hot flushes.[43] Investigators in the Multiple Outcomes of Raloxifene (MORE) trial of more than 7000 postmenopausal, osteoporotic women over three years showed a decreased breast cancer risk in those already at low risk for the disease.[44] The study results were analyzed separately for women presenting with pre-existing fracture. While treatment effectiveness was similar in both groups, the absolute risk of fractures in the group with pre-existing fractures was 4.5 times greater than in the group with osteoporosis but no pre-existing fracture (21% versus 4.5%). Thus, it is important to identify and treat patients at higher risk. Studies of women at higher risk for breast cancer are currently under way.

A summary of overall treatment strategies is given in Table 14.6, and guidelines for dosing of the pharmacologic agents are given in Table 14.7.

Complementary and alternative therapies

Evidence from animal studies suggests a beneficial effect of phytoestrogens on bone, but long-term human studies are lacking.[45] Epidemiologic evidence reporting that Asian women have a lower fracture rate than white women, even though the bone density of Asian women is less than that of African-American women, promotes consideration of the impact of nutrition. It is possible that high soy intake contributes to improved bone quality in Asian women. A study of a soy-protein diet high in isoflavones as compared with a milk-protein diet or medium-isoflavone and soy-protein diet demonstrated that those receiving the high-isoflavone preparation had improvement in trabecular (vertebral) bone rather than cortical (femoral) bone.[46]

A topical form of natural progesterone derived from diosgenin, which occurs in soy beans and Mexican wild yams, has been promoted as a treatment for osteoporosis, hot flushes, and premenstrual syndrome, and as a prophylactic against breast cancer. However, eating or applying wild yam extract or diosgenin does not produce increased progesterone levels in humans because humans cannot convert diosgenin into progesterone.[45]

Addressing glucocorticoid-induced osteoporosis

Glucocorticoids are used widely in the treatment of many chronic diseases, particularly asthma, chronic lung disease, and inflammatory and rheumatologic disorders, and in people who have undergone organ transplantation. The risk that oral steroid therapy poses to BMD, among other side effects, has been known for some time. As a result, clinicians have eagerly substituted inhaled steroids in an endeavor to partially protect the patient from unwanted negative steroid effects.

Recent evaluations of the effects of inhaled glucocorticoids on bone density in premenopausal women demonstrated a dose-related decline in bone density at both the total hip and the trochanter.[47] Women asthmatics were enrolled who were using no inhaled steroids, using four to eight puffs per day, or using more than eight puffs per day at 100 μg/puff. No dose-related effect was noted at the femoral neck or the spine. Serum and urinary markers of bone turnover and adrenal function did not predict the degree of bone loss. To achieve the best

Table 14.6 Summary of the risks and benefits of osteoporosis therapy

	Estrogen	Raloxifene	Calcitonin	Alendronate	Risedronate
Reduction of vertebral fracture	Yes	Yes	Yes	Yes	Yes
Reduction of non-vertebral fracture	Yes	No	No	Yes	Yes
Experience with long-term use	Large epidemiologic studies over decades	RCT three years in length	RCT five years in length	RCT four years in length	RCT three years in length
Administration	Orally: once daily any time Transdermally: weekly patches	Orally: once daily any time	Intranasally: once daily any time	Once daily in morning, 30 minutes before eating, with water while upright; or weekly	Once daily in morning, 30–60 minutes before eating, with water, while upright
Adverse effects	Breast tenderness, vaginal bleeding, thromboembolic disorders	Increased risk of venous thrombosis, hot flushes, leg cramps	Nasal irritation	Dyspepsia, esophagitis, avoid in patients with esophagheal disorders	Dyspepsia
Effect on cardiovascular mortality	Increased in those with pre-existing cardiovascular disease	No final-outcome data	None	None	None
Breast cancer	Increased	Possibly decreased risk of estrogen-receptor-positive breast cancer	None	None	None
Endometrial cancer	Increased if unopposed estrogen used	None	None	None	None
Dementia, Alzheimer's disease	Possible decreased incidence	Maybe?	None	None	None

Modified from Gueldner, S. H. *Managing Osteoporosis – Part 3: Prevention and Treatment of Postmenopausal Osteoporosis.* Chicago: AMA; 2002.

Table 14.7 Pharmacologic doses

Medication	Dosage	Route
Estradiol patch	0.05 mg/week	Topical
Conjugated estrogens	0.625–1.25 mg/day	Oral
Elemental calcium	1000–1500 mg/day	Oral
Calcitonin	140 IU/day or 50–100 IU/day	Intranasal or subcutaneous/ intramuscular
Vitamin D	400 IU/day (800 IU/day in winter in northern latitudes)	Oral
Alendronate	5 mg/day (prevention) 10 mg/day (treatment)	Oral
Raloxifene	60 mg/day	Oral

Table 14.8 Treatment strategies for patients on glucocorticoids

Lowest dose of a short-acting glucocorticoid or topical preparations whenever possible

Maintain a well-balanced, 2–3 g/day sodium diet

Weight-bearing and isometric exercise to prevent proximal muscle weakness.

Calcium intake of 1500 mg/day and vitamin D intake of 400–800 IU/day after hypercalciuria is controlled

Gonadal hormones in all postmenopausal women, premenopausal women with low levels of estradiol, and men who have low levels of testosterone (unless contraindicated)

Thiazide diuretic to control hypercalciuria

Measure BMD at baseline and every 6–12 months during the first two years of therapy to assess treatment efficacy

If bone loss occurs while being treated, or if HRT is contraindicated, treat with calcitonin or bisphosphonate.

From Lane, N.E., and Lukert, B. The science and therapy of glucocorticoid-induced bone loss. *Endocrinol. Metab. Clin. North Am.* 1998; **27**:465–83.

possible outcome for the patient, given the potentially devastating effects of systemic steroids, therapy to combat the steroids should begin as soon as the steroids are begun. See Table 14.8 for specific guidelines.

Summary

Osteoporosis is a silently progressive condition that is best managed through prevention. The strongest predictors of low bone density and subsequent fracture are clinical risk factors. Those clinical risk factors associated most consistently with low bone density and fracture in postmenopausal women include increasing age, white race, low weight or weight loss, non-use of estrogen replacement, history of previous fracture, family history of fracture, history of falls, and low scores on one or more measures of physical activity or function.

When the history suggests increased risk of low bone density and the patient is reluctant to adjust lifestyle, then obtaining BMD results indicating decreased bone mass can convince the patient to change their lifestyle and/or to begin therapy. Predictive value of BMD measurement is greatest at the site at which the measurement is done. Behavior modification remains the most important early intervention, while pharmacotherapy assists for prevention or treatment later in the disease process. Bisphosphonates increase BMD at the spine and hip in a dose-dependent manner in patients with osteoporosis. SERMs are beneficial in the treatment and prevention of osteoporosis. Pursuing a methodical evaluation minimizes the possibility of missing the diagnosis and can prevent many of the long-term, irreversible effects.

REFERENCES

1 Melton, L. J. How many women have osteoporosis? *J. Bone Miner. Res.* 1992; **7**:1005–10.

2 Cooper, C. and Melton, L. J., III. Epidemiology of osteoporosis. *Trends Endocrinol. Metab.* 1992; **314**:224–9.

3 www.nof.org/osteoporosis/stats.htm. Accessed March 2003.

4 Taxel, P. Osteoporosis: detection, prevention, and treatment in primary care. *Geriatrics* 1998; **53**:22–33

5 Finkelstein, J. S., Sowers, M., Greendale, D. A., *et al.* Ethnic variation in bone turnover in pre- and early perimenopausal women: effects of anthropometric and lifestyle factors. *J. Clin. Endocrinol. Metab.* 2002;. **87**:3051–6.

6 Cadogen, J. Eastell, R., Jones, N. and Barker, M. E. Milk intake and bone mineral acquisition in adolescent girls: randomised, controlled intervention trial. *Br. Med. J.* 1997; **315**:1255–60.

7 Eisman, J. Relevance of pregnancy and lactation to osteoporosis. *Lancet* 1998; **352**:504–5.

8 Hotta, M., Shibasaki, T., Sato, K. and Demura, H. The importance of body weight history in the occurrence and recovery of osteoporosis in patients with anorexia nervosa: evaluation by dual x-ray absorptiometry and bone metabolic markers. *Eur. J. Endocrinol.* 1998; **139**:276–83.

9 Ernst, E. Exercise for female osteoporosis. A systematic review of randomised clinical trials. *Sports Med.* 1998; **25**:359–68.

10 Dalsky, G. P., Stocke, K. S., Ehsani, A. A., *et al.* Weight-bearing exercise training and lumbar bone mineral content in postmenopausal women. *Ann. Intern. Med.* 1988; **108**:824–8.

11 Chow, R., Harrison, J. E. and Notarius, C. Effect of two randomized exercise programs on bone mass of healthy postmenopausal women. *Br. Med. J.* 1987; **295**: 1441–4.

12 Kohrt, W. M., Snead, D. B., Slatopolsky, E. and Birge, S. J. Additive effects of weight-bearing exercise and estrogen on bone mineral density in older women. *J. Bone Miner. Res.* 1995; **10**:1303–11.

13 Nelson, M. E., Fiatarone, M. A., Morganti, C. M., *et al.* Effects of high-intensity strength training on multiple risk factors for osteoporotic fractures. *J. Am. Med. Assoc.* 1994; **272**:1909–14.

14 Henderson, N. K., White, C. P. and Eisman, J. A. The role of exercise and fall risk reduction in the prevention of osteoporosis. *Endocrinol. Metab. Clin. North Am.* 1998; **27**:369–87.

15 Drinkwater, B. L. Physical exercise and bone health. *J. Am. Med. Womens Assoc.* 1990; **45**:91–97.

16 Kroger, H. and Reeve, J. Diagnosis of osteoporosis in clinical practice. *Ann. Med.* 1998; **30**:278–87.

17 World Health Organization. *Assessment of Fracture Risk and its Application to Screening for Postmenopausal Osteoporosis: Report of a WHO Study Group.* Geneva: WHO; 1994.

18 Arnaud, C. D. Osteoporosis: using "bone markers" for diagnosis and monitoring. *Geriatrics* 1996: **51**:24–30.

19 Genant, H. K. Current state of bone densitometry for osteoporosis. *Radiographics* 1998; **18**:913–18.

20 Blake, G. M. and Fogelman, I. Applications of bone densitometry for osteoporosis. *Endocrinol. Metab. Clin. North Am.* 1998; **27**:267–88.

21 Scientific Advisory Board, Osteoporosis Society of Canada. Clinical practice guidelines for the diagnosis and management of osteoporosis. *Can. Med. Assoc. J.* 1996; **155**:1113–33.

22 US Preventive Services Task Force. *Guide to Clinical Preventive Services.* Baltimore, MD: Williams & Wilkins; 1996.

23 Umland, E. M., Rinaldi, C., Parks, S. M. and Boyce, E. G. The impact of estrogen replacement therapy and raloxifene on osteoporosis, cardiovascular disease, and gynecologic cancers. *Ann. Pharmacother.* 1999; **33**:1315–28.

24 Ravn, P., Bidstrup, M., Wasnich, R. D. *et al.* Alendronate and estrogen–progestin in the long-term prevention of bone loss: four-year results from the early postmenopausal intervention cohort study: a randomized trial. *Ann. Intern. Med.* 1999; **131**:935–42.

25 Roussouw, J., Anderson, G. L., Prentice, R. L., *et al.* Risks and benefits of estrogen plus progestin in healthy postmenopausal women. *J. Am. Med. Assoc.* 2002; **288**: 32–33.

26 Colditz, G. A., Hankinson, S. E., Hunter, D. J., *et al.* The use of estrogens and progestins and the risk of breast cancer in postmenopausal women. *N. Engl. J. Med.* 1995; **332**:1589–93.

27 Reid, I. R. The role of calcium and vitamin D in the prevention of osteoporosis. *Endocrinol. Metab. Clin. North Am.* 1998; **27**:389–98.

28 Aloia, J. F., Vaswani, A., Yeh, J. K., *et al.* Calcium supplementation with and without hormone replacement therapy to prevent postmenopausal bone loss. *Ann. Intern. Med.* 1994; **114**:97–103.

29 Reid, I. R. The role of calcium and vitamin D in the prevention of osteoporosis. *Endocrinol. Metab. Clin. North. Am.* 1998; **27**:389–98.

30 Avioli, L. V. The role of calcitonin in the prevention of osteoporosis. *Endocrinol. Metab. Clin. North. Am.* 1998; **27**:411–18.

31 Overgaard, K., Hansen, M. A., Jansen, S. B. and Christiansen, C. Effect of salcatonin given intranasally on bone mass and fracture rates in established osteoporosis: a dose response study. *Br. Med. J.* 1992; **305**:556–61.

32 Chestnut, C. H., Silverman, S. L., Adriano, K., *et al.* Salmon-calcintonin nasal spray prevents vertebral fractures in established osteoporosis. Final world wide results of the "PROOF". *Calcif. Tissue Int.* 1999; **64** (supp 1):1–26.

33 Watts, N. B. Treatment of osteoporosis with bisphosphonates. *Endocrinol. Metab. Clin. North. Am.* 1998; **27**:419–39.

34 Devogelaer, J. P. A risk–benefit assessment of alendronate in the treatment of involutional osteoporosis. *Drug Saf.* 1998; **19**:141–54.

35 Black, D. M., Cummings, S. R., Karpf, D. B., *et al.* Randomised trial of effect of alendronate on risk of fracture in women with existing vertebral fractures. *Lancet* 1996; **348**:1535–41.

36 Saag, K. G., Enkey, R., Schnitzer, T. J., *et. al* Alendronate for the prevention and treatment of glucocorticoid-induced osteoporosis. *N. Engl. J. Med.* 1998; **339**: 292–9.

37 Reginster, J. Y., Minne, H. W., Sorensen, O. H., *et al.* Randomized trial of the effects of risedronate on vertebral fractures in women with established postmenopausal osteoporosis. *Osteoporos. Int.* 2000; **11**:83–91.

38 Harris, S. T., Watts, N. B., Genant, H. K., *et al.* Effects of residronate treatment on vertebral and nonvertebral fractures in women with postmenopausal osteoporosis. A randomized controlled trial. *J. Am. Med. Assoc.* 1999; **282**:1344–52.

39 McClung, M. Therapy for fracture prevention. *J. Am. Med. Assoc.* 1999; **282**; 687–9.

40 Kreig, M. A., Seydoux, C., Sandini, L., *et al.* Intravenous pamidonate as treatment for osteoporosis after heart transplantation: a prospective study. *Osteoporos. Int.* 2001; **12**:112–16.

41 Delmas, P. D., Bjarnason, N. H., Mitlak, B. H., *et al.* Effects of raloxifene on bone mineral density, serum cholesterol concentrations and uterine endometrium in postmenopausal women. *N. Engl. J. Med.* 1997; **337**:1641–7.

42 Draper, M. W., Flowers, D. E., Huster, W. J., *et al.* A controlled trial of raloxifene HCL: impact on bone turnover and serum lipid profile in healthy postmenopausal women. *J. Bone. Miner. Res.* 1996; **11**:835–42.

43 Willhite, S. L., Goebel, S. R. and Scoggin, J. A. Raloxifene provides an alternative for osteoporosis prevention. *Ann. Pharmacother.* 1998; **32**:834–7.

44 Ettinger, B., Black, D. M., Mitlak, B. H., *et al.* Reduction of vertebral fracture risk in postmenopausal women with osteoporosis treated with raloxifene. results from a 3 year randomized clinical trial." *J. Am. Med. Assoc.* 1999; **282**:637–45.

45 Fugh-Berman, A. Progesterone cream for osteoporosis. *Altern. Ther. Womens Health* 1999; **1**:33–40.

46 Potter, S. M., Baum, J. A., Teng, H., *et al.* Soy protein and isoflavones: their effects on blood lipids and bone density in postmenopausal women. *Am. J. Clin. Nutr.* 1998; **68**(supp):1375–9.

47 Israel, E., Banerjee, T. R., Fitzmaurice, G. M., *et al.* Effects of inhaled glucocorticoids on bone density in premenopausal women. *N. Engl. J. Med.* 1401; **345**:941–7.

15

Diabetes in mid-life women

Phillippa Miranda and Diana McNeill

Case: a 51-year-old woman who has had type 2 diabetes for five years is managed with metformin, diet, and exercise. She notes worsening hyperglycemia, but attention to diet and exercise does not seem to improve glycemic control as it has in the past. She mentions to her physician that she has missed her last two menstrual periods and that she seems to be a "bit more edgy." She wonders whether there is a correlation between her worsening diabetes control and her menstrual changes.

Definitions

Diabetes mellitus refers to a group of common metabolic disorders characterized by hyperglycemia. Diabetes may be type 1 (juvenile-onset or insulin-dependent diabetes mellitus – IDDM), type 2 (adult-onset or non-insulin-dependent diabetes mellitus – NIDDM), or gestational (during pregnancy). In type 1 diabetes, hyperglycemia is caused by an absolute deficiency of insulin secretion. In type 2 diabetes, hyperglycemia is caused by a combination of insulin resistance and inadequate compensatory insulin secretory response, with a relative, not absolute, insulin deficiency.

The most common type of diabetes in mid life is type 2 diabetes, often caused by a combination of inherited and environmental factors and lifestyle choices. *Type 2 diabetes is associated with numerous metabolic abnormalities, including reduced insulin secretion, increased hepatic glucose production, decreased glucose uptake by muscle and adipose tissue, and dyslipidemia.* These metabolic abnormalities underlie the complications of diabetes, including heart attack, stroke, blindness, end-stage renal disease, and lower-extremity amputation. With type 2 diabetes, there may be a long period without clinical symptoms but with elevated insulin levels and mild to moderate hyperglycemia, which can result in damage to target tissues before diabetes is diagnosed.

Epidemiology

The incidence and prevalence of diabetes is increasing worldwide. Using World Health Organization (WHO) diagnostic criteria, the worldwide prevalence of diabetes in adults was estimated to be 4.0% (135 million people) in 1995, rising to 5.4% (300 million people) by 2025. Diabetes is more prevalent in developed countries. The countries with the largest numbers of people with diabetes are India, China, and the USA. There are more women than men with diabetes, especially in developed countries.[1]

Applying American Diabetes Association (ADA) diagnostic criteria to those aged 40–74 years, the prevalence of diabetes (both diagnosed and undiagnosed) in the USA rose from 8.9% in 1976–1980 to 12.3% in 1988–1994.[2] In a cohort of US adults aged 25–74 years, who were followed from 1971 to 1993, the 5.1% of subjects who had diabetes experienced 10.6% of the observed mortality. *Median life expectancy was eight years lower for those aged 55–64 years with diabetes and four years lower for those aged 65–74 years with diabetes.*[3] In addition to the high rates of diabetes and associated mortality, mid-life women should be concerned about diabetes because of the implications for management of menopause. This chapter will examine the diagnosis, prevention, and management of diabetes in mid-life women.

Clinical course

Signs and symptoms

In mid life, type 2 diabetes is the most common type of diabetes. The diagnosis of type 2 diabetes is based on symptoms of hyperglycemia and the measurement of elevated blood-glucose readings. The classic symptoms of significant hyperglycemia include polyuria, polydipsia, weight loss, polyphagia, and blurred vision. Hyperglycemia may also cause fatigue, vaginitis, or other non-specific symptoms, which may be attributed to menopause. If the onset of hyperglycemia is gradual, then there may not be any symptoms, thus delaying the diagnosis of diabetes.

Screening of asymptomatic individuals

Since hyperglycemia can be asymptomatic, those individuals at increased risk for diabetes should be screened at regular intervals. Individuals at increased risk for type 2 diabetes include those with increasing age, obesity, and lack of physical activity. *Obesity is a major contributing factor to insulin resistance and diminished beta-cell reserve capacity in type 2 diabetes;* even those patients who are not overweight by standard criteria may have an increased percentage of body fat and/or an abnormal distribution predominantly in the abdominal

Table 15.1 Risk factors associated with type 2 diabetes

Increasing age
Obesity (BMI >25 kg/m^2)
Lack of physical activity
Prior gestational (pregnancy-related) diabetes
Delivery of a baby weighing >4.1 kg
Hypertension
Dyslipidemia
Family history of type 2 diabetes

BMI, body mass index.

Table 15.2 Indications for more frequent diabetes testing in asymptomatic individuals

Overweight (BMI >25 kg/m^2)
First-degree relative with diabetes
Member of a high-risk ethnic population
Diagnosed with gestational diabetes
Delivered a baby weighing over 4.1 kg
Hypertension with blood pressure ≥140/90 mmHg
HDL cholesterol ≤35 mg/dl
Triglycerides ≥250 mg/dl
Pre-diabetes, impaired glucose tolerance, or impaired fasting glucose

HDL, high-density lipoprotein.

viscera. Additional risk factors for type 2 diabetes include prior gestational (pregnancy-related) diabetes or delivery of a baby weighing over 4.1 kg, hypertension, dyslipidemia, family history of type 2 diabetes, and certain racial and ethnic groups (Table 15.1).

Screening for type 2 diabetes is important because as many as 50% of people with type 2 diabetes in the USA, or eight million people, are undiagnosed. Undiagnosed diabetes may be clinically significant because complications such as retinopathy may develop before diagnosis. Coronary heart disease, stroke, and peripheral vascular disease are common in people with undiagnosed diabetes. Thus, early detection of diabetes in those at risk has significant potential to impact morbidity and mortality from the disease.[4] *The ADA recommends that testing for diabetes in asymptomatic individuals should be considered for those age 45 years and older and should be repeated every three years.* In addition, testing should be considered at a younger age or more frequently for those women listed in Table 15.2. Testing may be performed using an oral glucose tolerance test (OGTT) or fasting plasma glucose (FPG). FPG is preferred because of ease of administration, convenience, acceptability to patients, and lower cost.

Table 15.3 ADA criteria for diagnosis of diabetes

Symptoms of diabetes (polyuria, polydipsia, or unexplained weight loss) plus
    random plasma glucose ≥ 200 mg/dl (11.1 mmol/l)
Fasting (no calories for at least eight hours) plasma glucose ≥126 mg/dl
    (7.0 mmol/l)
Two-hour plasma glucose ≥200 mg/dl (11.1 mmol/l) during an OGTT, with a 75-g
    glucose load, per WHO guidelines

Data from the Expert Committee on the Diagnosis and Classification of Diabetes
Mellitus. Report of the Expert Committee on the Diagnosis and Classification of
Diabetes Mellitus. *Diabet. Care* 2002; **25**(supp 1):S5–20.

Diagnostic criteria

Diagnostic criteria and classification schemes for diabetes have been proposed
and published by the ADA and the WHO.[5,6] In January 2002, the ADA published revised criteria for the diagnosis of diabetes, which state that diabetes
can be diagnosed by any one of three criteria (Table 15.3). In the absence
of unequivocal hyperglycemia with metabolic decompensation, the criteria
should be confirmed by repeat testing on a different day. The OGTT is not
recommended for routine clinical use, but it may be necessary when diabetes is
suspected despite normal fasting plasma glucose.[5] The ADA does not recommend glycosylated hemoglobin (hemoglobin A1c, HbA1c) for the diagnosis
of diabetes. Even though HbA1c is a reliable marker of glycemia over a period
of about two to three months, this test should not be used to diagnose diabetes
because too many different methods are used for the measurement of HbA1c,
and the correlations between fasting plasma glucose, two-hour post-load glucose, and HbA1c are imperfect.

In recent years, the levels at which plasma glucose is considered diagnostic of
diabetes have been revised downwards. The cut-off point of a two-hour post-
load glucose over 200 mg/dl (11.1 mmol/l) has been shown to correlate with
the level of hyperglycemia at which the prevalence of microvascular complications considered specific for diabetes increases dramatically.[5] The FPG has
been revised down from 140 mg/dl (7.8 mmol/l) to 126 mg/dl (7.0 mmol/l)
because this value better reflects the same degree of hyperglycemia responsible for the two-hour post-load glucose of over 200 mg/dl (11.1 mmol/l) on an
OGTT.

Blood glucose target levels

For the individual with diabetes, monitoring of blood glucose levels by the
patient and the healthcare provider is necessary to achieve glycemic control. Based on findings from the Diabetes Control and Complications Trial

Table 15.4 Target levels of blood glucose readings

Time of day	Plasma (mg/dl (mmol/l))	Whole blood (mg/dl (mmol/l))
Preprandial glucose	90–130 (5.0–7.2)	80–120 (4.4–6.7)
One- to two-hour postprandial glucose	<180 (<10.0)	<180 (<10.0)
Bedtime glucose	110–150 (6.1–8.3)	100–140 (5.5–7.8)

(DCCT), self-monitoring of blood glucose (SMBG) is recommended for most individuals with diabetes. The routine use of home blood glucose meters has replaced the use of urine glucose testing, which was previously the only method of home testing available to patients. Target preprandial, postprandial, and bedtime blood glucose levels, based on ADA recommendations, are given in Table 15.4.[7]

In addition to SMBG data, HbA1c is recommended for monitoring response to diabetes therapy. HbA1c testing should be performed at initial assessment and then as part of continuing care in all patients with diabetes. Because the test reflects average blood glucose over two to three months, testing every three months is required to determine whether glycemic control departs from the target range. Expert opinion recommends HbA1c testing at least twice a year in patients meeting treatment goals, and more frequently for those not at goal or whose therapy has changed.

Although reference ranges vary by laboratory and method used for measuring HbA1c, normal individuals without diabetes usually have HbA1c readings of 4–6%, corresponding to blood glucose levels of 60–120 mg/dl (3.3–6.7 mmol/l). For those with diabetes, the ADA recommends a target level for HbA1c of less than 7%, which corresponds to a blood glucose level of 150 mg/dl (8.3 mmol/l).[8]

Prevention of diabetes

In April 2002, the ADA published a position statement on the prevention or delay of type 2 diabetes.[9] This statement reviews the evidence for the benefits of prevention, which people to screen, and how to implement prevention programs. *Screening should occur during the regular office visit with either FPG or two-hour OGTT.* If impaired glucose tolerance (IGT, defined as glucose ≥ 140 mg/dl but <200 mg/dL on OGTT) or impaired fasting glucose (IFG, defined as FPG level of ≥ 110 mg/dl but <126 mg/dl) is found, then intervention should proceed, including counseling for weight loss and increase in physical activity. Follow-up counseling is vital, with rescreening for diabetes every one to two years.

Additional interventions to reduce other cardiovascular risk factors are appropriate, but drug therapy for glycemic control is not routinely recommended to treat IGT or IFG until more conclusive evidence is available. In addition, individuals at high risk for diabetes need to become aware of the benefits of weight loss and increased physical activity.

Risk factors

Risk factors for the development of type 2 diabetes include obesity, physical inactivity, age, and family history of type 2 diabetes. The Nurses' Health Study found that obesity, specifically adult weight change, was a risk factor for diabetes. In this prospective cohort study, more than 114 000 women aged 30–55 years in 11 US states were followed for 14 years, during which time 2204 cases of diabetes were diagnosed. Compared with women with a BMI of less than 22 kg/m², *women of average weight (BMI 24–24.9 kg/m²) had a relative risk for developing diabetes of 5.0 (95% confidence interval (CI) 3.6–6.6) and obese women (BMI >31.0 kg/m²) had a relative risk of 40.0 or greater.* This study also confirmed that family history is a predictor of risk for diabetes. However, family history did not alter the risks associated with weight gain.[10]

Another risk factor for type 2 diabetes is physical inactivity. The Iowa Women's Health Study Cohort was used to examine the relationship between physical activity and new diabetes in postmenopausal women. A series of mailed questionnaires were sent to a cohort of 34 257 postmenopausal women aged 55–69 years to assess the 12-year incidence of diabetes and level of physical activity. After adjusting for age, education, smoking, alcohol, estrogen use, diet, and family history, *women who reported any physical activity had a relative risk of diabetes of 0.69 compared with sedentary women.* When adjusted further for obesity, the relative risk reduction with physical activity decreased to 0.86. Any level of physical activity decreased diabetes risk; however, with increasing frequency or intensity of exercise, the diabetes risk showed an incremental decrease.[11]

Diabetes prevention program

Type 2 diabetes is a preventable disease for both men and women if obesity and physical inactivity can be modified with lifestyle changes. The Diabetes Prevention Program (DPP) research group conducted a large, randomized, controlled trial to compare directly the effects of lifestyle modification and medical therapy with metformin in the prevention of diabetes.[12] In this study, more than 3200 US adults at high risk for the development of type 2 diabetes were randomized to standard lifestyle recommendations plus placebo, standard lifestyle recommendations plus metformin, a biguanide antihyperglycemic agent, or an intensive lifestyle-modification program with goals of at least 7% weight loss and 150 minutes of physical activity per week. The participants had a mean age of 51 years, had a mean BMI of 34.0 kg/m^2, were 68% women, and were 45% racial minorities. Over the 2.8-year follow-up period, the intensive lifestyle-modification group had a 58% reduction in the incidence of diabetes, while the metformin group had a 31% reduction as compared with placebo. In order to prevent one case of diabetes during three years, seven people would have to undertake intensive lifestyle modification. This study demonstrates that *both intensive lifestyle modification and metformin can reduce the incidence of diabetes in men and women at increased risk of diabetes.*

Menopause and diabetes

Type 2 diabetes and menopause

Menopause is defined as the cessation of menses for one year. Erratic menses that may occur before that time is known as perimenopause. As the population ages, estimates suggest that by 2015, 45% of all women will be 45 years or older, an age often associated with changes in the menstrual cycle.[13] The decrease in endogenous estrogen associated with the onset of menopause can be associated with:

- fluctuations in sex hormone levels and increased relative androgen levels, which can contribute to increased fasting glucose;
- increasing hepatic glucose production, leading to increased fasting glucose;
- increased body fat, particularly central intra-abdominal fat, which can lead to increased insulin resistance and cardiovascular risk;[14]
- other changes in insulin metabolism and resistance.[15]

All of these physiologic changes can affect glycemic control in the menopausal woman with diabetes.

Evidence regarding the effects on glycemic control of hormone replacement therapy (HRT) used for the management of menopausal symptoms is inconclusive and conflicting. In the Postmenopausal Estrogen Progestin Intervention (PEPI) trial, *combination treatment with estrogen plus medroxyprogesterone increased two-hour postprandial glucose levels.*[16] Other studies have shown that estrogen alone may improve diabetes control in postmenopausal women by decreasing relative androgen levels, since androgens contribute to insulin resistance, as seen in patients with polycystic ovary syndrome.[17]

In the UK Prospective Diabetes Study (UKPDS), the seminal study of glycemic control in patients with type 2 diabetes, HbA1c improved by 0.5% in patients using HRT compared with those who did not use HRT. While this change may seem small, it is consistent with a 10% reduction in any diabetes complication and a 7% decrease in myocardial infarction for those taking

HRT.[18] The UKPDS results were supported further in an observational study of 15 435 women with type 2 diabetes and who were members of a health-maintenance organization. In the 25% who were using HRT, HRT use was associated independently with a decreased HbA1c, regardless of whether the HRT contained a progestin.[19] Further randomized studies are clearly needed to understand the full impact of HRT on glycemic control.

Women with diabetes have increased cardiovascular risk compared with women without diabetes, regardless of menopausal status. Controversy about the use of HRT generated by the data from the Women's Health Initiative (WHI) has made recommendations about HRT in the woman with diabetes less clear. In the WHI trial, 16 608 postmenopausal women with a uterus, of whom only 4.4% had diabetes, were randomized to placebo versus conjugated equine estrogen (0.625 mg) plus medroxyprogesterone acetate (2.5 mg). After 5.2 years, the trial was stopped due to concerns that the risks of invasive breast cancer and cardiovascular events outweighed the benefits of decreased colorectal cancer and improved bone health.[20]

Women who consider using HRT are more likely to modify other aspects of their health, monitor their blood glucose levels more often, exercise more regularly, and attempt weight management and control. The WHI has offered healthcare workers and patients an opportunity to discuss the relative risks and benefits of HRT on an individual basis. At present, there are no uniform recommendations for the use of HRT and the management of the postmenopausal woman with or without diabetes, except for avoiding HRT in the first year after myocardial infarction.[21]

In addition to cardiovascular disease prevention and glycemic control, what else should the mid-life woman with diabetes be told about the management of her health? Issues for the menopausal woman with diabetes include bone health and the risk of osteoporosis, depression, and macrovascular and microvascular complications of diabetes. Bone health should be assessed and a bone density evaluation considered for women over 50 years old or any woman with increased risk of osteoporosis from chronic thyroid hormone replacement, smoking, low body mass index, or a family history of osteoporosis.[22] *Depression is more common in women with diabetes, and depression also increases in postmenopausal women.* Since anxiety and depression can affect glycemic control adversely, stress management and pharmacologic treatment of severe depression may have a positive effect on glycemic control.[23]

Type 1 diabetes and menopause

The relationship between type 1 diabetes and menopause is even more complex, as menopause in patients with type 1 diabetes may occur at a younger age.[24.] Genetic factors, including haplotypes found in association with the DR4 haplotype (more common in type 1 diabetes), may increase the risk of early menopause two-fold. The long-term effects of premature menopause, in addition to a shorter time for childbearing, include a higher risk of cardiovascular disease, abnormal lipid profile, and increased risk of osteoporosis. Early menopause may occur in women with type 1 diabetes from autoimmune premature ovarian failure (similar to the autoimmune thyroiditis seen more commonly in patients with type 1 diabetes), from peripheral hyperinsulinemia and hyperandrogenemia seen in polycystic ovary syndrome, and from hypothalamic dysfunction from poorly controlled diabetes. A good menstrual history will help with the early detection of premature menopause in these women.

Glycemic control: therapeutic interventions

Once the diagnosis of diabetes has been made, each individual patient needs a diabetes management plan to control the disease and prevent complications. The diabetes management plan should include the following components:
• education about the disease;
• instruction in home SMBG;
• diet counseling and nutritional modification;
• exercise, and medications if needed.
    Oral agents, which can be used alone or in combination, include sulfonylureas, biguanides, thiazolidinediones, and others. Options for insulin therapy have increased in recent years with the introduction of insulin analogs, such as insulin lispro, insulin aspart, and insulin glargine.

Education

Education of the individual with diabetes about the disease and its management is the most important intervention in the diabetes management plan. Certified diabetes educators (CDEs) are excellent resources for providing diabetes education. Education may be provided through group classes, one-on-one counseling sessions, or both. The goal of education is to provide knowledge and understanding of the disease in order to improve motivation and compliance with other therapies, and thus improve outcomes and quality of life. Education programs should include:
• basic disease information and blood glucose targets;
• practical advice to implement lifestyle changes, including diet and exercise;
• instruction in SMBG;
• education on prevention of complications.
Each of these topics is discussed in more detail below.

Table 15.5 Nutrition guidelines for people with diabetes

Total amount of carbohydrate is more important than source or type of carbohydrate
Good carbohydrate sources include whole grains, fruits, vegetables, and low-fat milk
Sucrose does not need to be restricted because it does not increase glycemia more
   than starch, but it should be substituted for other carbohydrates
Less than 10% of energy should come from saturated fats
Dietary cholesterol should be less than 300 mg/day
Non-nutritive sweeteners are safe when consumed in recommended amounts

Data from American Diabetes Association. Evidence-based nutrition principles and recommendations for the treatment and prevention of diabetes and related complications. *Diabet. Care* 2002; **25**(supp 1):S50–60.

Diet

Diet therapy is central to the management of type 2 diabetes. Frequently, type 2 diabetes coexists with obesity. A reduction in calorie intake will not only facilitate weight loss but also improve metabolic parameters by decreasing insulin resistance, reducing hepatic glucose output, and enhancing insulin secretion from the pancreas. As little as a 5–10% reduction in body weight may improve glycemic control significantly. A well-balanced diet with a moderate calorie restriction (250–500 fewer calories per day) in combination with behavioral modifications and education is a safe and effective method for improving metabolic control.

Because of the complexity of nutritional issues, the ADA recommends that a registered dietitian who is knowledgeable about diabetes management and education provides medical nutrition therapy. All diabetes caregivers should be familiar with medical nutrition therapy and supportive of patient efforts to make lifestyle changes. Some specific nutritional recommendations are listed in Table 15.5.[25] Carbohydrate and monounsaturated fat together should provide 60–70% of energy intake for individuals with diabetes. There is no evidence to suggest that the usual protein intake of 15–20% should be modified, as long as renal function is normal.

Exercise

Middle-aged and older adults with diabetes should be encouraged to exercise and be physically active, as the potential health benefits of exercise for the individual with type 2 diabetes are substantial.[26,27] Exercise may improve insulin sensitivity and help to normalize blood glucose levels. Evidence also suggests that the progressive decline in fitness and strength seen with aging can be decreased with regular exercise, leading to an improved quality of life.

Although exercise is an important component of therapy in diabetes, the risks and benefits of exercise must be understood and analyzed for each individual patient. Before beginning an exercise program, each individual with diabetes should undergo a complete medical evaluation to screen for vascular disease with diagnostic studies, as appropriate. The history and physical examination should focus on the heart and blood vessels, eyes, kidneys, and nervous system. For those planning to participate in low-intensity exercise, such as walking, the physician should use clinical judgment in deciding whether a cardiac/exercise stress test is warranted. For those planning a moderate- to high-intensity exercise program, an exercise electrocardiogram or cardiac stress test is recommended for the following individuals:

- known or suspected coronary artery disease;
- older than age 30 years and with type 1 diabetes;
- greater than 15-year history of type 1 diabetes;
- older than 35 years old and with type 2 diabetes.[26]

A thorough ophthalmologic examination is also recommended, as impaired vision increases the risk of injury and proliferative retinopathy increases the risk of retinal or vitreous hemorrhage during certain activities.

Evidence from the Diabetes Prevention Program, discussed above, supports 30 minutes of moderate physical activity at least five days per week (150 minutes/week). Aerobic exercise is recommended, with precautionary measures taken if the activity involves the feet. For those individuals with loss of protective sensation in the feet, recommended exercises include swimming, bicycling, rowing, chair exercises, arm exercises, and other non-weight-bearing exercise. Regardless of the activity, exercise should include a proper warm-up and cool-down period. Warm-up should include five to ten minutes of low-intensity aerobic activity followed by five to ten minutes of gentle muscle stretching. After the exercise activity is complete, a cool-down period of five to ten minutes should be performed at a lower-intensity level to bring the heart rate down gradually to pre-exercise level. As for anyone who exercises, proper hydration is essential, especially if exercising in extreme temperatures. Individuals with diabetes should wear a diabetes identification bracelet or tag that is clearly visible when exercising.

Home blood glucose monitoring

Monitoring of blood glucose levels by the patient and the healthcare provider is a cornerstone of diabetes care. With the development of home blood glucose meters, the management of diabetes has changed dramatically. Based on findings from the DCCT, SMBG is recommended for individuals with diabetes to facilitate reaching goals for blood glucose levels.[28] The optimal frequency of blood glucose monitoring in type 2 diabetes is not known, and the role of monitoring in diet-controlled type 2 diabetes is not known. SMBG is recommended for all insulin-treated patients with diabetes, and the frequency of monitoring should be increased when adding or modifying any diabetes therapy, with insulin or oral hypoglycemic agents. Patients need instruction in SMBG, including:

Table 15.6 Oral agents for treatment of type 2 diabetes

Sulfonylureas	Biguanides	Thiazolidinediones	Other agents
Glipizide	Metformin	Pioglitazone	Acarbose
Glyburide		Rosiglitazone	Miglitol
Glimepiride			Repaglinide
			Nateglinide

- the use of the blood glucose meter;
- goal blood glucose levels (see Table 15.4);
- how to interpret and use SMBG data to modify diet, exercise, or medical regimen to maintain adequate glycemic control;
- recording blood glucose data in a logbook format that can be reviewed to determine patterns of abnormal blood glucose levels that can be corrected with changes to the diabetes management plan.

Medications
A summary of oral medications used to treat type 2 diabetes is given in Table 15.6.

Sulfonylureas
In the mid 1960s, the first generation of sulfonylureas was used to treat type 2 diabetes. Although use of sulfonylureas declined after tolbutamide was shown to increase cardiovascular risk in the University Group Diabetes Program (UGDP) study, a second generation of sulfonylureas with more potency and fewer side effects has emerged and is used widely. The second-generation sulfonylureas include glipizide, glyburide, and glimepiride. The mechanism of action of these compounds involves binding to the adenosine triphosphate (ATP)-dependent potassium channel of the pancreatic beta-cell, leading to sustained depolarization, calcium ion influx, and increased insulin secretion. The sulfonylureas have been shown to lower fasting plasma glucose by 50–70 mg/dl and to lower HbA1c by 0.8–1.7%. Despite these typical improvements in glycemic control, 20–25% of patients will have primary failure to obtain glycemic control with sulfonylurea therapy, while an additional 5–10% per year will experience secondary failure to maintain glycemic control.[29]

Initiation of sulfonylurea therapy should be considered if a patient has failed to achieve adequate blood glucose control with diet and exercise. Recommended doses and frequency of dosing vary by specific drug, but for many of these agents best results are obtained when taken 15–30 minutes before meals. The most common side effect from sulfonylurea therapy is hypoglycemia, which may be life-threatening. Because these drugs are metabolized by the liver and kidneys, they should be used with caution in patients with hepatic or renal dysfunction, which may increase the risk of hypoglycemia.

Biguanides
Metformin is the only biguanide currently available for clinical use. The mechanism of action of metformin, although understood incompletely, involves decreased hepatic glucose output, improved insulin sensitivity, and decreased gastrointestinal glucose absorption. The effects on hepatic glucose output appear to be the most important in reducing fasting plasma glucose and HbA1c. *Metformin reduces fasting plasma glucose by 22–26% and reduces HbA1c by 1.2–1.7%, without the risk of hypoglycemia seen with sulfonylureas.*

Although 5–10% of patients do not tolerate metformin because of gastrointestinal side effects, 80–90% of patients show improvement in overall glycemic control. The most serious potential side effect from metformin therapy is lactic acidosis, with an estimated incidence of 0.03 cases per 1000 patient-years. Contraindications to metformin therapy include renal dysfunction (creatinine >1.5 mg/dl), hepatic dysfunction, alcohol abuse, cardiac disease, peripheral vascular disease, pulmonary disease, and intercurrent illness. Metformin therapy should be discontinued temporarily when intravenous contrast studies are planned, as a transient decrease in renal clearance could lead to increased risk of lactic acidosis.

Thiazolidinediones
Thiazolidinediones (TZDs) are peroxisome proliferator-activated receptor (PPAR)-gamma ligands. They enhance insulin sensitivity directly, to improve glycemic control. Pioglitazone and rosiglitazone are the two members of this class that are currently available for clinical use. The mechanism of action of TZDs is understood incompletely, but it involves decreased insulin resistance in peripheral tissues and increased insulin-stimulated glucose uptake in skeletal muscle.

Controlled studies have shown that both rosiglitazone and pioglitazone reduce HbA1c by 1.5–1.6%. Side effects of TZDs include weight gain, edema, and anemia. Given the liver toxicity associated with troglitazone, which was withdrawn from clinical use, the US Food and Drug Administration (FDA) recommends periodic monitoring of liver function tests for all patients receiving TZDs. Patients with congestive heart failure and/or hepatic impairment should not receive TZDs. Several weeks of therapy are necessary to see improvement in glycemic control. These medications may be used alone or in combination with other agents; however, only pioglitazone is approved for use with insulin.[30]

Table 15.7 Insulins and insulin analogs*

Class	Onset	Peak(h)	Duration(h)	Members
Rapid-acting	5–15 min	1–2	4–6	Lispro, aspart
Short-acting	30–60 min	2–4	6–10	Regular
Intermediate-acting	1–2 h	4–8	10–20	NPH Lente
Long-acting	2–4 h	10–30	16–20	Ultralente
Very long-acting	1–2 h	Flat	24	Glargine

* *Note:* in addition to the insulins listed here, a variety of insulin mixtures, such as 70/30 or 75/25, which contain a combination of long- and short/rapid-acting insulins, are also available and are used widely.

Other oral agents

The alpha-glucosidase inhibitors, acarbose and miglitol, decrease the rate of breakdown of dietary polysaccharides, delaying the absorption of glucose from the gut and thus decreasing the postprandial glucose rise. These agents reduce fasting plasma glucose by 25–35 mg/dl and reduce HbA1c by 0.4–0.7%. However, for patients who consume less than 50% of calories as carbohydrates, there is little benefit on glycemic control. The non-sulfonylurea insulin secretagogs (meglitinides) have similar action to sulfonylureas and act by stimulating insulin production from the pancreas to control postprandial hyperglycemia. The two members of this class are the benzoic acid derivative repaglinide and the phenylalanine derivative nateglinide.

Insulin: types and profiles

Individuals with type 2 diabetes usually experience a progressive decline in endogenous insulin production as the duration of diabetes increases. Thus, many people with type 2 diabetes may become insulin-requiring. Insulin supplementation in type 2 diabetes may be necessary either on a temporary basis for stress-induced hyperglycemia or permanently after failure of oral agents to maintain adequate glycemic control.

A variety of insulin preparations are currently available, including human insulins and insulin analogs. Animal insulins, such as pork and beef insulin, are no longer used routinely in clinical practice. Each type of insulin has a unique profile of action, including onset of effect, time of peak effect, and duration of action (see Table 15.7).

The profile of action is dependent on absorption from the subcutaneous site of injection into the circulation. The timing of insulin injections and choice of type and dose of insulin must be made on an individual basis using home blood glucose monitoring data and HbA1c as a guide. Individuals with type 1 diabetes always require insulin therapy alone. For individuals with type 2 diabetes who do not reach a target HbA1c of less than 7.0% with a single oral agent or insulin, combination therapy can be helpful. The use of an oral agent, in particular an insulin sensitizer such as metformin or a TZD, in combination with insulin may improve glycemic control and decrease insulin requirements.

Depending on the level of glycemic control achieved and the patient's willingness and ability to use a multi-injection regimen, an intensive insulin regimen with three to four insulin injections per day may be appropriate. Referral to an endocrinologist for assistance with diabetes management is appropriate for patients with polypharmacy, continued poor glycemic control, progressive diabetic complications including hypoglycemia, and insulin pump therapy.

Diabetes complications

The complications of diabetes develop over many years and include microvascular disease (neuropathy, retinopathy, nephropathy) and macrovascular disease (myocardial infarction, stroke, peripheral vascular disease). Given the chronicity of diabetes, the increasing evidence that improving glycemic control in type 1 diabetes[31] and type 2 diabetes[32] can decrease microvascular complications and ameliorate macrovascular complications has been encouraging. Prevention and management of diabetes complications are now part of the standard of care in the management of all patients with diabetes.

Cardiovascular disease remains the major cause of morbidity and mortality for all patients with diabetes. Women with diabetes are five times more likely to develop coronary artery disease than women without diabetes.[33] The protective effect of female gender against cardiovascular disease before menopause is not true for any woman with diabetes. *Presentation of heart disease may be atypical in the woman with diabetes.* Fatigue, decreased exercise tolerance, or dyspepsia may be anginal equivalent symptoms in the woman with diabetes.[34] Routine evaluation with exercise stress testing may have up to a 54% false-positive rate in women, so other cardiac evaluations, such as a stress nuclear perfusion study or stress echo, may be necessary. Small-vessel disease is common in diabetes; therefore, revascularization procedures may be more difficult in women with diabetes. Risk-factor modification, including smoking cessation, aspirin use, blood pressure control (with consideration of an angiotensin-converting enzyme (ACE) inhibitor or an angiotensin-receptor blocking agent), and aggressive lipid management should be addressed.

Dyslipidemia in women is a powerful contributing factor to the macrovascular complications of diabetes, in particular the increasing cardiovascular morbidity and mortality. Subset analysis has shown that goal low-density lipoprotein (LDL) cholesterol of less than 100 mg/dl and triglycerides less than 200 mg/dl impact cardiovascular events in women with diabetes. In addition to diet and exercise, lipid-lowering medications such as the 3-hydroxy-3-methylglutaryl ceenzyme A (HMG CoA) reductase inhibitors (to lower LDL)

Table 15.8 Preventive care in diabetes

Serum blood glucose monitoring
HbA1c at least twice a year (target <7%)
Blood pressure target <130/80 mmHg
Annual test for urine microalbumin if urinalysis negative for protein
Annual dilated eye examination
Smoking cessation
Laboratory testing for lipid abnormalities, at least annually (target LDL <100 mg/dl)
Aspirin therapy (adult diabetes patients with macrovascular disease or age >40 years)
Medical nutrition therapy
Regular physical activity (goal of 30 min at moderate intensity five times/week)
Annual influenza vaccine
Lifetime pneumococcal vaccine (once)

or fibric acid derivatives (to lower triglycerides) may be necessary to achieve target lipid levels.

Microvascular disease affecting the eyes, kidneys, and feet can be devastating for the patient with diabetes. Annual dilated ophthalmology examinations, urine screening for protein or microalbumin, and a careful foot examination at each healthcare visit can help to detect complications early, allowing for stabilization and improved outcomes. Preventive care suggestions in the management of diabetes are outlined in Table 15.8.

Diabetes complications appear to be related to the level of glycemic control. The UKPDS showed a 14% reduction in all-cause mortality for every 1% lowering in HbA1c. HbA1c levels averaging below 7% are associated with fewer long-term microvascular complications than HbA1c levels over 7%.

With aggressive glucose lowering to meet HbA1c targets and prevent vascular complications, *increasing frequency and severity of hypoglycemia occur and should also be considered a diabetes complication.* One option to help achieve target HbA1c with less hypoglycemia is to monitor two-hour postprandial glucose levels, with target glucose less than 180 mg/dl (10.0 mmol/l).

Summary

The development of diabetes in mid life can make the management of both menopausal symptoms and diabetes more difficult. Good glycemic control, through education, self-blood glucose monitoring, diet, and exercise, as well as medications, is important to minimize the increased health risks associated with diabetes. Since the complications of diabetes, including heart attack, stroke, blindness, end-stage renal disease, and lower-extremity amputation, are more prevalent with advancing age and duration of diabetes, mid-life women with diabetes must advocate for their own healthcare management. Working with their healthcare providers, women with diabetes can participate in healthcare maintenance behavior that can prevent or identify diabetes complications earlier. As research toward understanding the cause and finding the cure for all types of diabetes continues, prevention and early treatment of diabetes are crucial to improve outcomes and quality of life for all who live with this disease.

Take-home points

- Physiologic changes of menopause can worsen glycemic control.
- Use of HRT in menopausal women with diabetes remains controversial.
- Women with diabetes are at increased risk for cardiovascular disease, which is the leading cause of death in menopausal women with diabetes.
- Osteoporosis and depression need to be addressed in the menopausal woman with diabetes.
- A diabetes management plan should include education, self-blood glucose monitoring, diet, and exercise, as well as medications and insulin if necessary.

For the 51-year-old woman with type 2 diabetes and symptoms suggestive of perimenopause, her worsening diabetes control is likely related to her menstrual changes. If her glycemic control remains inadequate with current diet, exercise, and metformin therapy, then she may require additional therapy with a second medication or insulin. She should discuss her individual risks and benefits from HRT with her primary care provider, and the decision to use HRT or not should be reassessed on a regular basis, as more evidence becomes available.

FURTHER RESOURCES

American Diabetes Association: www.diabetes.org
The Endocrine Society: www.endo-society.org
Information on diabetes and menopause: www.mayoclinic.com

REFERENCES

1 King, H., Aubert, R. E. and Herman, W. H. Global burden of diabetes, 1995–2025. *Diabet. Care* 1998; **21**:1414–31.
2 Harris, M. I., Flegal, K. M., Cowie, C. C., *et al.* Prevalence of diabetes, impaired fasting glucose, and impaired glucose tolerance in U.S. adults. *Diabet. Care* 1998; **21**:518–24.

3　Gu, K., Cowie, C. C. and Harris, M. I. Mortality in adults with and without diabetes in a national cohort of the U.S. population, 1971–1993. *Diabet. Care* 1998; **21**: 1138–45.

4　American Diabetes Association. Screening for diabetes. *Diabet. Care* 2002; **25**(supp 1):S21–4.

5　Expert Committee on the Diagnosis and Classification of Diabetes Mellitus. Report of the Expert Committee on the Diagnosis and Classification of Diabetes Mellitus. *Diabet. Care* 2002; **25**(supp 1):S5–20.

6　World Health Organization. *Diabetes Mellitus: Report of a WHO Study Group.* Geneva: World Health Organization; 1985.

7　American Diabetes Association. Standards of medical care for patients with diabetes mellitus. *Diabet. Care* 2002; **25**(supp 1):S33–49.

8　American Diabetes Association. Tests of glycemia in diabetes. *Diabet. Care* 2002; **25**(supp 1):S97–9.

9　American Diabetes Association and NIDDK. The prevention or delay of type 2 diabetes. *Diabet. Care* 2002; **25**:742–9.

10　Colditz, G. A., Willett, W. C., Rotnitzky, A. and Manson, J. E. Weight gain as a risk factor for clinical diabetes mellitus in women. *Ann. Intern. Med.* 1995; **122**:481–6.

11　Folsom, A. R., Kushi, L. H. and Hong, C. P. Physical activity and incident diabetes mellitus in postmenopausal women. *Am. J. Publ. Health* 2000; **90**:134–8.

12　Knowler, W. C., Barret-Connor, E., Fowler, S. E., *et al.* Reduction in the incidence of type 2 diabetes with lifestyle intervention or metformin. *N. Engl. J. Med.* 2002; **346**:393–403.

13　Poirier, L. and Coburn, K. *Women and Diabetes.* Alexandria, VA: American Diabetes Association; 1997.

14　Samaras, K., Hayward, C., Sullivan, D., Kelly, R. and Campbell, L. Effects of postmenopausal hormone replacement therapy on central abdominal fat, glycemic control, lipid metabolism, and vascular factors in type 2 diabetes. *Diabet. Care.* 1999; **22**:1401–7.

15　Matthews, K. A., Meilahn, E., Kuller, L. H., *et al.* Menopause and risk factors for coronary heart disease. *N. Engl. J. Med.* 1989; **321**:641–6.

16　The Writing Group for the PEPI Trial. Effects of estrogen or estrogen/progestin regimens on heart disease risk factors in postmenopausal women: the Postmenopausal Estrogen/Progestin Intervention (PEPI) trial. *J. Am. Med. Assoc.* 1995; **273**:199–208.

17　Andersson, B., Mattsson, L. A., Hahn, I., *et al.* Estrogen replacement therapy decreases hyperandrogenicity and improves glucose homeostasis and plasma lipids in postmenopausal women with noninsulin-dependent diabetes. *J. Clin. Endocrinol. Metab.* 1997; **82**:638–43.

18　Stratton, I. M., Adler, A. I., Neil, H. A., *et al.* Association of glycaemia with macrovascular and microvascular complications of type 2 diabetes (UKPDS 35): prospective observational study. *Br. Med. J.* 2000; **321**:405–12.

19　Ferrara, A., Karter, A., Ackerson, L., Liu, J. and Selby, J. Hormone replacement therapy is associated with better glycaemic control in women with type 2 diabetes. *Diabet. Care* 2001; **24**:1144–50.

20　Writing Group for the Women's Health Initiative Investigators. Risks and benefits of estrogen plus progestin in healthy postmenopausal women. *J. Am. Med. Assoc.* 2002; **288**:321–23.

21 Grady, D. and the HERS research group. Cardiovascular disease outcomes during 6.8 years of hormone therapy. *J. Am. Med. Assoc.* 2002; **288**:49–57.

22 Osteoporosis prevention, diagnosis, and therapy. *NIH Consens. Statement* 2000; **17**:1–36.

23 Surwit, R., Van Tilburg, M., Zucker, N., *et al.* Stress management improves long-term glycemic control in type 2 diabetes. *Diabet. Care* 2002; **25**:30–34.

24 Dorman, J., Steenkiste, A., Foley, T., *et al.* Menopause in type 1 diabetic women: is it premature? *Diabetes* 2001; **50**:1857–62.

25 American Diabetes Association. Evidence-based nutrition principles and recommendations for the treatment and prevention of diabetes and related complications. *Diabet. Care* 2002; **25**(supp 1):S50–60.

26 American Diabetes Association. Diabetes mellitus and exercise. *Diabet. Care* 2002; **25**(supp 1):S64–8.

27 Devlin, J. T. and Ruderman, N. *The Health Professional's Guide to Diabetes and Exercise.* Alexandria VA: American Diabetes Association; 1995.

28 American Diabetes Association. Implications of the Diabetes Control and Complications Trial. *Diabet. Care* 2002; **25**(supp 1):S25–7.

29 Feinglos, M. N. and Bethel, M. A. Treatment of type 2 diabetes mellitus. *Med. Clin. North Am.* 1998; **82**:757–90.

30 Inzucchi, S. E. Oral antihyperglycemic therapy for type 2 diabetes. Scientific review. *J. Am. Med. Assoc.* 2002; **287**:360–72.

31 Diabetes Control and Complications Trial research group. The effect of intensive treatment of diabetes on the development and progression of long-term complications in insulin-dependent diabetes mellitus. *N. Engl. J. Med.* 1993; **329**:977–86.

32 UK Prospective Diabetes Study Group. Intensive blood glucose control with sulfonylureas or insulin compared with conventional treatment and risk of complications in patients with type 2 diabetes (UKPDS 33). *Lancet* 1998; **352**:837–53.

33 Poirier, L. and Coburn, K. *Women and Diabetes.* Alexandria, VA: American Diabetes Association; 1997.

34 Howard, B., Cowan, L., Go, O., *et al.* Adverse effects of diabetes on multiple cardiovascular disease risk factors in women. *Diabet. Care* 1998; **21**:1258–65.

Part IV

Cancer prevention

16

Breast cancer: screening and prevention

Jo Ann Rosenfeld

Introduction

Breast cancer has the highest incidence and the third highest death rate for cancer in women in the USA. More than 200 000 women annually develop breast cancer in the USA.[1] The incidence of breast cancer increased between 1973 and 1998 by 40%, perhaps caused by an increase in early-stage breast cancer detection.[2] A woman in the USA has approximately a one in eight risk of developing breast cancer in her lifetime. The incidence of breast cancer increases with age, making screening more important in middle-aged women.

Unlike with lung cancer, screening programs and early detection for breast cancer have reduced its mortality. No studies have found a method to prevent breast cancer. Thus, early detection to reduce mortality is essential.[3] The fact that early detection with mammography reduces mortality in women aged 50–69 years has been accepted and established. However, controversies about the efficacy of screening with different methods and in different populations have occurred; newer studies may be reported in the near future that may reduce or increase these disputes. Evaluation of previous investigations is, thus, important.

Presentation

The most common presentation of breast cancer is no symptoms. The first symptom is often a small, painless nodule or pain. Other symptoms include skin changes, dimpling, and nipple discharge.

Case: a 48-year-old woman comes to the office for an episode of acute bronchitis. After history and examination, you notice that there is no note of any breast cancer screening, including mammography, on her chart. You suggest a mammogram, but she says, "Hasn't that proven lately not to be accurate?"

Screening

There are several methods of screening – self-breast examination (SBE), clinical breast examination (CBE) (by doctor or health worker), and mammography. None of these methods, except mammography, has been shown by randomized, controlled trials (RCTs) to be an effective tool for early detection (reducing mortality).[4] Combinations of these and newer methods such as ultrasound and computed tomography (CT) scanning are also used.

Self-breast exmination

Although SBE has been taught to women for years and its use widely encouraged, recent evidenced-based reviews have called into question its importance, efficacy, and even harmless nature. No RCTs have found a reduction in mortality from use of SBE alone. More than 30 non-randomized studies have produced conflicting results.[5]

Women who used SBE did not find smaller or more curable tumors than those who did not. In fact, there were significantly more biopsies that proved negative in women who used SBE.[6] Studies have found that tumors found in those women who used SBE were similar in size to those found in women who did not use SBE. The Canadian Task Force on Preventive Health Care has decided that there is no good evidence of benefit, and evidence of harm, in teaching SBE to women of all ages (grade D recommendation).[7]

Clinical breast examination

Whether health professional-performed CBE is an adequate, sufficient, or effective tool for screening by itself is disputed. *The efficacy of CBE is dependent on the amount of time the provider spends.* Its sensitivity has been estimated at 54%, with a specificity of 94%.[8] In women aged 50–59 years, one large RCT found that CBE alone was as effective as mammography, although mammography was more sensitive in detecting small cancers.[9] Other studies found that CBE diagnosed a percentage of breast cancers that were missed by screening mammography.[9,10]

Mammography

Mammography has been recommended as the most efficient method of screening in women over age 50 years. The Health Insurance Plan Breast Cancer Screening Project completed in 1963 after it had followed more than 60 000 women aged 40–64 for more than ten years was the first study to find that women in the screening group (four annual mammograms) had a 30% reduction in breast cancer mortality.[11] Six of seven subsequent large RCTs

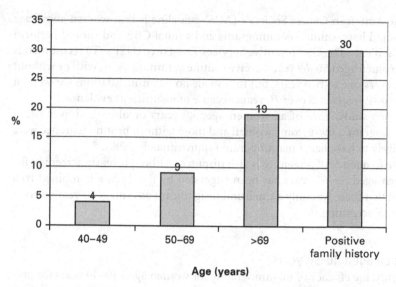

Figure 16.1 Positive predictive value of mammography by age. (From Kerlikowske, K., Grad, D. and Barclay, J. Positive predictive value of screening mammography by age and family history of breast cancer. *J. Am. Med. Assoc.* 1993; **270**:2444–50.

that differed somewhat in methods found significant reduction in mortality rates in those women who were screened with mammography (relative risk 0.69–0.97).[12,13]

Women aged 50–65 years

Multiple RCTs and case–control studies have shown a 20–30% reduction in mortality in women age 50–65. For women of this aged, mammography has a higher sensitivity than either CBE or SBE alone (75–94%).[14] The specificity is also high (83–98%).[5] The positive predictive value of mammography (Figure 16.1) increases with age and family history.[15] Efficacy of screening in women aged 40–50 and older than age 65 is less well documented.

Mammography does have risks as well as benefits. Radiation exposure, false-positives leading to subsequent tests with additional radiation and expense, biopsies, surgery, and emotional scarring are all risks. The risk of false-positives is higher in younger women than in older women. The rate of false-positives is 7.8% in women aged 40–49 years and 7.4% in women aged 50–59 years. *The cumulative rate for a false-positive rate is 49% after ten annual mammograms.*[16] Out of 10 000 women aged 50–65 and screened by mammography, approximately 500–700 will need to return for further X-rays. Fewer than 100 will receive biopsies, and approximately 50–60 cancers will be found.[4]

The American Cancer Society's (ACS) guideline is that women above age 40 should have annual mammograms and annual CBE and should perform annual BSE.[17] The US Preventive Services Task Force (USPSTF) recommends that women aged 50–69 years receive routine mammography, with or without CBE, every one to two years, but they made no recommendations for women aged 40–49 years and over 70 years because of insufficient evidence.[5]

In one study, 85% of all women aged 40 years or older had ever had a mammogram. Low-income women and those without health insurance were less likely to have had a mammogram (approximately 70%).[18]

The frequency of screening is also disputed. Although yearly screening for women aged 50–65 years has been suggested by the ACS, a combined trial found that there was only a small and insignificant advantage to yearly versus triennial screening.[19]

Women aged 40–50 years

Recently, the efficacy of mammography for women aged 40–49 years for preventing breast cancer mortality has been disputed. A Canadian study of more than 50 000 women followed for 13–16 years, either by one CBE and instruction in SBE, or by four or more annual mammographies, found no improvement in mortality or in detection of number of breast cancers in the annual mammography group.[20] The same group found similar findings when they studied 40 000 women aged 50–59 years, calling into question the efficacy of annual mammography.[21]

Further analysis finds benefit in screening. A meta-analysis of eight RCTs, all following women aged 40–49 years for more than 12 years, found an 18% reduction in mortality in screened women.[22] The USPSTF concluded in 2000, in a meta-analysis of RCTs, that mammography reduced breast cancer mortality in women aged 40–74 years, and the risk reduction was greater in older women.[23]

Women over age 65 years

Mammography has been found to be effective in reducing mortality from breast cancer in older women in some studies. In a meta-analysis of studies in which women older than age 65 were included, there was a non-significant reduction in mortality up to age 70.[24] In one population study, older women who had not used mammography at all within the two years prior to the study were more likely to have breast cancer diagnosed at a more serious stage and to have greater mortality from breast cancer. This difference persisted even up to age 85 years.[25] In another study, use of mammography in women older than 70 years was related significantly to smaller breast cancer size at detection.[26]

Table 16.1 Risk factors for breast cancer

High relative risk	Moderately increased relative risk	Increased risk
Personal history of breast cancer	One first-degree relative with breast cancer	Obesity
Two or more first-degree relatives with breast cancer at early age	Atypical hyperplasia	High socioeconomic status
Age >65 years		Early menarche (<12 years)
		Late menopause (>54 years)
		No full-term pregnancy
		Late age at first pregnancy
		Recent oral contraceptive use
		Recent hormone replacement therapy use

Other modalities

Ultrasonography, CT scanning, and magnetic resonance imaging (MRI) are being studied for their uses in delineating breast cancer and their efficacy in detecting early breast cancer. CT scans, especially helical CT scans, have been studied only for delineating the extent of cancer before surgery.[27] One study establishing normals for MRI found a 98% negative and a 50% positive predictive rate for breast cancer, making it a possible adjunct study to help delineate malignancy.[28]

Ultrasonography has been the radiologic examination of choice in evaluation of breast lumps and abnormalities in younger women, especially those under 25 years. Used with mammography, especially in women with dense breasts, ultrasound significantly increases the detection of small cancers and those at smaller size and lower stage.[29]

Prevention

Risk factors

Most of the risk factors (see Table 16.1) of breast cancer cannot be modified. Breast cancer incidence increases with age. Seventy-seven per cent of new cases occur in women older than age 50. Lack of health insurance is associated with a lower survival rate once cancer is diagnosed.

After the age of 40, white women are more likely to be diagnosed with breast cancer than African-Americans; the incidence is lower still in other racial groups (Figure 16.2). However, although the overall five-year survival rate is 86%, the rate is lower in African-American women (72% versus 87% in white women) (Figure 16.3).

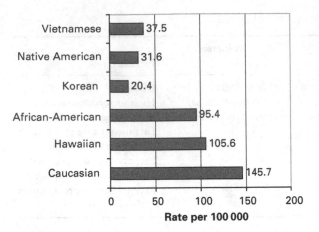

Figure 16.2 Incidence of breast cancer by ethnicity. (From Lawson, H., Hensen, R., Bobo, J. K. and Kaeser, M. K. Implementing recommendations for the early detection of breast and cervical cancer among low income women. *Morb. Mortal. Wkly Rep.* 2000; **49**: 37–55.)

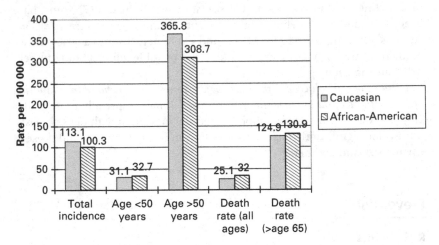

Figure 16.3 Incidence and death rate for breast cancer by ethnicity. (From Lawson, H., Hensen, R., Bobo, J. K. and Kaeser, M. K. Implementing recommendations for the early detection of breast and cervical cancer among low income women. *Morb. Mortal. Wkly Rep.* 2000; **49**: 37–55.)

In addition, family history, age at birth of first child, early menarche, and late menopause are risk factors. Women who had a first full-term pregnancy before age 20 are half as likely to develop breast cancer as those whose first pregnancy occurred after age 35.[30]

Modifiable risk factors include alcohol abuse/overuse, hormone replacement therapy, and obesity. Some studies have shown an inverse relationship between the level of physical activity and the risk of developing breast cancer. A history of active exercise has been associated with a 30–40% risk reduction.[31]

Diet

Reports have suggested that obesity and certain diets may increase the risk of breast cancer. Weight gain and obesity in the postmenopausal period have been linked to an increased risk of breast cancer.[32] Although a higher-fat diet has been associated with an increased risk of breast cancer in a few large population studies, a low-fat diet has not been proven to reduce the risk and meta-analysis fails to support the correlation.

Hormone replacement therapy

Hormone replacement therapy (HRT) (see Chapter 10) has been associated with an increased risk of breast cancer, especially in recent users. The risk may be dose-related.[33,34] The risk is greater in estrogen/progesterone users than in users of estrogen alone.

Hereditary factors

Case: R.W., a 28-year-old teacher, comes in with a request for breast cancer screening. Her 35-year-old sister is well, but her mother and maternal aunt have had breast cancer and mastectomies. She wants to know her risks and possibilities for prevention

Women with two first-degree relatives with breast cancer, especially if they developed it at an early age, are at higher risk for breast cancer. However, whether to screen women younger than age 50, including even those with a strong family history, and what method to use is disputed. One study of approximately 400 000 women found that cancer detection rates in women with a strong family history were similar to those in women a decade older without such a history. Age was the primary influence on the sensitivity of screening mammography.[35]

Fewer than 5% of breast cancers are associated with genetic syndromes of increased breast cancer risks. Some specific genes are linked to increased incidence of cancer, including BRCA1 and BRCA2. Women with these mutations have an increased risk of breast (56–85%),[36,37] ovarian, and colon cancer, while men with these mutations have an increased risk of breast and possibly prostate cancer.

In primary care, women may ask to be tested for the presence of these genes because of a positive family history for breast cancer. Discussion about the likelihood and requests that the index case (the relation who has breast cancer) be tested first may help to reassure many women.

No RCTs examining the efficacy of early screening for women with family histories of breast cancer have been carried out. Several large studies have shown no increase in cancer, whereas one shows an increase in the number of cancers found compared with women of a similar age but without histories.[38]

Pharmacotherapy prevention

The use of tamoxifen (a non-steroidal anti-estrogen) reduces the recurrence of breast cancer, while maintaining bone density, in women who use it as treatment for breast cancer. Ongoing trials are studying the use of tamoxifen and raloxifene to prevent breast cancer in high-risk women. One randomized double-blind trial of more than 13 000 women found a 49% reduction in the incidence of breast cancer in those women who received tamoxifen, with a concurrent reduction in fractures but an increased incidence of endometrial cancer and thromboses.[39] Other studies in Europe have not found similar prevention with tamoxifen.

Raloxifene, a selective estrogen receptor modulator (SERM), blocks estrogen at the breast and endometrium, unlike tamoxifen, which stimulates the uterus. The Multiple Outcomes of Raloxifene Evaluation (MORE) trial found that the incidence of estrogen-receptor-positive invasive breast cancer was reduced by 76% at 40 months' study.[40]

However, the general use of these agents for cancer chemoprevention is not yet approved or determined.

Summary

Breast cancer mortality may be reduced by early detection, especially in women older than age 50 with mammography. The use of other modalities is controversial. At the moment, there is no way to prevent breast cancer, although its prevention in high-risk women is under investigation.

FURTHER RESOURCES

National Cancer Institute information pages: www.nci.nih.gov/cancerinfo/pdq/prevention/breast/healthprofessional/
Harvard University information site for patients and for determining risk: www.yourcancerrisk.harvard.edu/

REFERENCES

1 Parker, S. L., Tong, T., Bolden, S. and Wingo, P. W. Cancer statistics, 1997. *CA Cancer J. Clin.* 1997; **47**:5–27.
2 Howe, H. L., Wingo, P. A., Thun, M. J., *et al.* Annual report to the nation on the status of cancer (1973 to 1998), featuring cancers with recent increasing trends. *J. Natl. Cancer Inst.* 2001; **93**:824–42.

3 Lawson, H., Henson, R., Bobo, J. K. and Kaeser, M. K. Implementing recommendations for the early detection of breast and cervical cancer among low income women. *Morb. Mortal. Wkly Rep.* 2000; **49**:37–55.

4 Blamey, R. W., Wilson, A. R. M. and Patnick, J. ABC of breast diseases: screening for breast cancer. *Br. Med. J.* 2000; **321**:689–93.

5 International Agency for Research on Cancer Working Group on the Evaluation of Cancer Preventive Strategies. Efficacy of screening by breast self-examination. In: H. Vaionio and F. Bianchini (eds.). *Breast Cancer Screening.* Lyon: IARC Press; 2002. pp. 107–13.

6 Semiglazov, V. R., Moisenyenko, V. M., Bavli, J. L., *et al.* The role of breast self-examination in early breast cancer detection. *Eur. J. Epidemiol.* 1992; **8**:498–502.

7 Baxter, N. and the Canadian Task Force on Preventive Health Care. Preventive health care, 2001 update: should women be routinely taught breast self-examination to screen for breast cancer? *Can. Med. Assoc. J.* 2001; **164**:1837–46.

8 Barton, M., Harris, R. and Fletcher, S. Does this patient have breast cancer? The screening clinical breast examination: should it be done? How? *J. Am. Med. Assoc.* 1999; **282**:1270–80.

9 Miller, A. B., To, T., Baines, C. J. and Wall, C. Canadian national breast screening study – 2: 13-year results of a randomized trial in women aged 50–59. *J. Natl. Cancer Inst.* 2000; **92**:1490–99.

10 Alexander, F. E., Anderson, T. J., Brown, H. K., *et al.* The Edinburgh randomized trial of breast cancer screening: results after 10 years follow-up. *Br. J. Cancer* 1994; **70**:542–8.

11 Shapiro, S., Venet, W., Strax, P., *et al.* Ten to fourteen year effect of screening on breast cancer mortality. *J. Natl. Cancer Inst.* 1982; **69**:349–55.

12 Brewster, A. and Davidson, N. Breast cancer screening. In: J. Rosenfeld (ed.). *Handbook of Women's Health.* Cambridge: Cambridge University Press; 2001. pp. 385–6.

13 Blanks, R. G., Moss, S. M., McGahan, C. E., Quinn, J. and Babb, B. J. Effect of NHS breast screening programme on mortality from breast cancer in England and Wales, 1990–8: comparison of observed with predicted mortality. *Br. Med. J.* 2000; **321**: 665–9.

14 US Preventive Services Task Force. *Guide to Clinical Preventive Services: Report of the US Preventive Services Task Force,* 2nd edn. Baltimore, MD: Williams & Wilkins; 1996.

15 Kerlikowske, K., Grad, D. and Barclay, J. Positive predictive value of screening mammography by age and family history of breast cancer. *J. Am. Med. Assoc.* 1993; **270**:2444–50.

16 Elmore, J., Barton, M., Moceri, V., *et al.* Ten year risk of false positive screening mammograms and clinical breast examinations. *N. Engl. J. Med.* 1998; **338**:1089–96.

17 American Cancer Society. *Cancer Prevention and Early Detection Facts and Figures, 2002.* Atlanta, GA: American Cancer Society; 2002.

18 Blackman, D. K., Bennett, E. M. and Miller, D. S. Trends in self-reported use of mammograms (1989–1997) and Papanicolaou tests (1991–1997) – behavioral risk factor surveillance system. *Morbid. Mortal. Wkly CDC Surveill. Summ.* 1999; **48**:1–22.

19 Kerlikowske, K., Grady, D., Barclay, J., Sickles, E. A. and Ernster, V. Effect of age, breast density, and family history on the sensitivity of first screening mammography. *J. Am. Med. Assoc.* 1996; **276**:33–8.

20 Miller, A. B., To, T., Baines, C. J. and Wall, C. The Canadian National Breast Screening Study-1: breast cancer mortality after 11 to 16 years of follow-up. A randomized screening trial of mammography in women age 40 to 49 years. *Ann. Intern. Med.* 2002; **137**:305–12.

21 Miller, A. B., To, T., Baines, C. J. and Wall, C. Canadian National Breast Screening Study-2: 13-year results of a randomized trial in women aged 50–59 years. *J. Natl. Cancer Inst.* 2000; **92**:1490–99.

22 Hendrick, R. E., Smith, R. A., Rutledge, J. H., III and Smart, C. R. Benefit of screening mammography in women aged 40–49: a new meta-analysis of randomized controlled trials. *J. Natl. Cancer Inst. Monogr.* 1997; **22**:87–92.

23 Humphrey, L. L., Helfand, M., Chan, B. K. and Woolf, S. H. Breast cancer screening: a summary of the evidence for the U.S. Preventive Services Task Force. *Ann. Intern. Med.* 2002; **137**:347–60.

24 Larson, L. G., Nystrom, L., Wall, S., *et al.* The Swedish randomized mammography screening trials: analysis of the effect on the breast cancer related excess mortality. *J. Med. Screen.* 1996; **3**:129–32.

25 McCarthy, E. P., Burns, R. B., Freund, K. M., *et al.* Mammography use, breast cancer stage at diagnosis and survival among older women. *J. Am. Geriatr. Soc.* 2000; **48**:2221–9.

26 Randolph, W. M., Goodwin, J. S., Mahnken, J. D. and Freeman, J. L. Regular mammography use is associated with elimination of age-related disparities in size and stage of breast cancer at diagnosis. *Ann. Intern. Med.* 2002; **137**:783–90.

27 Uematsu, T., Sano, M., Homma, K., Shiina, M. and Kobayashi, S. Three-dimensional helical CT of the breast: accuracy for measuring extent of breast cancer candidates for breast conserving surgery. *Breast Cancer Res. Treat.* 2001; **65**:249–57.

28 Gilhuijs, K. G., Deurloo, E. E., Muller, S. H., Peterse, J. L. and Schultz Kool, L. J. Breast MR imaging in women at increased lifetime risk of breast cancer: clinical system for computerized assessment of breast lesions initial results. *Radiology* 2002; **225**:907–16.

29 Kolb, T. M., Lichy, J. and Newhouse, J. H. Comparison of the performance of screening mammography, physical examination, and breast US and evaluation of factors that influence them: an analysis of 27,825 patient evaluations. *Radiology* 2002; **225**:165–75.

30 Brinton, L. A., Schairer, C., Hoover, R. N., *et al.* Menstrual factors and risk of breast cancer. *Cancer Invest.* 1988; **6**:245–54.

31 Thune, I., Brenn, T. and Lund, E. Physical activity and the risk of breast cancer. *N. Engl. J. Med.* 1997; **336**:1269–75.

32 Hirose, K., Tajima, K., Hamajima, N., *et al.* The effect of body size on breast cancer risk among Japanese women. *Int. J. Cancer* 1999; **80**:349–55.

33 Schairer, C., Lubin, J., Troisis, R., *et al.* Menopausal estrogen and estrogen–progestin replacement therapy and breast cancer risk. *J. Am. Med. Assoc.* 2000; **283**:485–91.

34 Colditz, F. A., Hankinson, S. E., Hunter, D. J., *et al.* The use of estrogens and progestins and the risk of breast cancer in post menopausal women. *N. Engl. J. Med.* 1995; **332**:1589–93.

35 Kerlikowske, K., Carney, P. A., Geller, B., *et al.* Performance of screening mammography among women with and without a first-degree relative with breast cancer. *Ann. Intern. Med.* 2000; **133**:855–63.

36 Easton, D. F., Bishop, D. T., Ford, D., *et al.* Genetic linkage analysis in familial breast and ovarian cancer: results from 215 familieis. *Am. J. Hum. Genet.* 1993; **52**:678–701.

37 Strueing, J. P., Hartge, P., Wacholder, S., *et al.* The risk of cancer associated with specific mutations of BRCA1 and BRCA2 among Ashkenazi Jews. *N. Engl. J. Med.* 1997; **336**:1401–8.

38 Macmillan, R. D. Screening women with a family history of breast cancer. Results from the British Familial Breast Cancer group. *Eur. J. Surg. Oncol.* 2000; **26**:149–52.

39 Fisher, B., Constatino, J. P., Wickerham, D. L., *et al.* Tamoxifen for prevention of breast cancer. Report of the National Surgical Adjuvant Breast and Bowel Project P-1 study. *J. Natl. Cancer Inst.* 1998; **90**:1371–88.

40 Cummings, S. R., Eckert, D., Kreuger, D. A., *et al.* The effect of raloxifene on risk of breast cancer in postmenopausal women. *J. Am. Med. Assoc.* 1999; **281**:2189–97.

17

Cervical cancer: prevention, screening, and early detection

Jo Ann Rosenfeld

Case: S.T. is a 45-year-old mother of two grown-up daughters. She comes in, complaining of fatigue. She is sleeping well and physical examination is normal, except for a 18-week-size uterus. She has not had a Pap test for 15 years. She complains of heavy and frequent menstrual periods, but considers this normal. Laboratory tests show a hematocrit of 21, with hemoglobin of 7.3 g/dl. Pap test reveals cells consistent with carcinoma.

Incidence

The incidence of cervical cancer has decreased since the 1950s and stabilized in the 1980s in the USA. Approximately 13 000 women will develop cervical cancer yearly, and approximately 4500 will die from it.[1] Because the incidence and mortality of cervical cancer have decreased by more than 40% since 1973 and the push for mass screenings, the Agency for Health Care Policy and Research (AHCPR) has given Pap tests an "A" recommendation, despite poor evidence for their efficacy.[2] In many cases, cervical cancer can be prevented.

The rate of cervical cancer varies widely with race. The highest incidence in the USA is among Vietnamese women, but the highest death rate is in African-American women, being approximately 50% higher than that of Caucasian Americans.[3] Death rates for cervical cancer increase with increasing age. Because stage I (invasive but localized) cancer has a 90% five-year survival rate, while stages III and IV (advanced invasive and/or metastatic) have a five-year survival rate of 12%, screening and early detection are possible, effective, and essential. Prevention may or may not be possible.

Screening and early detection

The Pap smear

The Pap test is one of the better tests for detecting precursors of cancer. If followed by evaluation and treatment, it significantly reduces the mortality from cervical cancer. The purpose of the Pap test is to detect and treat cervical intraepithelial neoplasia (CIN) and, thus, prevent invasive cancer. Of those women treated for CIN, the likelihood of cure and survival is nearly 100%.

Most women who develop cervical cancer have never had a Pap test, or have not had one in the past ten years. In the USA, more than half of those women who developed cervical cancer last year had never had a Pap test.[4] Another 10% have not had a Pap test within five years, and 10% have had ineffective follow-up for an abnormal Pap test.[5]

Case–control studies in the UK have found that cervical cancer screening by Pap test has changed the incidence of cervical cancer over the past 20 years. The incidence of cervical cancer has fallen since 1960, mostly in the group of women aged 40–69, who are "well-screened."[6] Most invasive cancer was found at stage I and these in women who had poor screening histories. Half had never been screened, and one-third had had only remote screening. There has been an increase in CIN III since 1982, occurring more often in women younger than 40 years and older than 70 years. There was a decrease in death from cervical cancer in all women and in women aged 45–64.[3]

Method

The specimen is obtained from the woman, not on her menses, by use of a wire brush and Ayre's speculum or plastic speculum if Thin Prep is used.

Over the past ten years, the standard slide and fixative has been replaced by the liquid preparations (Thin Prep) liquid method. These methods have more than a 100% increase in the detection of CIN lesions, a decrease in the false-negative rate, a decrease in the rate of atypical cells of unknown significance studies, and improvement in detection of high-grade squamous intraepithelial lesions (HGSIL),[7,8] although the sensitivity has been disputed.[9]

When and how often?

The frequency, initiation, and cessation of regular Pap tests are controversial. The 2003 American Cancer Society (ACS) guidelines are shown in Table 17.1.[10] Further modifications of these guidelines may include a test for human papilloma virus (HPV), which may delineate those women who need closer follow-up and evaluation. A study of more than 2000 women found that those with normal Pap tests but with positive detection of abnormal HPV were more likely to have subsequent abnormal Pap tests (odds ration 2.7):[11] fifteen per cent developed abnormal pap tests within five years.

Table 17.1 2003 American Cancer Society guidelines for frequency of Pap tests

Women begin regular Pap tests after three years of initiation of vaginal intercourse or
  at age 21 years
Pap tests performed annually if slide tests are used or every other year if liquid-based
  tests are used
After age 30 years, women with three normal Pap tests in a row may be screened less
  frequently (approximately every three years), unless there are increased risk factors
After age 70 years, women who have had three or more normal Pap tests and no
  abnormal tests for ten years may choose to stop cervical cancer screening
Women who have had a hysterectomy usually do not need cervical cancer screening

Data from American Cancer Society. American Cancer Society issues new cer-
vical cancer early detection guidelines. www.cancer.org/docroot/MED/content/
MED_2_1x_American_Cancer_Society_Issues_New_Cervical_Cancer_Early_Detection_
Guidelines. asp. Accessed March 6, 2003.

Evaluation of abnormal Pap test

Assuming an adequate specimen, normal or negative Pap test results can be
followed as in Table 17.1. Controversies and variation in consensus of the
evaluation of other readings occur.

Atypical cells of undetermine sequence (ASCUS) may be the reading that
causes much of the difficulty. One wants to neither overinvestigate with invasive procedures nor miss a cervical cancer before cure is possible. Use of
HPV testing, often done routinely by the laboratory if ASCUS is detected,
may determine a group of women with high-risk HPV infection who need
closer and more frequent evaluation. Women with readings of "ASCUS – favor
low-grade squamous intraepithelial lesion (LGSIL) or high-grade squamous
intraepithelial lesion (HGSIL)" are found to be more likely to be infected
with high-risk HPV.[12] Follow-up evaluation for ASCUS can include repeat
Pap testing in three months, HPV testing, and/or colposcopy, especially if the
woman is infected with high-risk HPV or has had previous abnormal Pap tests,
or a more definite diagnosis is wanted immediately by patient or physician.[13]
Because postmenopausal women have a much lower rate of HPV infection
and cervical cancer, ASCUS can be evaluated by a repeat cytology on Pap test
alone.[14]

Recent studies, including the Atypical Squamous Cell of Undetermined
Significance/Low-Grade Squamous Intraepithelial Lesions Triage Study
(ALTS), found that a positive high-risk HPV finding was more sensitive and
specific than repeat Pap test cytology in detecting HGSIL (sensitivity 96%).[15]
A single repeat cytology had only 44% sensitivity in detecting HGSIL.

Higher-grade abnormal Pap test results (LGSIL, HGSIL, cancer in situ
(CIS)) need rapid evaluation and verification by colposcopy. HPV testing
is not needed in these women, because 83–99% are positive for high-risk

infections.[3] Although only 15% of women with LGSIL will proceed to CIS, one-third to two-thirds will require colposcopy in the next two years. In one study, 15% of women with LGSIL on Pap smear had CIN III or invasive cancer on subsequent biopsy.[16] If these lesions are found on colposcopy, then treatment with cryosurgery, laser, loop excision by electrocautery procedure (LEEP), or further surgery may be needed.

Women in the perimenopausal years may have readings that include statements such as "Endometrial cells seen – clinical correlation necessary." While women are still menstruating, the appearance of endometrial cells is not pathologic and needs no further evaluation. If the woman is menopausal and this reading is given, then a vaginal ultrasound to examine for endometrial hyperplasia or cancer may be indicated.

The reading of "Atypical glandular cells (of unknown significance)" (AGUS) is more worrisome. Pap smears are less effective in detecting adenocarcinoma precursors, and have only a 50–75% sensitivity. Repeating the Pap test does not improve the sensitivity.[17]

AGUS is significant; 10–40% will be associated with a malignant or premalignant condition of the endocervix or endometrium.[18] A literature review found that of more than 1300 patients with AGUS, approximately one-third had abnormalities, most HGSIL, but one-third of these were adenocarcinoma.[19]

Prevention

Risk factors and etiology

The risk factors linked with cervical cancer include infection with certain subtypes of HPV, multiple sexual partners, sexually transmitted diseases, low socioeconomic status, and smoking.[20] Estrogen use, including hormone replacement therapy, is not a risk factor for cervical cancer and in fact may be protective.[21]

Most cases of squamous cervical cancers are caused by HPV. Approximately 90% of cervical carcinoma is caused by infection of one of 15 subtypes of HPV.[22] In one study that pooled data of case-controlled studies, including more than 200 women, HPV-DNA was detected in more than 90% of women with cervical cancer and in only 13% of control women.[23] The relative risk of death was increased in those women with cervical cancer and certain HPV subtypes.[24] Fifteen HPV subtypes are classified as high-risk types (16, 18, 31, 33, 35, 39, 45, 51, 52, 56, 58, 59, 68, 73, 82); three are classified as probable high-risk types (26, 53, 66); and 12 are classified as low-risk types (6, 11, 40, 42, 43, 44, 54, 61, 70, 72, 81, CP6108), by recent pooled data from case-controlled studies.[7] Infection with HPV may require synergism with other factors to produce intraepithelial neoplasia and cancer. Infection with HPV is related inversely to age.

Many studies have found no increase in the risk of cervical cancer in users of oral contraceptives. However, some have found a more rapid transition from dysplasia to CIS if the woman has used the oral contraceptive pill for more than six years. There is an increased risk of cervical cancer in users of progesterone-only contraception (relative risk 1.2 for ever used, 2.4 for use more than five years).[25]

Summary

Cervical cancer is a disease that can be prevented if precursors are detected early and treated appropriately. Although the incidence decreases with age, women aged 40–65 years still need cervical cancer screening, but perhaps less often than at younger ages.

REFERENCES

1 Greenlee, R. T., Murray, T., Bolden, S. and Wingo, P. A. Cancer statistics, 2000. *CA Cancer J. Clin.* 2000; **50**:7–33.
2 Agency for Health Care Policy and Research. *Evaluation of Cervical Cytology.* Evidence report/technology assessment No. 5. Rockville, MD: Agency for Health Care Policy and Research; 1999.
3 Ries, L. A. G., Kosary, C. L., Hankey, B. E., *et al.* (eds). *SEER Cancer Statistics Review, 1973–1996.* Bethesda, MD: US Department of Health and Human Services, National Institutes of Health, National Cancer Institute; 1999.
4 Nuovo, J., Melnikow, J. and Howell, L. P. New tests for cervical cancer screening. *Am. Fam. Physician* 2001; **64**:780–86.
5 Sawaya, G. F. and Grimes, D. A. New technologies in cervical cytology screening: a word of caution. *Obstet. Gynecol.* 1999; **94**:307–10.
6 Macgregor, J., Campbell, M. K., Mann, E. M. and Swanson, K. Y. Screening for cervical intraepithelial neoplasia in north east Scotland shows fall in incidence and mortality from invasive cancer with concomitant rise in preinvasive disease. *Br. Med. J.* 1994; **308**:1407–11.
7 Limaye, A., Connor, A. J., Huang, X. and Luff, R. Comparative analysis of conventional Papanicolaou tests and a fluid-based thin-layer method. *Arch. Pathol. Lab. Med.* 2003; **127**:200–204.
8 ACOG committee opinion. New Pap test screening techniques. Number 206, August 1998. Committee on Gynecologic Practice. American College of Obstetricians and Gynecologists. *Int. J. Gynecol. Obstet.* 1998; **63**:312–14.
9 Coste, J., Cochand-Priollet, B., de Cremoux, P., *et al.* Cross sectional study of conventional cervical smear, monolayer cytology, and human papillomavirus DNA testing for cervical cancer screening. *Br. Med. J.* 2003; **326**:733.

10 American Cancer Society. American Cancer Society issues new cervical cancer early detection guidelines. www.cancer.org/docroot/MED/content/MED_2_1x_American_Cancer_Society_Issues_New_Cervical_Cancer_Early_Detection_Guidelines.asp. Accessed March 6, 2003.

11 Castle, P. E. Absolute risk of a subsequent abnormal pap among oncogenic human papillomavirus DNA-positive, cytologically negative women. *Cancer* 2002; **95**:2145–51.

12 Hughes, S. A., Sun, D., Gibson, C., *et al.* Managing atypical squamous cells of undetermined significance (ASCUS): human papillomavirus testing, ASCUS subtyping, or follow-up cytology? *Am. J. Obstet. Gynecol.* 2002; **186**:2010–16.

13 Mitchell, M. F., Schottenfeld, D., Tortolero-Luna, G., *et al.* Colposcopy for the diagnosis of squamous intraepithelial lesions: a meta-analysis. *Obstet. Gynecol.* 1998; **91**:626–31.

14 Wright, T. C., Jr, Cox, J. T., Massad, L. S., *et al.* 2001 consensus guidelines for the management of women with cervical cytological abnormalities. *J. Am. Med. Assoc.* 2002; **287**:2120–29.

15 Solomon, D., Schiffman, M. and Tarone, R. Comparison of three management strategies for patients with atypical squamous cells of undetermined significance: baseline results from a randomized trial. *J. Natl. Cancer. Inst.* 2001; **93**:293–9.

16 Montz, F. J., Monk, B. J., Fowler, J. M. and Nguyen, L. Natural history of the minimally abnormal Papanicolaou smear. *Obstet. Gynecol.* 1992; **80**:385.

17 Shin, C. H., Schorge, J. O., Lee, K. R. and Sheets, E. E. Cytologic and biopsy findings leading to conization in adenocarcinoma in situ of the cervix. *Obstet. Gynecol.* 2002; **100**:271–6.

18 Solomon, D., Davey, D., Kurman, R., *et al.* The 2001 Bethesda system. *J. Am. Med. Assoc.* 2002; **287**:2114–19.

19 Geier, C. S., Wilson, M. and Creasman, W. Clinical evaluation of atypical glandular cells of undetermined significance. *Am. J. Obstet. Gynecol.* 2001; **184**:64–9.

20 Schiffman, M. H. and Brinton, L. A. The epidemiology of cervical carcinogenesis. *Cancer* 1995; **76**:1888–901.

21 Parazzini, F., La Vecchia, C., Negri, E., *et al.* Case–control study of oestrogen replacement therapy and risk of cervical cancer *Br. Med. J.* 1997; **315**:85–8.

22 Schiffman, M. H., Bauer, H. M., Hoove, R. R. N., *et al.* Epidemiological evidence showing that human papillomavirus infection causes most cervical intraepithelial neoplasia. *J. Natl. Cancer Inst.* 1993; **85**:958–64.

23 Munoz, N., Bosch, F. X., de Sanjose, S., *et al.* Epidemiologic classification of human papillomavirus types associated with cervical cancer. *N. Engl. J. Med.* 2003; **348**:518–27.

24 Lombard, I., Vincent-Salomon, A., Validire, P., *et al.* Human papillomavirus genotype as a major determinant of the course of cervical cancer. *J. Clin. Oncol.* 1998; **16**:2613–19.

25 Moodley, M., Moodley, J., Chetty, R. and Herrington, C. S. The role of steroid contraceptive hormones in the pathogenesis of invasive cervical cancer: a review. *Int. J. Gynecol. Cancer.* 2003; **13**:103–10.

18

Endometrial cancer: prevention, screening, and early detection

Ellen Sakornbut

Case: T.H. is a 48-year-old woman who has not had a menstrual period in seven months, when she comes into the office with a sudden heavy menstrual period that has already lasted ten days. She has had to use three boxes of pads, and up to one pad an hour at its most heavy flow. She has had no pain but wonders what is happening to her. She does not smoke, is moderately overweight (body mass index (BMI) 31.0), and had normal thyroid tests three months ago.

Introduction

Endometrial carcinoma is one of the most common cancers in women, with an incidence of 2.6%. It ranks behind breast cancer and colon cancer in incidence, but it is seen more commonly than ovarian cancer. Endometrial carcinoma may be preceded by endometrial hyperplasia. Hyperplasia, as a potentially pre-cancerous condition, and endometrial carcinoma meet criteria for conditions that benefit from early detection. Effective, reasonably tolerated treatments of endometrial hyperplasia and early-stage endometrial carcinoma are available. Early treatment has a significant impact on outcome.

Endometrial carcinoma and hyperplasia present most frequently with abnormal uterine bleeding, either in the premenopausal and perimenopausal age group, or in postmenopausal women. This is a common complaint in mid-life women. The presence of vaginal bleeding is also monitored in many women during mid life by clinicians concerned with the side effects of hormonal therapy or in high-risk women, such as those undergoing treatment with tamoxifen following breast cancer diagnosis.

This chapter will examine the effects of the woman's hormonal environment on the development of endometrial hyperplasia and endometrial carcinoma, additional risk factors, and preventive measures for this common malignancy. The use of screening and early detection modalities will be addressed and recommendations made for general and increased-risk women.

Classification and pathophysiology

Simple endometrial hyperplasia (formerly classified as "cystic") is associated with approximately 1% risk of progression to carcinoma. Complex hyperplasia is also fairly low risk, with only 3% of women progressing to endometrial carcinoma. Atypical hyperplasia, whether simple or complex, carries an 8% or 29% risk of progression to cancer, respectively.[1]

Other classification systems have been proposed, with a reduction in categories to two: endometrial hyperplasia (a benign lesion with very little risk of progression to cancer) and endometrial intraepithelial neoplasia (EIN) or endometrioid neoplasia.[2] Patients diagnosed with atypical complex hyperplasia carry a 29–45% risk of metachronous endometrial carcinoma.[3]

Endometrial polyps are present in 5–10% of women who undergo diagnostic work-up for abnormal uterine bleeding. Approximately one in four women display premalignant changes, and 1–2% undergo malignant degeneration.[4]

Endometrial carcinoma can be classified as one of two major histological types. Most (75%) endometrial carcinomas are endometrioid adenocarcinomas; a smaller percentage of carcinomas are classified as serous or papillary serous (10%), clear cell (4%), and squamous cell (very rare). *Endometrioid carcinomas arise from endometrial hyperplasia caused by relative estrogen excess.* These cancers and the precancerous hyperplasia are associated with microsatellite instability and ras and PTEN mutations. Endometrioid carcinoma has a slowly progressive course.

Conversely, serous carcinomas do not have hormonal influences and are associated with p53 mutations. They appear to develop from the endometrial surface epithelium (endometrial intraepithelial carcinoma) and can develop in an atrophic endometrium.[5] Carcinomas with p53 overexpression are characterized by high nuclear grade, high Federation International of Gynecologists and Obstetricians (FIGO) stage, and decreased patient survival.[6]

Clear-cell carcinomas of the endometrium are similar to those seen in the cervix, vagina, and ovary. They are generally very aggressive cancers.

Prevention

Risk factors

Most risk factors for endometrial cancer are not modifiable. Unopposed estrogen use is one risk factor that can be changed (Table 18.1).

Unopposed estrogen therapy

When hormone therapy consisted of unopposed estrogen, a higher incidence of endometrial hyperplasia and carcinoma was found in women on this therapy

Table 18.1 Risk factors for endometrial cancer

High estrogen states
   Unopposed estrogen use for hormone replacement
   Polycystic ovary disease
Obesity
Increasing age
Postmenopausal state
Diabetes
Breast cancer
   Genetic syndromes
   Tamoxifen use
Hereditary non-polyposis colon cancer

compared with non-treated women.[7] Most women who still use hormone therapy and have an intact uterus take a progesterone as well. Most studies report approximately 20% incidence of endometrial hyperplasia in women on unopposed estrogen therapy for one year.[8]

Age

Endometrial cancer is rare in women before the age of 40 years, and young women with endometrial cancer should be evaluated by family history for hereditary non-polyposis colon cancer (HNPCC) (see later in this chapter) and other genetic factors. *The average age at diagnosis for endometrial cancer is 60 years.*

However, carcinomas of the lower uterine segment occur predominately in women under 50 years of age, are more likely to be high-grade endometrioid tumors with deep myometrial invasion, and are less associated with endometrial hyperplasia than carcinomas of the uterine corpus.[9] A study of women with endometrial cancer under the age of 40 found a subset of women with low BMI (less than 25), all of whom had high-risk pathology and developed either serous or clear-cell carcinoma.[10]

Menopausal status

Endometrial carcinoma is more common in postmenopausal than pre-menopausal women. Endometrial hyperplasia is detected more frequently in women who enter menopause late.[11]

Obesity

Endometrial carcinoma is diagnosed more frequently in obese than non-obese women. *Women more than 22.7 kg over ideal weight have up to a ten-fold risk of this cancer.* Women who gain weight have a higher risk of endometrial cancer. This may be caused by higher endogenous levels of estrogen from conversion of androstenedione to estrone in peripheral adipose tissue. Studies comparing the highest quartile of women with the lowest quartile of women with respect to BMI demonstrate increasing risk between ages of 30 and 60 years with weight gain of more than 7.5 kg and increased risk with increased waste-to-hip ratio. In one study, the highest risk was seen with a gain of more than 15% of body weight between the ages of 40 and 50 years.

Diabetes mellitus

In a prospective cohort study with 12 years' follow-up of 24 664 post-menopausal women in Iowa (Iowa Women's Health Study), 1.4% of women in the cohort developed endometrial carcinoma, and diabetes was found to be a time-dependent variable. The relative risk for endometrial carcinoma in these women was 1.43 (95% confidence interval (CI) 0.98–2.1) and was confined to women in the upper two BMI quintiles.[12] Similarly, the odds ratio for development of endometrial hyperplasia in an Italian case–control study of diabetic women was 2.4 (95% CI 0.8–6.9) for diabetic women.[13]

Hypertension

Hypertension has historically been reported as a risk factor for endometrial carcinoma, although some of the attributed risk is due to its association with other risk factors, such as the metabolic syndrome and diabetes. A large population-based case–control study of Swedish women found increased risk of endometrial carcinoma only among hypertensive women who were obese.[14]

Breast cancer

Breast cancer survivors are at increased risk for endometrial carcinoma. This may be related in part to coexistent risk factors of obesity and higher circulating estrogen levels. Additionally, *women who have been treated with tamoxifen for prevention of breast cancer recurrence experience an increased risk of endometrial hyperplasia and carcinoma related directly to the duration of tamoxifen therapy,* with risk peaking for women taking tamoxifen as adjuvant therapy at two to five years of therapy in long-term population-based studies (odds ratio 5.1, 95% CI 2.1–13).[15] The risk increases from four to nine times in women who use tamoxifen for longer than five years.[16] Fewer data are available on other anti-breast-cancer drugs. Toremifene stimulates uterine tissues similarly to tamoxifen, whereas raloxifene has not been demonstrated to have any effect upon the endometrium in a randomized, double-blind trial.[17]

Hereditary non-polyposis colon cancer

The spectrum of malignancies associated with HNPCC includes colon, endometrial, renal-cell, ovarian, breast, stomach, pancreas, and brain malignancies. Endometrial carcinoma associated with HNPCC may be seen at an earlier age and in the premenopausal years. HNPCC has been associated with germ-line mutations in MSH2, MLH1, PMS1, PMS2, and MSH6 (the latter associated with more endometrial cancers than colon cancers in women). The mechanism of carcinogenesis associated with this syndrome is that of microsatellite instability.[18] The risk of endometrial carcinoma is approximately ten times that of the general population, with a cumulative incidence of 20% by age 70.[19]

Polycystic ovarian disease and anovulatory cycles
Long-term studies of women with polycystic ovary syndrome demonstrate an increased risk of endometrial cancer, presumably related to anovulatory status, obesity, high estrogen levels, and other features of the metabolic syndrome.[20] A case–control study of premenopausal women on antipsychotic medication also reported an increased risk for endometrial cancer in patients with hyperprolactinemia secondary to antipsychotic medication.[21]

Risk factors for endometrial hyperplasia
Large clinical series of endometrial hyperplasia in premenopausal women[22] and mixed series with pre- and postmenopausal women[23] confirm similar risk factors of age 45 years or older, high BMI, subfertility, family history of colon cancer, and nulliparity.

Prevention therapy

Oral contraceptives
Lower-dosage oral contraceptives currently in use have been associated with an overall reduction in the risk of endometrial carcinoma that is proportionate to the time that oral contraceptives have been used.[24]

Maintenance of ovulatory cycles or periodic progestin-induced endometrial shedding
Women with chronic anovulatory bleeding patterns and those with known polycystic ovarian disease[25] should, theoretically, benefit from periodic use of progestins to induce withdrawal bleeding. No outcome studies are available at the time of writing to demonstrate benefit.

Obesity treatment
Obesity is one of the main risk factors for chronic anovulatory cycles. Reduction in body fat is frequently associated with resumption of cyclical menses and should, therefore, lessen the risk for endometrial hyperplasia and endometrial carcinoma, although there is no strong evidence for this.

Hormone replacement therapy
Endometrial biopsies of women on sequential hormone replacement therapy (HRT) usually demonstrate weakly secretory features, while *women on*

continuous combined HRT are most likely to demonstrate endometrial atrophy or insufficient tissue for analysis, making endometrial hyperplasia and cancer less likely.[26] While initiation of continuous combined HRT may result in small amounts of irregular bleeding initially, this should resolve within the first six months of treatment.

A systematic review of randomized controlled trials found unopposed estrogen therapy in moderate to high doses to be associated with significant increases in rates of endometrial hyperplasia. Thus far, low-dose estrogen (such as 0.3 mg conjugated equine estrogens) has not been associated with effects on the endometrium.[27] The addition of progestins to estrogen therapy decreases the risk of endometrial hyperplasia, with the greatest protection noted with continuous combined therapy (odds ratio 0.3, 95% CI 0.1–0.97), followed by increasing risk of hyperplasia with monthly sequential therapy and greater risk in patients with long-cycle sequential therapy (progestin every three months).[28] Transdermal and oral routes of sequential hormonal therapy are equivalent in the control of bleeding and risk of hyperplasia.[29]

Prophylactic surgery

Prophylactic oophorectomy has been considered more frequently for prevention of ovarian cancer in women with BRCA 1/2 than prophylactic surgery in women with HNPCC. Women with HNPCC are at risk for both ovarian and endometrial cancer, and prophylactic hysterectomy and bilateral salpingoophorectomy may play a role in prevention in this high-risk group of women.

Summary

There is good evidence that the incidence of endometrial cancer of the endometrioid type can be reduced by one of several hormonal mechanisms: use of low-dose, estrogen–progestin balanced oral contraceptives in premenopausal women or continuous HRT with balanced estrogen–progestin regimes in postmenopausal women. While maintenance of ideal body weight carries a multitude of health benefits, there is no direct evidence that weight loss reduces the risk of endometrial cancer in an individual patient.

Secondary prevention

The risk of endometrial carcinoma in complex atypical hyperplasia is approximately 25%, and warrants surgical management with hysterectomy and salpingoophorectomy. In addition, progression to endometrial carcinoma with myometrial invasion within one to five years occurs in about one-third of patients with atypical hyperplasia, whether simple or complex. Therefore, hysterectomy should be considered as the treatment of choice. Hyperplasia without atypia may be managed hormonally.

Screening

Pap smears

Although the major reason for periodic Papanicolaou (Pap) smear screening is the detection of cervical dysplasia and squamous cervical carcinoma, endometrial pathology may be detected by cytologic examination on routine Pap smears. Benign endometrial cells are detected in Pap smears more frequently in women on HRT than in women who are not on HRT, and abnormal endometrial histology is less frequent in follow-up of women on HRT than in women with endometrial cells who are not on HRT.[30] Endometrial-type cells on cervicovaginal smears are associated with significant endometrial pathology in less than 9% of patients.[31]

Atypical glandular cells of undetermined significance (AGUS) are noted on less than 1% of Pap smears. Follow-up studies of patients with AGUS on Pap smears have demonstrated that between 25% and 60% of patients with follow-up biopsies have preneoplastic or neoplastic squamous or glandular lesions on biopsy, with squamous lesions being more common in premenopausal women and glandular lesions being more common in postmenopausal women.[32,33] The Bethesda system recommends qualification of AGUS with regard to their possible origin (endocervical or endometrial). In women diagnosed with AGUS-EM (favor endometrial origin), approximately one-third have been found with abnormal endometrial histology on biopsy. Most of these women are postmenopausal.[34]

Pelvic bimanual examination

Endometrial carcinoma and hyperplasia are not generally detectable by bimanual pelvic examination alone, but bimanual examination provides useful information to the clinician regarding the size, shape, and consistency of the uterus. This information should be recorded periodically when performing a pelvic examination on any woman, making comparison possible with changes in physical symptoms or in the case of abnormal findings. Other causes of abnormal uterine bleeding, such as uterine fibroids, may be diagnosed with bimanual examination. Bimanual examination should be considered a prerequisite before uterine instrumentation to decrease the likelihood of uterine perforation and facilitate greater success at retrieving adequate tissue on endometrial biopsy.

Routine use of endometrial biopsy

Mass sampling for endometrial cancer has been conducted in Japan since 1987. Patients judged at risk for endometrial cancer and who are undergoing cervical cancer screening are offered screening by endometrial smears. The procedure is offered to women with abnormal genital bleeding in the previous six months and who are also older than 50 years of age, postmenopausal, or nulligravidas with irregular menstrual cycles. Positive or suspicious smears are followed by fractional curettage. In this group of women, with an incidence of endometrial cancer of 7.3 per 100 000, patients participating in screening were diagnosed at an earlier stage and had a significantly improved five-year survival rate. The hazard ratio of dying of endometrial cancer in screened women was reduced by more than half.[35] However, this may be more clearly considered to be case-finding, since, by definition, all women who were "screened" were symptomatic (i.e. had abnormal uterine bleeding).

Studies of routine endometrial biopsy in asymptomatic women in the general population do not demonstrate any benefit from routine biopsy for screening or early detection. Studies of more than 4000 asymptomatic menopausal and perimenopausal women with endometrial sampling before initiation of HRT found an average incidence of 67.7% atrophic endometrium, 15.6% proliferative, 0.39% atypical hyperplasia, and 0.25% endometrial carcinoma.[36–38] Because tissue obtained was insufficient for diagnosis in approximately 10% of these women, it is likely that a good number of these women had atrophic endometrium as well.

Targeted use of endometrial biopsy in selected populations

A prospective study of routine sequential endometrial biopsy in asymptomatic but high-risk women on tamoxifen failed to demonstrate clinical benefit over monitoring periods between three and five years.[39]

There is no evidence at the time of writing of benefit to normal-risk asymptomatic women from routine endometrial biopsy. Little information is available about routine endometrial biopsy in high-risk asymptomatic women.

Transvaginal ultrasound and measurement of endometrial thickness

Technique and normal values

The endometrium is measured for its thickest dimension in the sagittal long-axis view, including both the anterior and posterior layers by transvaginal ultrasound. Endometrial thickness measurements are acceptably reproducible in studies of intraobserver and interobserver differences.[40] Transabdominal measurements of the endometrium are not precise enough and are frequently unsatisfactory on a technical basis. In addition, irregularities of the endometrial cavity and areas of cystic appearance or other abnormal morphology can be assessed by the transvaginal approach.

An observational study of asymptomatic postmenopausal women determined a mean endometrial thickness of 2.3 +/− 1.8 mm (range 1–10 mm). Women with a higher BMI and higher circulating levels of estrone and estradiol had an endometrium thicker than 5 mm.[41] Women with no endometrial hypertension had a thickness of less than 5 mm. Besides endometrial thickness measurements, *endometrial morphology should demonstrate no irregularity of echo pattern, focal increase or diffuse increase in echogenicity, or irregularity of the endometrial border. An appearance of an endoluminal mass is clearly abnormal and warrants investigation.*

Screening

A large prospective study of asymptomatic postmenopausal women not on HRT utilized a cut-off value of endometrial thickness of 6 mm or less, as measured by transvaginal ultrasound.[42] It found that women with this thin endometrial stripe value were very unlikely to have endometrial hyperplasia or cancer, giving this measure a very high negative predictive value, greater than 99%. The Postmenopausal Estrogen/Progestin Interventions (PEPI) trial, following asymptomatic women on placebo, unopposed estrogen, sequential HRT, and combined continuous HRT, used a cut-off value of 5 mm or less and obtained similar results.[43] However, this study was critical of the use of transvaginal ultrasound for this purpose, since over half the women studied were subjected to additional procedures (endometrial biopsy) with a yield of only 4% with serious disease. Therefore, both studies found the positive predictive value of transvaginal ultrasound as a screening test to be quite low (2% and 9%, respectively).

A retrospective European study compared symptomatic postmenopausal women with endometrial carcinoma with asymptomatic postmenopausal women with a suspicious endometrium, detected by transvaginal ultrasound. In this study, symptomatic women were found to be older, more frequently obese and hypertensive, and more likely to live in a rural area or seek gynecologic care infrequently. The asymptomatic women had no better survival outcomes if they had an ultrasound diagnosis within eight weeks onset of uterine bleeding.[44]

There is no evidence that transvaginal ultrasound is of benefit as a screening tool in asymptomatic women in the general population or that screening offers a survival advantage over early diagnosis in symptomatic women.

Screening with transvaginal ultrasound in high-risk populations

Screening for endometrial disease in women treated with tamoxifen remains controversial. Treatment with tamoxifen results in an increase in normal measured endometrial thickness, with mean thicknesses reported from

9.2 to 13.7 mm. Additionally, treatment with tamoxifen is associated with an increased risk of endometrial polyps and hyperplasia and approximately two times the risk of endometrial carcinoma, depending on duration of treatment.[45] Therefore, a cut-off of 5 mm endometrial thickness, appropriate in a postmenopausal woman who is not on HRT, results in an additional diagnostic procedure in 41% of women on tamoxifen. Of these, 46% will demonstrate an atrophic endometrium despite apparent endometrial thickening (false-positive).[46] Additionally, a study comparing transvaginal ultrasound and hysteroscopy using a cut-off value of 6 mm found a very high negative predictive value for both procedures (96%), but a very low positive predictive value for transvaginal sonography (TVS) compared with hysteroscopy (8% versus 65%).[47]

Using cut-off values of 10 mm measured endometrial thickness, approximately one in four women on tamoxifen and without symptoms of vaginal bleeding displayed endometrial abnormalities. Another study comparing symptomatic women with asymptomatic women found a similar incidence of abnormalities in women without bleeding and found up to 93% of women who were symptomatic to have endometrial hyperplasia, polyps, or carcinoma.[48]

The International Collaborative Group on Hereditary Nonpolyposis Colon Carcinoma recommends endometrial ultrasound surveillance of these high-risk women, but prospective studies thus far have demonstrated no obvious clinical benefit.[49] The approach to screening high-risk women remains controversial. *Because the risk of endometrial carcinoma appears to be dependent on duration of use of estrogen, screening of asymptomatic women should probably be considered only in women who have been on tamoxifen for more than two years, whereas diagnostic work-up should be initiated immediately in all symptomatic women.* There is insufficient information at this time to determine how women with HNPCC should be monitored for endometrial carcinoma risk.

Transvaginal ultrasound for diagnosis in symptomatic women

Large studies of postmenopausal women evaluated with transvaginal ultrasound because of postmenopausal bleeding demonstrate *very low rates of endometrial carcinoma (0.6–3.9%) in women with an endometrial thickness of 5 mm or less.*[50,51] Accuracy of transvaginal ultrasound is improved by combining endometrial thickness cut-off values of 5 mm with endometrial morphology and the assessment of the regularity of the endometrial border,[52,53] producing a sensitivity of 97%, specificities of 61–65%, and a positive predictive value of 72–80%.

In women with postmenopausal bleeding and with an endometrial thickness of less than 5 mm on ultrasound, both those randomized to expectant management and those managed initially with dilation and curettage experienced a recurrent episode of bleeding approximately 20–33% of the time. An isolated incident of recurrent uterine bleeding was not associated with endometrial pathology, but growth of the endometrium to a thickness of greater than 5 mm on repeat ultrasound was associated with a 33% risk of endometrial pathology.[54]

US consensus statements on assessment of uterine bleeding recommend either transvaginal ultrasound or endometrial biopsy as an initial approach to post-menopausal bleeding.[55] A European consensus statement advocates initial cytologic evaluation to exclude cervical carcinoma, followed by transvaginal ultrasound, with or without saline infusion sonohysterograghy, with invasive procedures (endometrial biopsy) only if the endometrial thickness is greater than 4 mm or if bleeding recurs. The choice of technique to be used initially should depend on individual patient factors, clinician experience, and the availability of high-quality clinical services.

A cost-analysis model comparing ultrasound and endometrial biopsy as the initial step in evaluating postmenopausal bleeding found slight cost savings for ultrasound in populations with 10% or less incidence of endometrial cancer and atypical hyperplasia, and with endometrial biopsy being a more cost-effective approach in populations with a higher incidence of malignancy.[56] This method utilized US Medicare reimbursement methods and did not account for costs other than real value unit (RVU) reimbursement, such as patient travel to facilities.

Other diagnostic modalities, such as hysteroscopy and saline sonohysteroscopy (saline infusion into the endometrial cavity during transvaginal ultrasound), have been recommended to improve accuracy in assessment of focal lesions of the endometrial cavity. Hysteroscopy carries the benefit of allowing directed biopsy of focal abnormalities. Although some series have reported as high as 34.5% of missed diagnoses in endometrial carcinoma,[57] a systematic quantitative review including more than 26 000 women determined diagnostic accuracy to be very high, with a negative result reducing the probability of cancer to less than 1%.[58] Hysteroscopy is more expensive than either transvaginal ultrasound or endometrial biopsy, is invasive, and is less widely available than non-selective endometrial biopsy.

Saline infusion sonohysterography provides information about focal lesions of the uterine cavity, but it carries a disadvantage in that a second procedure is needed for tissue diagnosis if an abnormality is found. It is not available as widely as non-contrast ultrasound and endometrial biopsy.

Summary

The work-up of abnormal uterine bleeding in peri- and postmenopausal women may be initiated with either transvaginal ultrasound or endometrial biopsy. In women without other risk factors, an endometrial thickness of less than 5 mm may be followed initially without biopsy, but rebleeding with an increase in endometrial thickness or persistent bleeding should be investigated in a timely manner with biopsy or dilation and curettage. HRT should not be initiated without diagnostic work-up in women with postmenopausal uterine bleeding.

Endometrial biopsy

Endometrial biopsy may be performed non-selectively, using one of several methods to sample all parts of the endometrial cavity, or it may be performed under direct visualization during hysteroscopy to selectively biopsy suspicious areas. The accuracy of endometrial biopsy as compared with dilation and curettage in detection of endometrial carcinoma ranges from 91 to 99.6% with sampling devices such as the Pipelle™.[59] Comparisons of flexible, disposable polypropylene sampling devices versus biopsies taken with the reusable Novak's curette reveal similar rates of efficacy in adequacy of specimen obtained, although efficacy rates for all devices are lower in postmenopausal women (approximately 75%).[60] The decrease in efficacy of obtaining adequate specimens for histologic examination in postmenopausal women is caused by two factors: an increase in cervical stenosis in this age group and atrophic endometrium with scant tissue available to sample.

Technique

Non-selective endometrial biopsy (EMB) or sampling is learned easily and can be performed safely and conveniently in ambulatory settings. It is useful to keep several biopsy instruments in the office setting, since different patients may require different methods for obtaining a good sampling of tissue. The procedure carries an extremely low incidence of complications, the most important being uterine perforation. Since bacteremia is possible with the procedure, patients needing bacterial endocarditis prophylaxis should receive antibiotics in the manner usual for any genitourinary procedure.[61]

A sterile speculum is inserted and good visualization of the cervix accomplished. The cervix is cleansed with povidone–iodine solution. The cervix may be sufficiently stabilized and the cervical os open sufficiently to readily pass a sterile uterine sound through the endocervix and to the uterine fundus. If the cervix is not well fixed by the speculum, or if relative difficulty is encountered in passing the uterine sound, then a single-toothed tenaculum may be placed on the anterior cervical lip. Placement of a tenaculum may be made less uncomfortable by *slow* closure of the handle grip.

A uterine sound should be passed with exertion of steady pressure past the mild to moderate resistance usually encountered at the internal cervical os and inserted to the depth of the uterine fundus. The sound will pass to at least 6–7 cm in most patients. If the sound does not pass readily, then one of several problems may be responsible. Cervical stenosis may render passage of a uterine sound difficult or impossible with usual amounts of traction on the tenaculum (see below). A retroflexed or strongly anteflexed uterus may present resistance to insertion of a straight sound. A pliable sound may be curved gently and passed in the appropriate manner, facilitated by some straightening of the uterus with steady, gentle traction on the tenaculum. A fibroid projecting into the lower uterine segment or endometrial cavity may impede complete insertion of the uterine sound.

Several types of endometrial sampling devices are available. Generally they consist of a thin, 3–4-mm flexible plastic tube with a rounded tip and a distal collection port, and contain a flexible guide or stylet. After inserting to the full depth of the uterus, the guide is withdrawn partially, creating a vacuum, and the instrument is withdrawn with a rotating motion, thus sampling the endometrial cavity on all walls and from fundus to lower uterine segment. The rounded end of the instrument is clipped off before expelling the tissue into the preservative.

The Novak curette is a metal biopsy curette with a rounded distal portion and a toothed collection port. It may or may not contain a stylet, depending on the size. The proximal end has a hub, which is attached to a syringe for suction. Novak curettes range in diameter from 2 to 4 mm. The 2-mm curette is a good choice for women who have significant cervical stenosis, because it is thinner than a sound, but rigid. The curette should be passed in a four-quadrant (anterior, posterior, right, and left walls of the uterus) pattern, each time sweeping from fundus to lower uterine segment with firm pressure and suction exerted by the syringe. A mild scraping sensation should be felt as the curette passes over the myometrium.

Several techniques have been utilized to decrease the discomfort, which may be perceived as anything from minor transient cramping to intolerable sharp pain. Most women benefit from a dose of short-acting non-steroidal anti-inflammatory medications (ibuprofen or naproxen sodium) 30–60 minutes before the procedure. Visual analog pain scores in a randomized, controlled trial comparing intrauterine instillation of 2% lidocaine or saline showed that there was an approximately 50% decrease in pain in women receiving lidocaine with no decrease in ability to interpret histologic specimens.[62] A randomized, double-blinded, controlled trial of paracervical block comparing 10 ml 1.5% mepivicaine with saline placebo also found significant reductions in pain and vasovagal reactions to the procedure.[63]

Summary

Endometrial cancer and its precursors are relatively common problems encountered in mid-life women. *There is not any benefit to implementation of any screening modality (other than continuance of Pap smears and pelvic examination) in asymptomatic women.* Nonetheless, women in their forties and with abnormal uterine bleeding and all women with postmenopausal bleeding should undergo diagnostic work-up unless slight irregular bleeding occurs in the first months of therapy with combined continuous HRT in a previously asymptomatic woman.

Screening protocols are available for high-risk asymptomatic women, such as those on tamoxifen therapy and those women with HNPCC. Their management remains controversial. Women who have been on tamoxifen for more than two years may benefit from screening. Very little information is available on women with HNPCC regarding the benefits of screening versus prophylactic surgery as a strategy.

Endometrial biopsy and transvaginal ultrasound are both appropriate initial modalities when investigating postmenopausal bleeding. Diagnostic work-ups should be initiated without delay. Women with a tissue diagnosis of atypical hyperplasia carry a high-risk of metachronous endometrial carcinoma and should be managed as such. Other modalities, such as saline infusion sonohysterography and hysteroscopy, are superior for assessment of endoluminal masses and focal lesions, but are more expensive and more invasive. They may be of benefit in selected patients for diagnosis.

REFERENCES

1 Kurman, R. J., Kaminski, P. F. and Norriss, H. J. The behavior of endometrial hyperplasia. A long-term study of "untreated hyperplasia" in 170 patients. *Cancer* 1985; **56**:403.

2 Dietel, M. The histological diagnosis of endometrial hyperplasia. Is there a need to simplify? *Virchows Arch.* 2001; **439**:604–8.

3 Horn, L. C., Bilek, K. and Schnurrbusch U. [Endometrial hyperplasias: histology, classification, prognostic significance, and therapy.] *Zentralbl. Gynakol.* 1997; **119**: 251–9.

4 Anastasiadis, P. G., Koutlaki, N. G., Skaphida, P. G., *et al.* Endometrial polyps: prevalence, detection, and malignant potential in women with abnormal uterine bleeding. *Eur. J. Gynaecol. Oncol.* 2000; **21**:180–83.

5 Sherman, M. E. Theories of endometrial carcinogenesis: a multidisciplinary approach. *Mod. Pathol.* 2000; **13**:295–308.

6 Sung, J., Zheng, Y., Quddus, M. R., *et al.* p53 as a significant prognostic marker in endometrial carcinoma. *Int. J. Gynecol. Cancer* 2000; **10**:119–27.

7 Effects of hormone replacement therapy on endometrial histology in postmenopausal women The Postmenopausal Estrogen/Progestin Interventions Trial. The Writing Group for the PEPI trial. *J. Am. Med. Assoc.* 1996; **275**:370–75.

8 Woodruff, J. D. and Pickar, J. H. Incidence of endometrial hyperplasia in postmenopausal women taking conjugated estrogens (Premarin) with medroxyprogesterone acetate or conjugated estrogens only. *Am. J. Obstet. Gynecol.* 1994; **170**: 1213–23.

9 Hachisuga, T., Fukada, K., Iwasaka, T., *et al.* Endometrioid adenocarcinomas of the uterine corpus in women younger than 50 years of age can be divided into two distinct clinical and pathologic entities based on anatomic location. *Cancer* 2001; **92**:2578–84.

10 Duska, L. R., Garrett, A., Rueda, B. R., *et al.* Endometrial cancer in women 40 years of age and younger. *Gynecol. Oncol.* 2001; **83**:388–93.

11 Ricci, E., Moronia, S., Parazzini, F., *et al.* Risk factors for endometrial hyperplasia: results from a case-control study. *Int. J. Gynecol. Cancer* 2002; **12**:257–60.

12 Anderson, K. E., Anderson, E., Mink, P. J., *et al.* Diabetes and endometrial cancer in the Iowa women's health study. *Cancer Epidemiol. Biomarkers Prev.* 2001; **10**:611–16.

13 Ricci, E., Moroni, S., Parazinni, F., *et al.* Risk factors or endometrial hyperplasia: results from a case–control study. *Int. J. Gynecol. Cancer* 2002; **12**:257–60.

14 Weidepass, E., Persson, I., Adami, H. O., *et al.* Body size in different periods of life, diabetes mellitus, hypertension, and risk of postmenopausal endometrial cancer (Sweden). *Cancer Causes Control* 2000; **11**:185–92.

15 Bernstein, L., Deape, D., Cerhan, J. R., *et al.* Tamoxifen therapy for breast cancer and endometrial cancer risk. *J. Natl. Cancer Inst.* 1999; **91**:1654–62.

16 Pukkal, E., Kyyronen, P., Sankila, R. and Holli, K. Tamoxifen and toremifene treatment of breast cancer and risk of subsequent endometrial cancer: a population-based case–control study. *Int. J. Cancer* 2002; **100**:337–41.

17 Neven, P., Lunde, T., Benedetti-Panici, P., *et al.* A multicentre randomized trial to compare uterine safety of raloxifene with a continuous combined hormone replacement therapy containing oestradiol and norethisterone acetate. *Br. J. Obstet. Gynaecol.* 2003; **110**:157–67.

18 Lynch, H. T. and Lynch, J. Lynch syndrome: genetics, natural history, genetic counseling, and prevention. *J. Clin. Oncol.* 2000; **18**(21 supp):19–31S.

19 Watson, P., Vasen, H. F., Mecklin, J. P., Jarvinen, H. and Lynch, H. T. The risk of endometrial cancer in hereditary nonpolyposis colorectal cancer. *Am. J. Med.* 1994; **96**:516–20.

20 Wild, S., Pierpoint, T., Jacobs, H. and McKeigue, P. Long-term consequences of polycystic ovary syndrome: results of a 31 year follow-up study. *Hum. Fertil. (Camb.)* 2000; **3**:101–5.

21 Yamazawa, K., Matsui, H., Seki, K. and Sekiya, S. A case–control study of endometrial cancer after antipsychotics exposure in premenopausal women. *Oncology* 2003; **64**:116–23.

22 Farquhar, C. M., Lethaby, A., Sowter, M., Verry, J. and Baranyai, J. An evaluation of risk factors for endometrial hyperplasia in premenopausal women with abnormal menstrual bleeding. *Am. J. Obstet. Gynecol.* 1999; **181**:525–9.

23 Anastasiadis, P. G., Skaphida, P. G., Koutlaki, N. G., *et al.* Descriptive epidemiology of endometrial hyperplasia in patients with abnormal uterine bleeding. *Eur. J. Gynaecol. Oncol.* 2000; **21**:131–4.

24 Thomas, D. E. The WHO Collaborative Study of Neoplasia and Steroid Contraceptives: the influence of combined oral contraceptives on risk of neoplasms in developing and developed countries. *Contraception* 1991; **43**:695–710

25 Balen, A. Polycystic ovary syndrome and cancer. *Hum. Reprod. Update* 2001; **7**: 522–5.

26 Feeley, K. M. and Wells, M. Hormone replacement therapy and the endometrium. *J. Clin. Pathol.* 2001; **54**:435–40.

27 Pickar, J. H., Yeh, I., Wheeler, J. E., Cunnane, M. F. and Speroff, L. *Fertil. Steril.* 2001; **76**:25–31.

28 Lethaby, A., Farquhar, C., Sarkis, A., *et al.* Hormone replacement therapy in post-menopausal women: endometrial hyperplasia and irregular bleeding. *Cochrane Database Syst Rev* 2000; CD000402.

29 Sendag, F., Terek, M. C. and Karadadas, N. Sequential combined transdermal and oral postmenopausal hormone replacement therapies: effects on bleeding patterns and endometrial histology. *Arch. Gynecol. Obstet.* 2001; **265**:209–13.

30 Mount, S. L., Wegner, E. K., Eltabbakh, G. H., Olmstead, J. I. and Drejet, A. E. Significant increase of benign endometrial cells on Papanicolaou smears in women using hormone replacement therapy. *Obstet. Gynecol.* 2002; **100**:445–50.

31 Karim, B. O., Burroughs, F. H., Rosenthal, D. L. and Ali, S. Z. Enodmetrial-type cells in cervico-vaginal smears: clinical significance and cytopathologic correlates. *Diagn. Cytopathol.* 2002; **26**:123–7.

32 Chhieng, D. C., Elgert, P. A., Cangiarella, J. F. and Cohen, J. M. Clinical significance of atypical glandular cells of undetermined significance. A follow-up study from an academic medical center. *Acta Cytol.* 2000; **44**:557–66.

33 Vhin, A. B., Bristow, R. E., Korst, L. M., Walts, A. and Lagasse, L. D. The significance of atypical glandular cells on routine cervical cytologic testing in a community-based population. *Am. J. Obstet. Gynecol.* 2000; **182**:1278–82.

34 Chhieng, D. C., Elgert, P., Cohen, J. M. and Cangiarella, J. F. Clinical implications of atypical glandular cells of undetermined significance, favor endometrial origin. *Cancer* 2001; **93**:351–6.

35 Nakagawa-Okamura, C., Sato, S., Tsuiji, I., *et al.* Effectiveness of mass screening for endometrial cancer. *Acta Cytol.* 2002; **46**:277–83.

36 Gol, K., Saracoglu, F., Ekici, A. and Sahin, I. Endometrial patterns and endocrinologic characteristics of asymptomatic menopausal women. *Gynecol. Endocrinol.* 2001; **15**:63–7.

37 Korhonen, M. O., Symons, J. P., Hyde, B. M., Rowan, J. P. and Wilborn, W. H. Histologic classification and pathologic findings for endometrial biopsy specimens obtained from 2694 perimenopausal and menopausal women undergoing screening for continuous hormones as replacement therapy (CHART 2 Study). *Am. J. Obstet. Gynecol.* 1997; **176**:377–80.

38 Archer, D. F., Mc-Intyre Seltman, K., Wilborn, W. W., Jr, *et al.* Endometrial morphology in asymptomatic postmenopausal women. *Am. J. Obstet. Gynecol.* 1991; **165**:317–20.

39 Barakat, R. R., Gilewski, T. A., Almadrones, L., *et al.* Effect of adjuvant tamoxifen on the endometrium in women with breast cancer: a prospective study using office endometrial biopsy. *J. Clin. Oncol.* 2000; **18**:3459–63.

40 Epstein, E. and Valentin, L. Intraobserver and interobserver reproducibility of ultrasound measurements of endometrial thickness in postmenopausal women. *Ultrasound Obstet. Gynecol.* 2002; **20**:486–91.

41 Andolf, E., Dahlander, K. and Aspenberg, P. Ultrasonic thickness of the endometrium correlated to body weight in asymptomatic postmenopausal women. *Obstet. Gynecol.* 1993; **82**:936–40.

42 Fleischer, A. C., Wheeler, J. E., Lindsay, I., *et al.* An assessment of the value of ultrasonographic screening for endometrial disease in postmenopausal women without symptoms. *Am. J. Obstet. Gynecol.* 2001; **184**:70–75.

43 Langer, R. D., Pierce, J. J., O'Hanlan, K. A., *et al.* Transvaginal ultrasonography compared with endometrial biopsy for the detection of endometrial disease. Postmenopausal Estrogen/Progestin Interventions Trial. *N. Engl. J. Med.* 1997; **337**:1792–8.

44 Gerber, B., Krause, A., Muller, H., *et al.* Ultrasonograhic detection of asymptomatic endometrial cancer in postmenopausal patients offers no prognostic advantage over symptomatic disease discovered by uterine bleeding. *Eur. J. Cancer.* 2001; **37**:64–71.

45 Neven, P. and Vernaeve, J. Guidelines for monitoring patients taking tamoxifen treatment. *Drug Saf.* 2000; **22**:1–11.

46 Love, C. D., Muir, B. B., Scrimgeour, J. B., *et al.* Investigation of endometrial abnormalities in asymptomatic women treated with tamoxifen and an evaluation of the role of endometrial screening. *J. Clin. Oncol.* 1999; **17**:2050.

46 Gerber, B., Krause, A., Muller, H., *et al.* Effects of adjuvant tamoxifen on the endometrium in postmenopausal women with breast cancer: a prospective long-term study using transvaginal ultrasound. *J. Clin. Oncol.* 2000; **18**:3464–70.

47 Giorda, G., Crivellari, D., Veronesi, A., *et al.* Comparison of ultrasonography, hysteroscopy, and biopsy in the diagnosis of endometrial lesions in postmenopausal tamoxifen-treated patients. *Acta Obstet. Gynecol. Scand.* 2002; **81**:975–80.

48 Cohen, I., Perel, E., Flex, D., *et al.* Endometrial pathology in postmenopausal tamoxifen treatment: comparison between gynecologically symptomatic and asymptomatic breast cancer patients. *J. Clin. Pathol.* 1999; **52**:278–82.

49 Dove-Edwin, I., Boks, D., Goff, S., *et al.* The outcome of endometrial carcinoma surveillance by ultrasound scan in women at risk for hereditary nonpolyposis colorectal carcinoma and familial colorectal carcinoma. *Cancer* 2002; **94**:1708–12.

50 Gull, B., Carlsson, S., Karlsson, B., *et al.* Transvaginal ultrasonography of the endometrium in women with postmenopausal bleeding: is it always necessary to perform an endometrial biopsy? *Am. J. Obstet. Gynecol.* 2000; **182**:509–15.

51 Karlsson, B., Granberg, S., Wikland, M., *et al.* Transvaginal ultrasonography of the endometrium in women with postmenopausal bleeding – a Nordic multicenter study. *Am. J. Obstet. Gynecol.* 1995; **172**:1488–94.

52 Weber, G., Merz, E., Bahlmann, F. and Rosch, B. Evaluation of different transvaginal sonographic parameters in women with postmenopausal bleeding. *Ultrasound Obstet. Gynecol.* 1998; **12**:265–70.

53 Randelzhofer, B., Prompeler, H. J., Sauerbrei, W., Madjar, H. and Emons, G. Value of sonomorphological criteria of the endometrium in women with postmenopausal bleeding: a multivariate analysis. *Ultrasound Obstet. Gynecol.* 2002; **19**:62–8.

54 Epstein, E. and Valentin, L. Rebleeding and endometrial growth in women with postmenopausal bleeding and endometrial thickness <5 mm managed by dilation and curettage or ultrasound follow-up: a randomized controlled study. *Ultrasound Obstet. Gynecol.* 2001; **18**:499–504.

55 Goldstein, R. B., Bree, R. L., Benson, C. B., *et al.* Evaluation of the woman with postmenopausal bleeding: Society of Radiologists in Ultrasound-Sponsored Consensus Conference statement. *J. Ultrasound Med.* 2001; **20**:1025–36.

56 Medverd, J. R. and Dubinsky, T. J. Cost analysis model: US versus endometrial biopsy in evaluation of peri- and postmenopausal abnormal uterine bleeding. *Radiology* 2002; **222**:619–27.

57 Deckardt, R., Lueken, R. P., Gallinat, A., *et al.* Comparison of transvaginal ultrasound, hysteroscopy, and dilation and curettage in the diagnosis of abnormal vaginal bleeding and intrauterine pathology in perimenopausal and postmenopausal women. *J. Am. Assoc. Gynecol. Laparosc.* 2002; **9**:277–82.

58 Clark, T. J., Gupta, J. K., Hyde, C., Song, F. and Khan, K. S. Accuracy of hysteroscopy in the diagnosis of endometrial cancer and hyperplasia: a systematic quantitative review. *J. Am. Med. Assoc.* 2002; **288**:1610–21.

59 Dijkhuizen, F. P., Mol, B. W., Brolmann, H. A. and Heintz, A. P. The accuracy of endometrial sampling in the diagnosis of patients with endometrial carcinoma and hyperplasia: a meta-analysis. *Cancer* 2000; **89**:1765–72.

60 Larson, D. M. and Broste, S. K. Histopathologic adequacy of office endometrial biopsies taken with the Z-sampler and Novak curette in premenopausal and postmenopausal women. *J. Reprod. Med.* 1994; **39**:300–303.

61 Livengood, C. H., 3rd, Land, M. R. and Addison, W. A. Endometrial biopsy, bacteremia, and endocarditis risk. *Obstet. Gynecol.* 1985; **65**:678–81.

62 Trolice, M. P., Fishburne, C., Jr. and McGrady, S. Anesthetic efficacy of intrauterine lidocaine for endometrial biopsy: a randomized double-masked trial. *Obstet. Gynecol.* 2000; **95**:345–7.

63 Cicinelli, E., Didonna, T., Schonauer, L. M., *et al.* Paracervical anesthesia for hysteroscopy and endometrial biopsy in postmenopausal women. A randomized, double-blind, placebo-controlled study. *J. Reprod. Med.* 1998; **43**:1014–18.

19

Ovarian cancer: prevention, screening, and early detection

Jo Ann Rosenfeld

Introduction

Despite advances in screening for other forms of cancer, ovarian cancer remains one of the most challenging illnesses encountered in women because of its poor cure rate and minimally available preventive strategies. *Seventy per cent of ovarian cancers are discovered when disease has spread beyond the ovaries.* Because of late diagnosis and limited long-term survival in stage 3 and 4 disease, the overall five-year survival rate is approximately 30–40%. Ovarian cancer is the leading cause of death from gynecologic malignancies and the fifth leading cause of cancer-associated death in women.

Awareness of ovarian cancer has increased among women. Women seeking routine care, as well as those experiencing pelvic or abdominal pain or diagnosed with a pelvic mass, may be concerned about their risk of cancer. This chapter will address risk factors for ovarian cancer, known and potential prevention strategies, screening methods, early diagnosis, and specific strategies for high-risk populations.

Prevention

Risk factors for ovarian cancer

The risk of ovarian cancer has been linked to overall number of lifetime ovulations, with increasing risk among women of low parity and late menopause and decreasing risk in women using oral contraceptives and in women of high parity. The overall lifetime risk in the general population is 1.6%. These risk factors are unlikely to be of help to the clinician for purposes of screening. However, historical information can be of benefit in delineating women at higher risk for ovarian cancer.

Both personal medical history and a detailed family history for malignancy are of use in identifying those women who are likely to benefit from additional

Table 19.1 Risk factors for ovarian cancer

Risk factor	Estimated lifetime incidence of ovarian cancer (general population 1.6%)
Personal history of breast cancer and age < 50 years	7%
First-degree relative with ovarian cancer	3.5–7%
Two first-degree relatives with ovarian cancer	15%
Other malignancies – endometrium, cervix, colon, melanoma, especially before age 50 years	Incidence not available, but observed/expected (O/E) ratios 3.5–17.9
BRCA1 mutation	16–63%
BRCA2 mutation	12–27%
HNPCC	3.5–2%
Infertility – idiopathic, PCOS, endometriosis	Some inconsistencies in information; lifetime incidence not available
Smoking	Mucinous carcinoma and borderline mucinous tumors only; incidence not available

HNPCC, hereditary non-polyposis colon cancer; PCOS, polycystic ovarian syndrome.

screening or preventive interventions. Table 19.1 summarizes the risk factors for ovarian cancer.

Genetic risk factors

Family history for specific malignancies is the most important risk factor. If one first-degree relative has been diagnosed with ovarian cancer, then a woman's lifetime risk of ovarian cancer increases to 3.5–7%. With two first-degree relatives, lifetime risk increases to 7–15%.[1,2] The relative risk of developing ovarian cancer is increased if family members developed this cancer at a younger age.[3]

Familial ovarian cancer appears in three types: (1) familial history of ovarian cancer only, (2) familial history of breast and ovarian cancer, and (3) family history of non-polyposis colorectal, endometrial, urologic, prostate, lung, and ovarian cancers (Lynch II syndrome or hereditary non-polyposis colon cancer, HNPCC). The first two groups account for 90% of familial ovarian cancer and are caused by germ-line mutations in tumor suppressor genes (*BRCA1* and *BRCA2*) in an autosomal dominant pattern. The Lynch II syndrome accounts for 10% of hereditary ovarian cancer and is associated with mutations in DNA mismatch repair genes, including *hMLH1* and *hMSH2*. Women with familial ovarian cancer are four times more likely to carry a *BRCA1* mutation than a *BRCA2* mutation. *Cancers associated with BRCA1 are more likely to manifest in younger women than cases of sporadic ovarian cancer or those associated with*

Table 19.2 Genetic cancer syndromes that include ovarian cancer

Syndrome	Mutation	Associated cancers	Defect
BRCA	BRCA1	Breast, ovarian, fallopian tube, peritoneal	
	BRCA2	Same as for BRCA1, but incidence of ovarian cancer is less	
HNPCC	MSH2, MLH1	Colon, endometrial, ovarian, renal, brain, gastric, biliary tract, small intestine	DNA mismatch repair

BRCA2. Risk estimates for ovarian cancer have varied with the population studied, from 16–63% for BRCA1 to 11–27% for BRCA2.[4] Table 19.2 shows the characteristics of these genetic cancer syndromes.

Breast cancers in patients carrying BRCA1 mutations tend to be higher-grade lesions that are steroid-hormone-receptor-negative and are more likely to be an atypical or medullary subtype. No specific types are more common with ovarian malignancies in carriers of either BRCA1 or BRCA2 mutations.[5] BRCA1 and BRCA2 are thought to act as tumor suppressor genes and to operate in a DNA damage response pathway implicated in double-strand repair. It is postulated that different BRCA1/2 mutations are more or less likely to be associated with ovarian cancer, but little information is available at this time.

Personal history of other malignancies
A study of second non-breast cancer malignancies in women with a diagnosis of breast cancer at less than 50 years of age found more than three times the incidence of ovarian cancer when compared with cohorts (relative risk 7 versus 1.96, $P = 0.0004$). The increased risk for ovarian cancer was not observed in women who were older than 50 years at the time of breast cancer diagnosis.[6]

Women with other malignant diagnoses are at increased risk. Analyzed data from cancer registries participating in the Surveillance, Epidemiology, and End Results program for women diagnosed with invasive cancer between 1973 and 1996 showed a significantly increased risk of ovarian cancer in women younger than 50 years and diagnosed with melanoma, cancer of the breast, cervix, or endometrium, colon, or previous ovarian cancer.[7] Whether any of these women were genetically predisposed because of an HNPCC mutation is not known.

Smoking
Data from population-based, case–control studies in the USA[8] and Australia[9] indicate that there is more than a doubled risk of mucinous and borderline mucinous adenocarcinoma of the ovary in women who smoke and in former smokers.

Hormonal therapy

Recent studies provide a link of hormone replacement therapy (HRT) to ovarian cancer, but these findings are inconsistent. *Oral contraceptive pills (OCPs) have been well-documented to decrease the risk of ovarian cancer.* The protective effect continues for many years following their discontinuance. Since OCPs suppress gonadotropin secretion, this mechanism of action might also be supposed to provide a benefit in menopausal HRT.

A large prospective cohort study, the American Cancer Society Cancer Prevention Study II, found an increased rate of death from ovarian cancer (64.4 versus 26.4 per 100 000) among women using estrogen for ten years or more as compared with non-users.[10] Other meta-analyses of case–control studies have not found an increased risk for ovarian cancer with estrogen use.[11] Another large cohort study in the USA found an increased risk of ovarian cancer in women using estrogen-only replacement therapy, and that risk was related to duration of therapy, while women using estrogen and progestin combined therapy demonstrated no increase in risk of ovarian cancer.[12] Similar results were obtained in a Swedish case–control study.[13]

Infertility

A pooled analysis of eight case–control studies of more than 5000 women from the USA, Denmark, Canada, and Australia demonstrated increased risk of borderline serous tumors with fertility drug use (odds ratio 2.43, 95% confidence interval (CI) 1.01–5.88). There was an increased risk of ovarian cancer in women with infertility compared with controls (odds ratio 2.67, 95% CI 1.91–3.74), but no increase in invasive ovarian cancer associated with fertility drugs.[14] Polycystic ovary syndrome has also been associated with an increased risk of ovarian cancer,[15] but this risk has not been confirmed with the same consistency as its association with endometrial carcinoma.[16]

A prospective, population-based study (the Iowa Women's Health Study) did not find an increased risk of ovarian cancer in women with endometriosis,[17] but endometrioid and clear-cell ovarian carcinomas may originate in endometriosis,[18] probably caused by somatic mutations in the PTEN tumor-suppressor gene.[19]

Inflammation and environmental causes

Conflicting information is available from case–control studies in Italy[20] and Canada[21] regarding the risk of ovarian cancer in women who have been diagnosed with pelvic inflammatory disease. Early retrospective case–control studies linking perineal application of talcum powder to ovarian cancer have not been supported by causality.[22] A long-term prospective study (the Nurses' Health Study) found no increase in ovarian cancer risk for women who used talc (ever users or increasing use), although a modest increase was present for invasive serous ovarian cancer and ever using talc.[23]

Table 19.3 Characteristics of ovarian cysts that are reassuring in premenopausal women

Size <5 cm,
Liquid (anechoic) contents
Less than three fine septations (<3 mm)
Thin cyst wall (<3 mm)
No vegetations or papillary structures
Normal color-flow-Doppler studies

A review of 48 epidemiologic studies on possible occupational and environmental risk factors for ovarian cancer found that studies lacked quantitative exposure-response data, were vulnerable to bias, and did not have sufficient power to assess adequately the risk of exposure to specific agents.[24]

Clinical findings

Unfortunately, ovarian cancer does not frequently manifest at an early stage with clinical symptoms or easily detected findings. Patients may experience any number of vague abdominal or pelvic symptoms, with pain or discomfort and gastrointestinal or genitourinary complaints. An adnexal mass may be palpable. Ascites is usually a late finding. Even when ovarian cancer appears visibly confined to one ovary (stage I disease) at the time of surgery, the incidence of lymph-node metastases with sampling of bilateral pelvic and paraaortic nodes may be as high as 15% in high-grade tumors.[25]

In contrast, ovarian cysts are relatively common and usually benign findings in premenopausal women. Ovarian cysts are also common incidental findings on pelvic ultrasound. In the menopausal or postmenopausal woman, functional cysts (follicular and corpus luteum) should not be seen. Characteristics of ovarian cysts that are reassuring are listed in Table 19.3.

Screening

Effective screening for ovarian cancer would ideally be performed as a noninvasive or minimally invasive test or as a procedure easily incorporated into well-woman care at a low cost with the lowest possible false-positive rate and high sensitivity. The positive predictive value of the test would be high, preventing the need for many costly and anxiety-provoking follow-up diagnostic procedures. The screening procedure would allow early diagnosis of ovarian cancer, since women with early stage I or II ovarian cancer experience a five-year survival of 50–90%, compared with 20% if diagnosis is made at stage

III or IV. Unfortunately, no such screening procedure currently exists. The following procedures may lead to a diagnosis of ovarian cancer.

History and pelvic examination

Retrospectively, symptoms have been reported by 78% of patients with early tumor diagnosis, including abdominal/pelvic pain (35%), bloating (32%), and vaginal bleeding (19%).[26] Clinicians providing primary care to women will recognize that abdominal and pelvic complaints are common. Diagnostic investigations in the setting of the above symptoms may be more properly considered case-finding than screening, and the yield of an ovarian cancer diagnosis may be low compared with other diagnoses. The finding of a symptomatic or asymptomatic pelvic mass on routine examination always bears further investigation, but confounding factors that may make detection of masses difficult include obesity and coexisting uterine fibroids. In general, ovaries should not be readily palpable in the menopausal woman, and any ovarian enlargement should be considered suspicious until proven otherwise.

Routine use of transvaginal ultrasound in the general population

Transvaginal ultrasound is relatively expensive as a screening procedure applied to a general population of women and requires specialized training, but it would be considered minimally invasive. It is not uncomfortable, causing approximately the same or less sensation of pelvic pressure as performance of a speculum exam. General observational studies of transvaginal ultrasound to exclude disease of the pelvis report negative predictive values greater than 90%, but these studies include both pre- and postmenopausal women who were evaluated for a wide range of pelvic complaints.[27] There are no data at the time of writing that indicate transvaginal ultrasound to be an effective screening modality in the general population.

CA-125

The tumor marker CA-125 is elevated in approximately 85% of patients with ovarian cancer. It has been used extensively to follow women for tumor recurrence following resection of an ovarian cancer. Its use as a screen is limited by several factors: patients with non-malignant pelvic conditions (uterine fibroids, pelvic inflammatory disease, endometriosis, pregnancy, menstruation, ovarian cyst) and other malignancies (pancreatic, breast, colon, lung) may demonstrate elevated CA-125.[28] Additionally, women with stage I ovarian cancer will not demonstrate elevation in CA-125 in up to 50% of cases. Some types of ovarian cancer (mucinous cystadenocarcinoma) are less likely to demonstrate elevation of CA-125. CA-125 II was developed using monoclonal antibodies and exhibits less day-to-day variation in levels. Protocols using single threshold values frequently utilize values of 30 or 35 units/ml for postmenopausal women and 25 units/ml for premenopausal women.

Baseline CA-125 levels vary in normal postmenopausal women with several factors, including race, history of previous hysterectomy, history of previous cancer other than ovarian cancer, smoking, age at menarche, and age at menopause. Thus, screening algorithms might be developed with increased sensitivity and specificity using these more complex factors, but no outcome data are available to indicate that this is effective.[29]

Combined CA-125 and transvaginal ultrasound

Although some authors have concluded only limited value to the use of CA-125 and transvaginal ultrasound for screening in the general population,[30] large multicenter trials sponsored by the National Cancer Institute are currently in progress, with more than 150 000 patients, and may provide more information combining these modalities for general screening.[31] A smaller randomized trial involving 11 000 normal-risk women utilized CA-125 as the initial screen, followed by transvaginal sonography (TVS) for elevated CA-125 values. Women with abnormal TVS findings were referred for gynecologic investigation. This study found six cancers and 23 false-positives in the screened group, with a positive predictive value of 20.7%. Survival of patients in the screened group versus controls was increased signicantly, but there was no significant difference in deaths between the two groups.[32] Additionally, ten women who developed cancer were missed with screening.

A systematic review of 16 studies in normal-risk women and nine studies in high-risk women determined that between 2.5 and 60 women would undergo surgery for every ovarian cancer detected, assuming an incidence of 40 per 100 000.[33] Given the low prevalence of ovarian cancer in the general population and the cost of screening modalities, there is no evidence at this time that routine use of these modalities should be incorporated into well-woman care for the general population.

Other tumor markers

New methods of identifying tumor markers employ complementary DNA (cDNA) microarray data to identify up-regulated genes in cancer cells whose products may be used as biomarkers for tumors. One such marker, osteopontin, has been isolated and measured in plasma from healthy women, women with benign ovarian disease, and women with ovarian cancer, but no data from screening trials are available.[34]

Screening in high-risk women: combined CA-125 and transvaginal ultrasound in high-risk women

In women at high risk for ovarian cancer, combined screening regimens, starting at age 25–35 years, have been recommended by expert panels, but they have not been demonstrated to improve outcomes.[35] In a small retrospective study of more than 300 high-risk women followed with CA-125 and TVS every six months for up to seven years and for one to 17 visits, nine went to surgery because of abnormal findings, and one patient was diagnosed with ovarian cancer.[36] Larger prospective studies will be compiled in 2004.

Summary of recommendations on screening

There is insufficient evidence to recommend screening modalities other than pelvic examination in asymptomatic women of average risk. Additionally, there is insufficient evidence at this time that combined screening programs decrease mortality rates in women with a genetic predisposition to ovarian cancer, but combined screening programs do result in increased numbers of women being diagnosed with stage I disease.

Prevention

Oral contraceptives

Epidemiologic studies over several decades have reported *a protective effect of oral contraceptives on ovarian cancer risk.* Meta-analysis of case–control studies demonstrates both a reduced odds ratio for ever-users of oral contraceptives compared with non-users (0.66, 95% CI 0.56–0.79) and a greater reduction in risk if OCPs were used for more than five years (0.5, 95% CI 0.33–0.76). This reduction in risk apparently persists for more than 20 years.[37] The protective effect of oral contraceptives appears to be independent of the dose of estrogen used, but controversy remains whether progestins of higher potency produce a greater effect than-low progestin formulations.[38,39]

Prophylactic oophorectomy at the time of hysterectomy

Prophylactic oophorectomy for all women undergoing hysterectomy at age 40 years or older has been proposed as a means of preventing ovarian cancer in normal-risk women. Retrospective studies of women undergoing hysterectomy for benign disease predicted that 5–10% of ovarian cancers could have been prevented by oophorectomy at the time of their surgery.[40] Oophorectomy has not been included as a standard of care with hysterectomy for benign disease because of considerations of endocrine functions. However, about one-third of patients undergoing hysterectomy with preservation of ovaries experience onset of menopausal symptoms within one to two years.[41] A significant portion of these women also experience decreased bone density.[42] This consideration makes oophorectomy more attractive in women aged 40 years or older and seeking hysterectomy for other conditions.

Dietary factors

Dietary factors have been postulated as a means of risk reduction in multiple common malignancies. One Chinese case–control study found a significantly reduced odds ratio for ovarian cancer in women who drank green tea, which was dependent on frequency and duration.[43] A US case–control study of women in Hawaii and Los Angeles found a significant reduction in the odds ratio for ovarian cancer in women with the highest quartile of dietary calcium intake compared with the lowest quartile, with a non-significant trend also found with calcium supplement intake.[44] A meta-analysis of five observational studies of beta-carotene intake determined a modest but statistically significant reduction in summary relative risk for ovarian cancer with a diet high in beta-carotene.[45] Another study found reduced risk with alpha-carotene and lycopene.[46]

Case–control data are also available suggesting some protective effect from a diet high in fiber from vegetable sources.[47] Information regarding dietary factors is thus somewhat scanty at this time, and the evidence is insufficient to recommend dietary intervention as a means of prevention of ovarian cancer, but there is no evidence of risk to individuals who choose to modify their diets to include these foods.

Non-hormonal chemoprophylaxis

Non-steroidal anti-inflammatory agents (cyclo-oxygenase 2 (COX-2) inhibitors) have been observed to decrease growth of cell lines of human ovarian cancer in vitro.[48] A protective effect has not been documented in retrospective case–control studies at this time.[49]

Summary

There is good evidence that oral contraceptives, especially when used for periods of five years or longer, have a prolonged protective effect against the development of ovarian cancer. This is a class B recommendation, since the use of oral contraceptives may be associated with other negative health effects in women, such as the development of thromboembolic disease. Thus, the use of oral contraceptives should be considered as primarily indicated for those women seeking family planning or other health benefits, such as regulation of menses, and the patient should be evaluated as would otherwise be indicated for all possible risks and benefits.

There is insufficient evidence to recommend the use of dietary measures, such as alpha- or beta-carotene, lycopene, a calcium-rich diet, green tea, or vegetable-source fiber for the prevention of ovarian cancer, but there is no evidence suggesting a deleterious effect.

There is good evidence that oophorectomy at the time of hysterectomy in women aged 40 years or older is of benefit in reducing the risk of ovarian cancer in the general population. This is a class B recommendation, given concerns regarding the possible benefit of natural hormonal function beyond the age at which hysterectomy is performed.

High-risk populations

The identification of a woman at high risk for ovarian cancer holds some promise for both prevention and early detection. The most important aspect of this risk stratification relies on a thorough family history, with elicitation of any family members diagnosed with cancer. The degree of relationship, type of cancer(s), and age at onset of malignancy are also important. Although awareness among families with genetic cancer syndromes may be increasing, not all families will communicate well about cancer diagnoses. Clinicians, thus, cannot count upon self-referral from patients who should be considered at risk for genetic cancer syndromes.

Women who may carry a cancer mutation include those with previous early-onset breast or ovarian cancer. These women should be considered as candidates for genetic counseling, especially if a family history is present. More frequently, a family history will reveal a pattern of family members with breast and/or ovarian cancer or other malignancies, or patients will inquire as to their risk of cancer because of concerns about a friend or family member. Formal genetic evaluation should be considered with a positive family history of two or more second-degree relatives with breast and/or ovarian cancer, especially if early-onset, or one first-degree relative with early-onset breast and/or ovarian cancer.

While members of families with breast and ovarian cancer may be recognized more readily as potential carriers of *BRCA1/2* mutations, carriers of HNPCC mutations may not be recognized as readily because of the diverse types of malignancies encountered in this syndrome and the lesser degree of medical and public awareness. The genetic risk scoring systems used with HNPCC or Lynch cancer syndrome are based on multiple diagnoses in a three-generation family history of colon cancer, one or more cases of early-onset colon or endometrial cancer (younger than age 45), and other more complex criteria present in the Amsterdam[50] or Bethesda criteria.[51]

Genetic counseling and testing
Genetic testing results in useful information about a mutation if the testing is performed with an affected individual in the family. Once the presence of a

mutation is established, genetic testing may be offered to the rest of the family to determine whether other individuals carry the mutation.

Several considerations that may make counseling or testing unacceptable to a woman include a fear of stigmatization or discrimination by insurance companies (health or life),[52] lack of health insurance coverage for genetic services, emotional factors, and health beliefs about potential treatments. An appropriate cancer counseling service includes consideration of these concerns, family communication, issues of fertility, ethical issues, and concerns that women may have about disfigurement or loss of body functions.

Small prospective studies have demonstrated a greater proportion of early-stage diagnoses of breast and ovarian/fallopian-tube malignancies for high-risk patients enrolled in comprehensive counseling and screening programs.[53] Whether earlier diagnoses will result in reduced cancer mortality has not been shown.

Management options in *BRCA*1/2

Preventive measures that have been offered include chemoprevention and prophylactic oophorectomy, generally performed after completion of childbearing but before age 40 years. These options may be combined or substituted by surveillance programs for early detection (see the previous section on screening). A study of French, British, and Canadian women suggests that cultural background may significantly affect acceptability of screening and prevention modalities.[54]

Oral contraceptives have been proposed as a means of decreasing risk of ovarian cancer in women with *BRCA1/2*. Although results of early studies are somewhat conflicting, a case–control study of patients with known genetic cancer syndromes and their sisters demonstrated *reduced risk of ovarian cancer for patients with both* BRCA1 *and* BRCA2 *with the use of oral contraceptives*.[55] Population-based studies in Israel seem to indicate a protective effect with greater parity.[56] No other effective chemoprevention is known at this time.

Studies of prophylactic oophorectomy in patients with known *BRCA1/2* status demonstrate approximately 2–12% incidence of early (stage I or II) ovarian or fallopian cancer at the time of surgery, approximately 1% incidence of late-onset peritoneal carcinomatosis, and a decrease from two to four times in the incidence of breast cancer.[57,58]

Decision analysis models incorporating prophylactic surgery (mastectomy and/or oophorectomy) versus screening demonstrate the greatest gain in life expectancy with prophylactic mastectomy and oophorectomy, but a strong advantage to breast screening and prophylactic oophorectomy when quality-adjusted life expectancy is considered, especially if prophylactic oophorectomy is performed before age 40,[59] or with the addition of tamoxifen to prophylactic oophorectomy.[60] These projections have not, as yet, been supported by observational studies or clinical trials.

Disadvantages of prophylactic oophorectomy include possible lack of insurance coverage,[61] emotional and quality-of-life issues, and possible failure of prophylactic surgery to prevent peritoneal cancer, presumably from unrecognized metastatic disease at the time of surgery.

Reduction of anxiety has been associated strongly with an interest in prophylactic oophorectomy in genetic counseling programs, independent of actual risk classification.[62] Conflicting information is available regarding the psychological impact of prophylactic oophorectomy. A prospective study of women in a familial cancer clinic compared women who did and did not undergo prophylactic oophorectomy; it found significant reduction in ovarian cancer anxiety and a high degree of satisfaction with the decision to undergo the prophylactic procedure.[63] Another small study compared utilized responses to the Short-Form (SF)-36 Health Status Questionnaire and the General Health Questionnaire (GHQ); women undergoing oophorectomy for prevention scored poorer functioning on the role-emotional and social functioning subscales, with a trend to report more menopausal symptoms, and reported higher scores on the GHQ. There were no significant differences in the groups with respect to cancer worry or sexual functioning.[64]

Summary

The actual risk status of women with a family history of ovarian or breast and ovarian cancer can be best determined by a complete genetic history. All clinicians providing primary care to women should obtain a family history containing cancer diagnoses of family members and age at onset of disease.

If a high risk of a genetic cancer syndrome is suspected, then it is preferable to perform genetic testing initially with an affected individual in the family rather than an individual not known to have the disease. Genetic counseling for the patient and/or family members includes a comprehensive approach to all issues associated, including quality-of-life and ethical issues, concerns about insurance, and possible options if a diagnosis is made. If testing occurs and a mutation is found, then further genetic testing of other family members may proceed.

Women who are known to carry *BRCA1* or *BRCA2* mutations should be offered a comprehensive approach, including the options of monitoring, chemoprevention, and prophylactic surgery. This is a class B recommendation, since there is fair evidence that risk of ovarian cancer can be reduced and ovarian cancer can be diagnosed at an earlier stage.

There is fair evidence that oral contraceptives and higher parity offer some protection for women carrying the *BRCA1/2* mutations (class B recommendation).

There is good evidence that prophylactic oophorectomy offers a reduction in risk for ovarian cancer for women carrying the *BRCA1/2* mutation, but it is not 100% preventive for the development of ovarian or primary peritoneal cancer (class B recommendation). There is good evidence that prophylactic oophorectomy reduces risk of breast cancer in women with *BRCA1/2* mutations.

There is currently no evidence as to whether oral contraceptives are protective in women with Lynch cancer syndrome (HNPCC). There is insufficient evidence regarding prophylactic opphorectomy in this small group of women. Nonetheless, women with these mutations and undergoing other pelvic surgery (hysterectomy) should be strongly considered for oophorectomy.

REFERENCES

1 Werness, B. A. and Eltabbakh, G. H. Familial ovarian cancer and early ovarian cancer; biologic, pathologic, and clinical features. *Int. J. Gynecol. Pathol.* 2001; **20**:48–63.

2 Stratton, J. F., Pharoah, P., Smith, S. K., Easton, B. and Ponder, B. A. A systematic review and meta-analysis of family history and risk of ovarian cancer. *Br. J. Obstet. Gynaecol.* 1998; **105**:493–9.

3 Ziogas, A., Gildea, M., Cohen, P., *et al.* Cancer risk estimates for family members of a population-based family registry for breast and ovarian cancer. *Cancer Epidemiol. Biomarkers Prev.* 2000; **9**:103–11.

4 Liede, A., Karlan, B. Y., Baldwin, R. L., *et al.* Cancer incidence in a population of Jewish women at risk of ovarian cancer. *J. Clin. Oncol.* 2002; **20**:1570–77.

5 Chang, J. and Elledge, R. M. Clinical management of women with genomic BRCA1 and BRCA2 mutations. *Breast Cancer Res. Treat.* 2001; **69**:101–13.

6 Galper, S., Gelman, R., Recht, A., *et al.* Second nonbreast malignancies after conservative surgery and radiation therapy for early-stage breast cancer. *Int. J. Radiat. Oncol. Biol. Phys.* 2002; **52**:406–14.

7 Hall, H. I., Jamison, P. and Weir, H. K. Secondary primary ovarian cancer among women diagnosed previously with cancer. *Cancer Epidemiol. Biomarkers Prev.* 2001; **10**:995–9.

8 Marchbanks, P. A., Wilson, H., Bastos, E., *et al.* Cigarette smoking and epithelial ovarian cancer by histologic type. *Obstet. Gynecol.* 2000; **95**:255–60.

9 Green, A., Purdie, B., Bain, C., Siskind, V. and Webb, P. M. Cigarette smoking and risk of epithelial ovarian cancer (Australia). *Cancer Causes Control* 2001; **12**:713–19.

10 Rodriguez, C., Pal, A. V., Calle, E. E., Jacob, E. J. and Thun, M. J. Estrogen replacement therapy and ovarian cancer mortality in a large prospective study of US women. *J. Am. Med. Assoc.* 2001; **285**:1460–65.

11 Coughlin, S. S., Giustozzi, A., Smith, S. J. and Lee, N. C. A meta-analysis of estrogen replacement therapy and risk of epithelial ovarian cancer. *J. Clin. Epidemiol.* 2000; **53**:367–75.

12 Lacey, J. V., Mink, P. J., Lubin, J. H., *et al.* Menopausal hormone replacement therapy and risk of ovarian cancer. *J. Am. Med. Assoc.* 2002; **288**:334–41.

13 Riman, T., Dickman, P. W., Nilsson, S., *et al.* Risk factors for invasive epithelial ovarian cancer: results from a Swedish case–control study. *Am. J. Epidemiol.* 2002; **156**:363–73.

14 Ness, R. B., Cramer, D. W., Goodman, M. T., *et al.* Infertility, fertility drugs, and cancer: a pooled analysis of case-control studies. *Am. J. Epidemiol.* 2002; **155**:217–24.

15 Schildkraut, J. M., Schwingl, P. J., Bastos, E., Evanoff, A. and Hughes, C. Epithelial ovarian cancer risk among women with polycystic ovary syndrome. *Obstet. Gynecol.* 1996; **88**:554–9.

16 Balen, A. Polycystic ovary syndrome and cancer. *Hum. Reprod. Update* 2001; **7**: 522–5.

17 Olson, J. E., Cerhan, J. R., Janney, C. A., *et al.* Postmenopausal cancer risk after self-reported endometriosis diagnosis in the Iowa Women's Health Study. *Cancer* 2002; **94**:1612–18.

18 Modesitt, S. C., Tortolero-Luna, G., Robinson, J. B., Gershenon, D. M., and Wolf, J. K. Ovarian and extraovarian endometriosis-associated cancer. *Obstet. Gynecol.* 2002; **100**:788–95.

19 Swiersz, L. M. Role of endometriosis in cancer and tumor development. *Ann. N. Y. Acad. Sci.* 2002; **955**:281–92.

20 Parazzini, F., La Vecchia, C., Negir, E., *et al.* Pelvic inflammatory disease and the risk of ovarian cancer. *Cancer Epidemiol. Biomarkers Prev.* 1996; **5**:667–9.

21 Risch, H. A., and Howe, G. R. Pelvic inflammatory disease and the risk of epithelial ovarian cancer. *Cancer Epidemiol. Biomarkers Prev.* 1995; **4**:447–51.

22 Wehner, A. P. Cosmetic talc should not be listed as a carcinogen: comments on NTP's deliberations to list talc as a carcinogen. *Regul. Toxicol. Pharmacol.* 2002; **36**:40–50.

23 Gertig, D. M., Hunter, D. J., Cramer, D. W., *et al.* Prospective study of talc use and ovarian cancer. *J. Natl Cancer Inst.* 2000; **92**:249–52.

24 Shen, N., Weiderpass, E., Antilla, A., *et al.* Epidemiology of occupational and environmental risk factors related to ovarian cancer. *Scand. J. Work Environ. Health* 1998; **24**:161–4.

25 Cass, I., Li, A. J., Runowicz, C. D., *et al.* Patterns of lymph node metastases in clinically unilateral stage I epithelial ovarian carcinoma. *Gynecol. Oncol.* 2001; **80**:56–61.

26 Elktabbakh, G. H., Yadev, P. R. and Morgan, A. Clinical picture of women with early stage ovarian cancer. *Gynecol. Oncol.* 1999; **75**:476–9.

27 Barloon, T. J., Brown, B. P., Monzer, M. A., and Warnock, N. Predictive value of normal endovaginal sonography in excluding disease of the female genital organs and adnexa. *J. Ultrasound Med.* 1994; **13**:395–8.

28 Bast, R. C., Xu, F. J., Yu, Y. H., *et al.* CA125: the past and future. *Int. J. Biol. Markers* 1998; **13**:179–87.

29 Pauler, D. K., Menon, U., McIntosh, M., *et al.* Factors influencing serum CA-125 levels in healthy postmenopausal women. *Cancer Epidemiol. Biomarkers Prev.* 2001; **10**:489–93.

30 Schwartz, P. E. Nongenetic screening of ovarian malignancies. *Obstet. Gynecol. Clin. North Am.* 2001; **28**:637–51,vii.

31 Simpson, N. K., Johnson, C. C., Ogden, S. L., *et al.* Recruitment strategies in the Prostate, Lung, Colorectal, and Ovarian (PLCO) Cancer Screening Trial: the first six years. *Control. Clin. Trials* 2000; **21**(6 supp):356–78S.

32 Jacobs, I. J., Skates, S. J., Macdonald, N., *et al.* Screening for ovarian cancer: a pilot randomised controlled trial. *Lancet* 1999; **353**:1207–10.

33 Bell, R., Pettigrew, M. and Sheldon, T. The performance of screening tests for ovarian cancer: results of a systematic review. *Br. J. Obstet. Gynecol.* 1998; **105**:1136–47.

34 Kim, J. H., Skates, S. J., Uede, T., *et al.* Osteopontin as a potential diagnostic biomarker for ovarian cancer. *J. Am. Med. Assoc.* 2002; **287**:1671–9.

35 Burke, W., Daly, M., Garber, J., *et al.* Recommendations for follow-up care of individuals with an inherited predisposition to cancer. II: BRCA 1 and BRCA2. *J. Am. Med. Assoc.* **277**:997–1003.

36 Laframboise, S., Nedelcu, R., Murphy, J., Cole, D. E., and Rosen, B. Use of CA-125 and ultrasound in high-risk women. *Int. J. Gynecol. Cancer* 2002; **12**:86–91.

37 Bosetti, C., Negri, E., Trichopoulos, D., *et al.* Long-term effects of oral contraceptives on ovarian cancer risk. *Int. J. Cancer* 2002; **102**:262–5.

38 Ness, R. B., Grisso, J. A., Klapper, J., *et al.* Risk of oral contraceptives in relation to estrogen and progestin dose and use characteristics of oral contraceptives. SHARE Study Group. Steroid Hormones and Reproduction. *Am. J. Epidemiol.* 2000; **152**:233–41.

39 Shildkraut, J. M., Calingaert, B., Marchbanks, P. A., Moorman, P. G. and Rodriguez, G. C. Impact of progestin and estrogen potency in oral contraceptives on ovarian cancer risk. *J. Natl Cancer Inst.* 2002; **94**:32–8.

40 Piver, M. S. Prophylactic oophorectomy: reducing the U. S. death rate from epithelial ovarian cancer. A continuing debate. *Oncologist* 1996; **1**:326–30.

41 Siddle, N., Sarrell, P. and Whitehead, M. The effect of hysterectomy on the age at ovarian failure: identification of a subgroup of women with premature loss of ovarian function and literature review. *Fertil. Steril.* 1987; **47**:94–100.

42 Watson, N. R., Studd, J. W., Garnett, T., *et al.* Bone loss after hysterectomy with ovarian conservation. *Obstet. Gynecol.* 1995; **86**:72–7.

43 Zhang, M., Binns, C. W. and Lkee, A. H. Tea consumption and ovarian cancer risk: a case control study in China. *Cancer Epidemiol. Biomarkers Prev.* 2002; **11**:713–18.

44 Goodman, M. T., Wu, A. H., Tung, K. H., *et al.* Association of dairy products, lactose, and calcium with risk of ovarian cancer. *Am. J. Epidemiol.* 2002; **156**:148–57.

45 Huncharek, M., Klassen, H. and Kupelnick, B. Dietary beta-carotene intake and the risk of epithelial ovarian cancer: a meta-analysis of 3,782 subjects from five observational studies. *In Vivo* 2001; **15**:339–43.

46 Cramer, D. W., Kuper, H., Harlow, B. L. and Titus-Ernstoff, L. Carotenoids, antioxidants, and ovarian cancer risk in pre- and postmenopausal women. *Int. J. Cancer* 2001; **94**:128–34.

47 Pelucchi, C., La Vecchia, C., Chatenoud, L., *et al.* Dietary fibres and ovarian cancer risk. *Eur. J. Cancer* 2001; **37**:2235–9.

48 Rodriguez-Burford, C., Barnes, M. N., Oeschlager, D. K., *et al.* Effects of nonsteroidal anti-inflammatory agents (NSAIDs) on ovarian carcinoma cell lines: preclinical evaluation of NSAIDs as chemopreventive agents. *Clin. Cancer Res.* 2002; **8**:202–9.

49 Meier, C. R., Schmitz, S. and Jick, H. Association between acetaminophen or nonsteroidal anti-inflammatory drugs and risk of developing ovarian, breast, or colon cancer. *Pharmacotherapy* 2002; **22**:303–9.

50 Vasen, H. F. A., Mecklin, J.-P., Khan, M. P. and Lynch, H. T. The International Collaborative Group on Hereditary Non-Polyposis Colorectal Cancer (ICG-HNPCC). *Dis. Colon Rectum* 1991; **34**:424–5.

51 Syngal, S., Fox, E. A., Eng, C., *et al.* Sensitivity and specificity of clinical criteria for hereditary non-polyposis colorectal cancer associated mutations in *MSH2* and *MLH1*. *J. Med. Genet.* 2000; **37**:641–5.

52 Peterson, E. A., Milliron, K. J., Lewis, K. E., Goold, S. D. and Merajver, S. D. Health insurance and discrimination concerns and BRCA 1 and 2 testing in a clinic population. *Cancer Epidemiol. Biomarkers Prev.* 2002; **11**:79–87.

53 Scheuer, L., Kauff, N., Robson, M., *et al.* Outcome of preventive surgery and screening for breast and ovarian cancer in BRCA mutation carriers. *J. Clin. Oncol.* 2002; **20**:1260–68.

54 Julian-Reynier, C. M., Bouchard, L. J., Evans, D. G., *et al.* Women's attitudes toward preventive strategies for hereditary breast or ovarian carcinoma differ from one country to another: differences among English, French, and Canadian women. *Cancer* 2001; **92**:959–68.

55 Narod, S. A., Risch, H., Moslehi, R., *et al.* Oral contraceptives and the risk of hereditary ovarian cancer. Hereditary Ovarian Cancer Clinical Study Group. *N. Engl. J. Med.* 1998; **339**:424–8.

56 Modan, B., Harge, P., Hirsch-Yechezkel, G., *et al.* Parity, oral contraceptives, and the risk of ovarian cancer among carriers and non-carriers of a BRCA1 or BRCA2 mutation. *N. Engl. J. Med.* 2001; **345**:235–40.

57 Lu, K. H., Garber, J. E., Cramer, D. W., *et al.* Occult ovarian tumors in women with BRCA1 or BRCA2 mutations undergoing prophylactic oophorectomy. *J. Clin. Oncol.* 2000; **18**:2728–32.

58 Rebbeck, T. R., Lynch, H. T., Neuhausen, S. L., *et al.* Prophylactic oophorectomy in carriers of BRCA1 or BRCA 2 mutations. *N. Engl. J. Med.* 2002; **346**:1616–22.

59 Van Roosmalen, M. S., Verhoef, L. C., Stalmeier, P. F., Hoogerbrugge, N. and van Daal, W. A. Decision analysis of prophylactic surgery or screening for BRCA1 mutation carriers: a more prominent role for oophorectomy. *J. Clin. Oncol.* 2002; **20**:2092–100.

60 Grann, V. R., Jacobson, J. S., Thomason, D., Hershman, D., Heitjan, D. F. and Neugut, A. L. Effect of prevention strategies on survival and quality-adjusted survival of women with BRCA1/2 mutations: an updated decision analysis. *J. Clin. Oncol.* 2002; **20**:2520–29.

61 Kuerer, H. M., Hwang, E. S., Anthony, J. P., *et al.* Current national health insurance coverage policies for breast and ovarian cancer prophylactic surgery. *Am. Surg. Oncol.* 2000; **7**:325–32.

62 Hurley, K. E., Miller, S. M., Cosatlas, J. W., Gillespie, D. and Daly, M. B. Anxiety/uncertainty reduction as a motivation for interest in prophylactic oophorectomy in women with a family history of ovarian cancer. *J. Womens Health Gend. Based Med.* 2001; **10**:189–99.

63 Tiller, K., Meiser, B., Butow, P., *et al.* Psychological impact of prophylactic oophorectomy in women at increased risk of developing ovarian cancer: a prospective study. *Gynecol. Oncol.* 2002; **86**:212–19.

64 Fry A, Busby-Earle C, Rush R, Cull A. Prophylactic oophorectomy versus screening: psychosocial outcomes in women at increased risk of ovarian cancer. *Psychooncology* 2000 May–Jun;**10**(3):231–41.

20

Colon, lung, and skin cancer: screening and prevention

Jo Ann Rosenfeld

Colorectal cancer: prevention and screening

Epidemiology

Colorectal cancer is the second most common cancer and the third most common cause of cancer death in women (Figure 20.1). Although breast and gynecological cancers may be mentioned more commonly, colon cancer causes 55 000 deaths yearly in the USA[1] (28 000 in women)[2] and 15 000 deaths yearly in the UK.[2] It may be prevented.[3] A person at age 50 has about a 5% lifetime risk of being diagnosed with colorectal cancer and a 2.5% chance of dying from it; the average patient dying of colorectal cancer loses 13 years of life (Table 20.1).[1] Ninety per cent of colon cancers occur after age 50 years. More men than women over age 50 develop colon cancer, but because more women live longer, the total number of cases is higher in women.[2]

Because most colorectal cancers arise from adenomatous polyps, removal of these polyps during colonoscopy and sigmoidoscopy can prevent colon cancer. Ten per cent of adenomatous polyps larger than 1 cm will develop into cancer within ten years.[4] Colonoscopic removal of polyps results in a 76–90% reduction in colon cancer over six years.[5] Primary prevention by reduction of risk factors may decrease the risk. In addition, screening is effective in reducing or preventing morbidity and mortality.

Screening

The US Preventive Services Task Force (USPSTF) has made an A recommendation that *all individuals over age 50 years should be screened for colon cancer.* There is a variety of methods of screening, most of which are equally effective, but they carry different risks and benefits. Fecal occult blood testing (FOBT), sigmoidoscopy, colonoscopy, and a combination of these three methods are all considered valid screening methods (Table 20.2). However,

Table 20.1 Lifetime risk of colon cancer

Risk factor	Lifetime risk
Two first-degree relatives affected	1/6
One first-degree relative with colon cancer before age 45 years	1/10
One first-degree and one second-degree relative affected	1/12
One first-degree relative (any age)	1/17
No first-degree relatives	1/50

Data from Cole, T. R. P. and Sleightholme, H. V. The role of clinical genetics in management: ABC of colorectal cancer. *Br. Med. J.* 2000; **321**:943–6.

Table 20.2 Effective methods of screening for colon cancer

Method	Frequency	Note
FOBT (three specimens done at home)	Yearly	Produces more false-positives
	Twice a year	Fewer false-positives, less sensitivity
Sigmoidoscopy	Every 5–10 year	
Colonoscopy	Every 10 years	Exact data supporting the best interval not yet known
Double-contrast barium enema	Every 5–10 years	Less sensitive than colonoscopy
CT scan		Not yet proven to be effective
Digital rectal examination		Ineffective

CT, computed tomography.

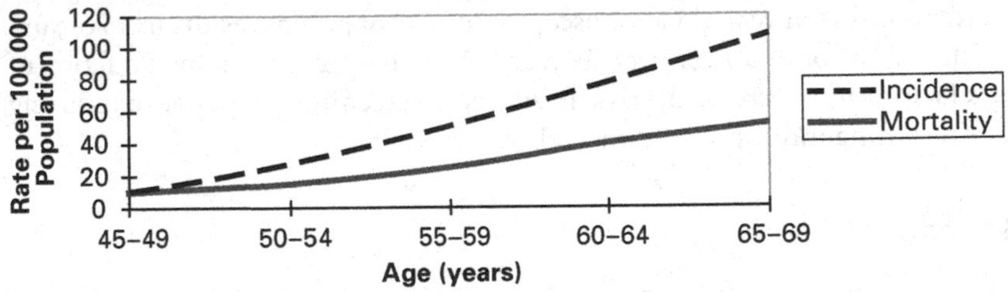

Figure 20.1 Cancer of the colon: incidence and mortality in women 1994–1998. (From American Cancer Society. *Cancer Facts and Figures 2002.* Atlanta, GA : American Cancer Society; 2002.)

less than 40% of women over age 50 years have had sigmoidoscopy or colonoscopy.[6]

Screening after the age of 50 is suggested because of the prevalence of colon cancer in this age group. In individuals with first-degree relatives with colon cancer before the age of 60, and in people with familial polyposis, hereditary non-polyposis, or ulcerative colitis, more frequent screening starting at a younger age is suggested.[1]

FOBT (three specimens done at home) yearly reduces mortality from colon cancer the greatest but produces more false-positives than twice-yearly testing. It has been suggested that sigmoidoscopy be carried out every ten years, although some evidence suggests that every five years may be more effective. It has been suggested that colonoscopy for screening be carried out every ten years, but exact data supporting the best interval have not yet been developed. Double-contrast barium enemas are less sensitive than colonoscopy, and other radiological tests such as computed tomography (CT) scans have not yet been proven effective as screening tools. Digital rectal examination with or without one-card occult blood screening in the office is ineffective in detecting colon cancer. Less than 10% of colon cancers occur within range of the digital examination, and 42% of occult bleeding is missed with just one card.[7]

Combining FOBT with sigmoidoscopy for screening detects more cancers. A positive FOBT test is an indication for colonoscopy rather than sigmoidoscopy. Colonoscopy is the most sensitive but the most expensive and risky option, requiring anesthesia, trained personnel, bowel preparation and longer recovery time, which may necessitate transportation for the patient. It is not certain whether the potential added benefits of colonoscopy relative to screening alternatives are large enough to justify the added risks and inconvenience for all patients. However, recent studies have shown that adenomatous polyps are often found beyond the splenic flexure, out of reach of the sigmoidoscope. Between 46% and 52% of patients had adenomatous polyps beyond the splenic flexure, with no polyps in the terminal and descending colon.[4,8] If these patients had sigmoidoscopy alone, then their polyps would have been missed.

Data have not determined what interval is best for colonoscopy. One study in which patients had two colonoscopies within 24 hours found that 24% of adenomas were missed with only colonoscopy, but only 6% of those greater than 1 cm were missed. Of those patients with negative colonoscopies, 16% had polyps on the second screening.[9] Consensus panels support screening with colonoscopy every ten years for normal-risk patients.

The American Cancer Society's recommendations are similar, with screening of individuals beginning at 50 years of age by FOBT annually, flexible sigmoidoscopy every five years, double-contrast barium enema every five years, or colonoscopy every ten years.[10]

Prevention and risk factors

Genetic factors

Between 5% and 10% of colon cancer has an inherited base, although only a few mutated genes are known.[11] Most familial clusters of colon cancer have no defined gene for their expression. However, *the risk of colon cancer is increased in those individuals with first-degree relatives with colon cancer* (Table 20.1).

Two well-defined colon cancer syndromes are described. Familial adenomatous polyposis, an autosomal dominant disorder, was the first colorectal cancer syndrome recognized, but this accounts for less than 1% of all colon cancers. Usually, individuals with this syndrome have more than 100 tubovillous adenomas in their colon, with malignant transformation inevitable. Other tumors are associated with this. Hereditary non-polyposis colon cancer is autosomal dominant, with colonic and extracolonic tumors. There must be three or more cases of colon cancer in two generations, with aggregations in first-degree relatives.

Diet

Changes in diet may prevent up to 80% of bowel cancer.[12] Diets high in fruits, vegetables, and fibers are linked to a decreased risk of colon cancer, as compared with diets high in red meats. Ingestion of two portions of red and processed meats daily was associated with an increased risk of 1.8 in two large studies of professionals. Alcohol use increases the risk, while appropriate dietary intake of folate may decrease the risk.[13] Constipation and low stool weights are related to an increased risk of cancer.

Inflammatory bowel disease

Individuals with inflammatory bowel disease, particularly those with ulcerative colitis, have an increased risk of colon cancer and need more frequent and ongoing follow-up. Cancer in this setting develops from dysplastic mucosa rather than polyps and, thus, evaluation by colonoscopy is more difficult. In addition, random biopsies every 10 cm and biopsies of suspicious areas are suggested throughout the colon during colonoscopy, although the efficacy of this screening is uncertain.[14] Risk of cancer is greatest in those individuals at younger age at diagnosis, with extensive disease, and with primary sclerosing cholangitis.

Clinical symptoms

Colon cancer can be asymptomatic or may appear as iron-deficient anemia, gastrointestinal hemorrhage, change of bowel habits or size of stool, or constipation. Between 4% and 11% of those patients over age 60 who present with iron-deficiency anemia will have colon cancer, even when an addition upper-gastrointestinal disease is discovered.[15]

Lung cancer: prevention and screening

Lung cancer is the most common cancer in men. In women, it is the third most common cancer, but the most common cancer cause of death. It is estimated to have caused more than 65 700 deaths in women in the USA in 2002.[2] In the UK, lung cancer accounts for one out of 6.5 deaths from cancer – more than 30 000 in 1996.[6,16] Because women have recently been smoking cigarettes in greater numbers, quitting in smaller numbers, and smoking for 30 years or more, the incidence of lung cancer in women may continue to grow. In the UK, the incidence of lung cancer for women between 1971 and 1996 has increased by 9%, while it declined by 28% in men.[6]

During the past two decades, there has been little improvement in survival; almost half of those with diagnosed lung cancer are dead within one year.[7] Thus, prevention is important. However, methods of screening have not been promising or effective.

Prevention

The most common cause of lung cancer is smoking, which accounts for 90% of lung cancers. Occupational exposures, including asbestos, pollutants, radon, and radiation exposure from occupational and medical sources, account for the other risk factors. Some dietary changes may reduce the risk of lung cancer. Vegetables containing beta-carotene may act as antioxidants and reduce the risk of lung cancer.[6]

Early detection

There is no good method for detecting lung cancer early enough and sensitively enough to reduce mortality. Chest X-rays, sputums for cytology, and even bronchosopy have not been shown to be effective screening tools. Helical CT scanning may become a screening tool in the future.

Ten studies have examined the efficacy of various methods and CT scans in detecting lung cancer, without showing any improvement in mortality.[17] The Mayo Lung Project found that intensive following with cytology and chest X-rays of men who smoked found more treatable lung cancers but the same number of untreatable cancers, and the mortality actually increased in the intensively studied group.[18] The Early Lung Cancer Action Project (ELCAP) studied 1000 40–64-year-old men smokers; it found that yearly CT scanning was more effective than chest X-rays for detecting early lung cancer, that repeat scans were more effective than just one scan, and that semi-solid and non-solid nodules were more likely to be cancer than solid nodules.[19]

Prognosis and treatment

Surgery, radiation, and chemotherapy are the treatments, with surgery being the treatment of choice if the cancer is local. The one-year survival rate is 41% but the five-year survival rate is only 15%.[2]

Skin cancer

There are approximately 23 500 cases of melanoma in women yearly in the USA, making it the sixth most common cancer in women, with more than one million cases of basal-cell and squamous-cell cancers identified yearly. Melanoma is ten times more likely in Caucasians than African-Americans.

Excessive exposure to radiation, excessive tanning and burning, and fair complexion are risk factors. Occupational exposures to coal tar, arsenic, radium, pitch, and creosote also increase the risk of skin cancer. Prevention includes limiting exposure to the sun by covering up with a hat and clothes, wearing sunglasses, and using sunscreen.

Any skin growth that is changing shape or color is suspicious for skin cancer. Asymmetry, border irregularity, non-uniform pigmentation, and diameter greater than 6 mm increases the likelihood of a malignancy. Treatment is surgery for basal-cell or squamous-cell carcinoma, and cure is likely. Melanoma needs more aggressive surgery and treatment.

REFERENCES

1 Loren, D. E., Lewis, J. and Kochman, M. L. Colon cancer: detection and prevention: *Gastroenterol. Clin.* 2000; 31:1–19.
2 American Cancer Society. *Cancer Facts and Figures 2002.* Atlanta, GA: American Cancer Society; 2002 p. 10.
3 Winawer, S. J., Fletcher, R. H., Miller, L., *et al.* Colorectal cancer screening: clinical guidelines and rationale. *Gastroenterology* 1997; 112:594–642.
4 Stryker, S. J., Wolff, B. G., Culp, C. E. *et al.* Natural history of untreated colonic polyps. *Gastroenterology* 1987; 93:1009–13.
5 Winawer, S. J., Zauber, A. G., Ho, M. N., *et al.* Prevention of colorectal cancer by colonoscopic polypectomy. The National Polyp Study Workgroup. *N. Engl. J. Med.* 1993; 329:1977–81.
6 National Centre for Chronic Disease Prevention and Health Promotion. *Behavioral Risk Factor Surveillance System.* Atlanta, GA: National Center for Disease Prevention and Health Promotion/Center for Disease Control and Prevention; 2000.

7 Yamamoto, M. and Nakama, H. Cost-effectiveness analysis of immunochemical occult blood screening for colorectal cancer among three fecal sampling methods. *Hepatogastroenterology* 2000; **47**:396–9.

8 Imperiale, T. F., Wagner, D. R., Lin, C. Y., *et al.* Risk of advanced proximal neoplasms in asymptomatic adults according to the distal colorectal findings. *N. Engl. J. Med.* 2000; **343**:169–74.

9 Rex, D. K., Cutler, C. S., Lemmel, G. T., *et al.* Colonoscopic miss rates of adenomas determined by back to back colonoscopies. *Gastroenterology* 1997; **112**:24–8.

10 Byers, T., Levin, B., Rothenberger, D., Dodd, G. D. and Smith, R.A. American Cancer Society guidelines for screening and surveillance for early detection of colorectal polyps and cancer: Update 1997. American Cancer Society Detection and Treatment Advisory Group on Colorectal Cancer. *CA Cancer J. Clin.* 1997; **47**:154–60.

11 Cole, T. R. P. and Sleightholme, H. V. The role of clinical genetics in management: ABC of colorectal cancer. *Br. Med. J.* 2000; **321**:943–6.

12 Cummings, J. H. and Binham, S. A. Diet and the prevention of cancer. *Br. Med. J.* 1998; **317**:1636–40.

13 Chief Medical Officer's Committee on Medical Aspects of Food. *Nutritional Aspects of the Development of Cancer.* London: Stationery Office; 1998.

14 Karlen, P., Kornfeld, D., Brostrom, O., *et al.* Is colonscopic surveillance reducing colorectal cancer mortality in ulcerative colitis? A population based case control study. *Gut* 1998; **42**:711–14.

15 Till, S. H. and Grundman, M. J. Lesson of the week: prevalence of concomitant disease in patients with iron deficiency anaemia. *Br. Med. J.* 1997; **314**:206.

16 Sethi, T. Science, medicine, and the future: lung cancer. *Br. Med. J.* 1997; **314**:652.

17 Reich, J. M. Improved survival and higher mortality. the conundrum of lung cancer screening. *Chest* 2002; **122**:329–37.

18 Fontana, R. S., Sanderson, D. R., Woolner, L. B., *et al.* Lung cancer screening: the Mayo program. *J. Occup. Med.* 1986; **28**:746–50.

19 Henschke, C. I., Yankelevitz,, D. F., Mertcheva, R., *et al.* CT screening for lung cancer: frequency and significance of part-solid and nonsolid nodules. The ELCAP Group. *Am. J. Roentgenol.* 2002; **178**:1053–7.

21

Common gastrointestinal and urinary problems

Jo Ann Rosenfeld

Common gastrointestinal problems

The most common gastrointestinal (GI) complaints are constipation, diarrhea, and irritable bowel syndrome (IBS). Although often limited and innocent, a change in bowel habits or blood in or around the stool can be linked to an increased risk for colon cancer, and is therefore serious.

Constipation

Constipation is the most common GI complaint, accounting for 2.5 million visits in the USA yearly.[1] Approximately 2–13% of individuals complain of constipation, with higher incidences in women, African-Americans, people older than 60 years, and those with less activity, low income, and less leisure activity.

Each individual's normal bowel pattern is different. However, constipation can be defined as no bowel movement in more than three days, hard stools, difficulty or pain with evacuation, abdominal pain, and bloating. Most episodes are limited.

Etiology

Low fiber intake and poor diet can cause constipation. Medications also can lead to constipation (Table 21.1). Constipation is associated with many metabolic and endocrine disorders, including hypocalcemia, renal failure, hypothyroidism, hyperparathyroidism, and diabetes.[1] Neurological disorders can impede normal GI movement; multiple sclerosis, strokes, and spinal cord injury can cause constipation. Malfunction or anatomical abnormalities, including colitis, cancer, diverticular disease, and rectal prolapse, can cause constipation.

Table 21.1 Medications that can lead to constipation

Antacids
Anticholinergics – antihistamines
Anticonvulsants
Antidepressants
Antihypertensives, especially calcium-channel blockers
Antiparkinson drugs
Diuretics
Iron
Laxative abuse
Narcotics

Evaluation

Evaluation of constipation is necessary if it is new, associated with cramps, severe pain, or fever, or if the stool contains blood or mucus. Evaluation includes a white blood count and hematocrit, C reactive protein or erythrocyte sedimentation rate, and either a double-contrast barium enema or colonoscopy. Often, constipation is chronic, with periodic worsening. In this case, an additional evaluation besides preventive colon cancer screening is not indicated.

Treatment

Treatment entails first of all changes in diet and lifestyle; only if these measures do not work should pharmocotherapy be instigated.

Increasing the bulk and fiber is primary. Increased intake of vegetables, fruit, and fiber, including cereals and wholemeal breads, is essential. Second, increased intake of water to 2 l a day may be very helpful. Use of vegetable fiber from psyllium or other sources (e.g. methylcellulose) twice daily until stools are soft will solve many episodes of constipation.

Changes in lifestyle are important. Change of medication and decreasing the use of anticholinergic medication or narcotics will help. Exercise is very important, and necessary. If these methods have failed, then further evaluation is necessary and pharmocotherapy can be considered. Behavioral therapy has been used with 50–80% success rates.[2]

Pharmacotherapy

A variety of classes of laxatives can help induce more normal bowel movements. If an immediate effect is not needed and a long-term treatment is required, then bulk laxatives, which are a form of non-starch polysaccharides, are useful.[2] These include wheat, plant-seed mucilage, and methylcellulose. Ispaghula, plant-seed mucilage, and psyllium are available in a variety of formulations that are swallowed with water. They ferment in the colon and can quadruple fecal bulk.

More immediate therapy or relief, within two to three days, may be obtained by osmotic laxatives. Lactulose, sorbitol, and other non-absorbed sugars create an osmotic load. The dose of lactulose is 15 ml twice a day, reduced as needed; this can also be used for chronic diarrhea. Magnesium and sulfate salts are not absorbed and can be used chronically and safely. The dose of magnesium hydroxide is 1.2–3.6 g daily.[2] Combinations may work more efficaciously, especially in the older women.

Stimulant laxatives should be used for single or only a few doses and should work within 24 hours. These include anthranoid compounds, including those with senna, aloe, and cascara, which are all plant-derived. They may cause adverse chronic changes in the gut, thus they should be used only for temporary constipation.[2] Phenolphthalein, docusate sodium, and bisacodyl products should also be used only temporarily. Enemas and suppositories, including gylcerin and bisacodyl suppositories, can be useful but should not be used chronically.

Chronic diarrhea

Chronic diarrhea can be a significant problem, medically, socially, and economically. Stool frequency varies widely among many people. The definition of diarrhea can be used for increased number and decreased consistency and form of stools, or more than the average of 200 g of stool daily. Many infectious agents may cause acute diarrhea, but chronic diarrhea is defined as lasting more than four weeks. The prevalence of chronic diarrhea, occurring at least 25% of the time in one study, was 14–18%.[3]

Etiology
In the USA and UK, the most common causes of chronic diarrhea are irritable bowel syndrome, malabsorption, chronic infections, and inflammatory bowel disease (Table 21.2).[4] Inflammatory bowel disease is usually discovered in young adulthood and can certainly cause chronic diarrhea. IBS (see below), chronic infections, including giardiasis and amebiasis, and some endocrinopathies, such as diabetes and hyperthyroidism, can cause diarrhea that does not respond to fasting. Malabsorptive diarrheas, including lactose deficiency and other carbohydrate malabsorption symptoms, should resolve when the patient stops eating.

Evaluation
First, a precise definition of bowel pattern is necessary, including number of stools, color, associated blood or mucus, consistency, and whether the stool is fatty, foul-smelling, and floats in the toilet. A history of travel, ownership of pets, chronic or frequent use of antibiotics, the duration of the diarrhea, its

Table 21.2 Common causes of chronic diarrhea

Irritable bowel syndrome
Inflammatory bowel disease
Endocrine causes
   Diabetic diarrhea
   Hyperthyroidism
Chronic infectious diarrhea (especially parasites and worms, e.g. giardiasis, amebiasis)
Bacterial overgrowth
Malabsorptive causes (respond to fasting)
   Lactose deficiency and other carbohydrate malabsorption
   Bile acid diarrhea
   Food allergy
   Laxative overuse or abuse

response to different foods or fasting, and whether it has occurred before is important.

Stool for culture and the presence of white blood cells is indicated if the diarrhea is sudden, of new onset, or associated with pain, or if infectious diarrhea is possible. The usefulness of stool cultures is disputed, and their yield is quite low.[5] Usually, however, most infectious diarrheas are viral. Even if infectious organisms are identified, they are seldom treated with antibiotics. If the woman has traveled or family members also have diarrhea, then stool for ova and parasites should be obtained. Stool positive for white blood cells suggests the presence of inflammatory or infectious diarrhea.

Elimination diets may be needed. Elimination of all milk products is a first step. Sometimes, after an acute viral gastroenteritis, a chronic lactose deficiency may worsen, causing a chronic diarrhea. If the diagnosis is unclear, the diarrhea is bloody, and/or the diarrhea persists, then a sigmoidoscopy or colonoscopy is indicated.

Laboratory analysis for white blood count, hematocrit/hemoglobin, electrolytes to evaluate for hypokalemia and dehydration, fasting glucose, and thyroid functions are indicated.

Treatment

First treatment is hydration. If the diarrhea is infectious, then a consensus practice guideline suggests that there is good evidence that antibiotic therapy should be initiated only for traveler's diarrhea, shigellosis, or campylobacter, but not necessarily other infectious diarrheal agents.[6] In the case of traveler's diarrhea, empirical treatment with fluoroquinolone may reduce the duration of an illness from three to five days to less than one or two days. Other causes of traveler's diarrhea that lasts more than ten days may necessitate empiric treatment for giardiasis.[7] Treatment for patients with fever and suspected

Table 21.3 Rome II criteria for diagnosis of irritable bowel syndrome

Lasting 12 or more weeks (need not be consecutive)
Two of the following pain problems:
  Relief with defecation
  Onset associated with change in frequency of stool
  Onset associated with change in form or appearance of stool

Data from Borum, M. L. Irritable bowel syndrome. *Prim. Care* 2001;
28:147–62.

infectious invasive diarrhea includes a quinolone antibiotic or trimethoprim/
sulfa.[8]

Dysmotility agents can be used in most chronic diarrheas, but they should be
avoided with bloody diarrhea or proven infection with Shiga toxin-producing
Escherichia coli.

Irritable bowel syndrome

IBS is an ill-defined syndrome consisting of abdominal pain, bloating, cramping and a change of bowel habits – constipation or diarrhea, or both – without
any other diagnosed gastrointestinal condition and without evidence of other
organic or anatomic disease.[9] It accounts for 12% of visits to primary-care
physicians and 28% of visits to gastroenterologists, accounting for 30 million
individuals in the USA.[10,11] It has been considered a diagnosis of exclusion. Criteria for diagnosis of IBS have been developed (the Rome II) (see Table 21.3).[12]
The prevalence in women is twice that in men.[11] The symptoms are often
transient; many individuals who describe symptoms at one point do not have
symptoms a year later.[11]

IBS may be thought to be a dysmotility disorder. Some evidence exists that
patients with IBS have visceral hypersensitivity with increased reaction to pain
stimuli.[13] Some IBS patients have increased rectosigmoid motor activity and
exaggerated gastrocolic response.[14] In addition, IBS often presents like lactose
deficiency, and malabsorption has been suggested as a cause.

Clinical symptoms

IBS can present as abdominal pain of variable intensity and position, although
often it is in the lower abdomen or left lower quadrant and often it is crampy.
Usually there is a change or alteration in bowel habits – diarrhea, constipation,
or a combination. Other symptoms may include nausea, vomiting, and gas.
Weight loss is usually not a symptom and suggests other causes. Women with
IBS may have other chronic pain syndromes, including headaches, dyspepsia,

and chronic pelvic pain, and fatigue and malaise. *IBS patients should not exhibit bloody diarrhea, weight loss, acute pain, or fever.*

Psychological features
Approximately 40–80% of individuals with IBS have a concomitant psychiatric diagnosis, depending on the population studied.[15] A significant percentage of women with IBS will report a recent or remote episode of sexual abuse or violent sexual episode.[16]

Evaluation
With symptoms suggestive of IBS, a few laboratory and radiologic tests are needed to eliminate other causes. A complete blood count, electrolytes, glucose, thyroid studies, and stool examination for blood, ova, and parasites are necessary. If diarrhea is the primary complaint, then stool cultures can also be requested. In women over age 50 years, a colonoscopy or barium enema should be performed to eliminate masses or colitis and will show normal findings or spasms.

Treatment
Treatment can be challenging for the woman and physician. However, working together, expecting improvement but not necessarily cure, with a prescription of diet, exercise, and medication, should produce a reduction in symptoms in most women.

Dietary changes are the first step. Some patients with IBS, especially those with excessive gas, may have significant improvement with the elimination of all dairy products or addition of lactose supplements. Addition of fiber, naturally and with supplements (as discussed in the section on constipation, above), is necessary and may be needed for a long time. Additional fiber decreases GI transit time and bile salt concentration, which may cause colonic contractions. Mild to moderate exercise should help the stooling pattern.

Various pharmacological therapies have been used (Table 21.4), with various strength of evidence. Antidiarrheal agents, such as loperamide and combined diphenoxylate and atropine (co-phenotrope), can help, especially if diarrhea is a major symptom. However, co-phenotrope can be addictive and cause drowsiness. Both drugs can worsen constipation caused by narcotics and lengthen the course of infectious diarrhea. The antispasmodics (anticholinergics) hyoscyamine and dicyclomine have been used extensively with some effectiveness. Calcium-channel blockers and peppermint oil have been used, but evidence of their efficacy is mixed. Antidepressants such as tricyclics have been used, but no double-blinded studies have tested their effects.

Controversies have arisen over a class of GI prokinetic agents, type 3 serotonin ($5-HT_3$) receptor antagonists, such as alosetron, because they were reported to produce 84 instances of ischaemic colitis, 113 of severe constipation, 143 admissions to hospital, and seven deaths. The US Food and Drug

Table 21.4 Medications for irritable bowel syndrome

Medication	Form and dose	Notes
Hyoscyamine	Tablet (three to four times a day), extended-release (long-acting) capsule (twice a day), liquid to be taken by mouth (three to four times a day), injectable form	Antispasmodic
Dicyclomine	10 mg – capsule, tablet, oral liquid four times a day	
Diphenoxylate and atropine	2.5 mg – oral liquid two to four times a day	May be habit-forming or addictive; may make overflow incontinence worse; may cause drowsiness
Loperamide	2 or 4 mg – liquid, tablet, capsule two to four times a day	May worsen constipation caused by narcotics
Tricyclic antidepressants	Amitryptilene 25–100 mg qhs	Sedation

Administration (FDA) suspended the sale of alosetron but then allowed its sale again.[17] Tegaserod (a 5-HT$_4$ antagonist) and cilansetron (a 5-HT$_3$ antagonist), two similar drugs, are trying to gain FDA approval. These drugs promote increased GI motility and reduce visceral sensation and should be used in patients with constipation-predominant IBS. Whether they are safer than alosetron is not yet known.[18] Although some GI prokinetic agents produce cardiac effects, tegaserod may be free from these serious side effects.[19]

Psychotherapy, especially for those with long-term issues and diagnoses with or without biofeedback can be helpful.

Urinary problems

Incontinence

Impact
The evidence for effective preventive strategies is very limited, but evidence for valuable and effective therapy is available. Although it affects millions of women, urinary incontinence (UI) is still one of the more invisible complaints. Fewer than half of women with intermittent incontinence mention it to their physicians, and few physicians feel comfortable in methods of helping women manage this problem.

The incidence of UI is high. In several studies of women aged 42–50 years, more than 60% reported urine loss at some time, and more than 30% reported UI regularly. More than 35 % of these women reported having to change their

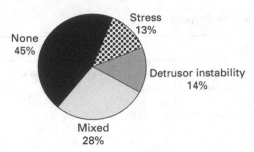

Figure 21.1 Percentage of postmenopausal women with urinary incontinence. (Form Brown, J. S., Grad, D., Ouslander, J. G., *et al.* Prevalence of urinary incontinence and associated risk factors in postmenopausal women. *Obstet. Gynecol.* 1999; **94**:66–70.)

garments. Only one-quarter sought treatment.[20] In one survey of more than 2700 postmenopausal women, with an average age of 67 years, 56% reported UI at least weekly, and fewer than 50% of these had consulted a physician.[21]

The social and personal costs are massive. The total US cost may be more than 26 million dollars yearly, and UI may affect more than 14 million Americans. In the UK, more than 2.5 million women and men may have intermittent UI. Its prevalence is increasing with the increasing aging of the population.

Personally, UI may lead to social isolation, loss of independence, and poor sexual health and self-esteem.[22,23] Medically, UI can lead to urinary-tract and vaginal infections, pressure ulcers, and even renal failure and sepsis. The evidence for effective preventive strategies is very limited, but evidence for valuable and effective therapy is available. Treatment is achievable, and significant improvement and cure are possible if the physician and patient work together.[24]

Primary prevention and risk factors

Although men experience UI, women are twice as likely to suffer the symptoms (Figure 21.1). The risk of UI increases with age, but it should not be considered a natural part of aging. Young women may also have incontinence during physical activity and postpartum. The risk of UI is related to body mass and race, but not to parity, caffeine or alcohol intake, smoking, physical activity, or previous gynecological surgery.[25]

Pregnancy complications have been related positively to later UI, including loss of pelvic support, perhaps caused by multiple and large pregnancies and instrumented deliveries.[26]

No good evidence exists that stress incontinence can be prevented by any particular therapy, including antenatal pelvic-floor (Kegel) exercises.[27] Postnatal exercises have been shown by one randomized clinical trial (RCT) to reduce stress incontinence, but only for a short time.[7]

Evaluation

History

The history often leads to the definition of type of UI (see below). The amount, frequency, and situations under which incontinence occurs should be discussed. Any inciting factors should be noted, such as exercise, sneezing, coughing, or sex. A gynecological and surgical history is important. Recent symptoms or changes, such as increased frequency, dysuria, hematuria, or nocturia, should be questioned. Medications and concomitant diseases, including diabetes, should be considered as causative factors.

Any medication with an anticholinergic effect (see Table 21.1), including antispasmodics, antihistamines, antipsychotics, antidepressants, and antiparkinsonian drugs, can induce urinary retention and overflow incontinence. Diuretics, and caffeine and alcohol through their diuretic effects, can increase urine flow and induce or worsen any form of incontinence. Sedatives, antipsychotics, and alcohol can cause sedation, worsening the woman's ability to respond to urinary urges.

Recent changes in urinary symptoms tend to suggest medication effects or urinary-tract infections as the cause.

Physical examination

A physical examination is necessary, but it rarely provides additional clues to diagnosis and treatment. A general and pelvic examination is sufficient. Pelvic examination may show prolapse or atrophic vaginal mucosa. Fever and suprapubic or costovertebral angle tenderness might be consistent with a urinary tract infection. Pelvic masses from tumors or cysts and uterine prolapse could affect urinary continence.

Bedside urinary tests with q-tips or other instruments are not necessary and can be painful. If overflow incontinence is a possibility, then a post-void residual measurement with a single catheterization may help define the diagnosis and treatment. A post-void residual of more than 200–300 cm^3 is significant.

Laboratory tests

A fasting blood sugar test to evaluate for diabetes is important. Urine analysis and culture are essential. They will eliminate urinary-tract infections as a cause or might suggest diabetes.

Definitions

The definition of type of UI is important because treatment differs by type. However, women often have mixed forms, and precise definition may not be available. In the middle-aged women, in the Hormone–Estrogen Replacement Study (HERS) study, 55% complained of incontinence (13% stress incontinence, 14% urge incontinence, 28% mixed) (Figure 21.2).[6]

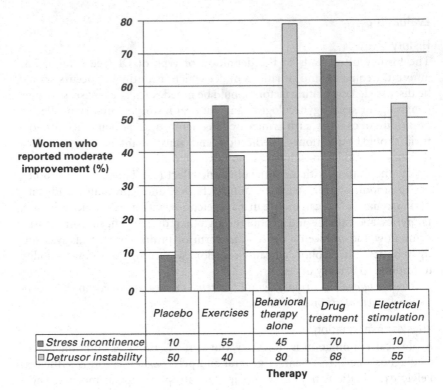

	Placebo	Exercises	Behavioral therapy alone	Drug treatment	Electrical stimulation
Stress incontinence	10	55	45	70	10
Detrusor instability	50	40	80	68	55

Therapy

Figure 21.2 Improvement of urinary incontinence reported with different therapies.

Stress urinary incontinence (SUI) is the most common form of incontinence. It is described as the loss of small amounts of urine with increased abdominal pressure, such as with sneezing, coughing, grunting, and exercise.

Urge incontinence or *detrusor instability* (DI) is usually described as the sudden urge and loss of moderate amounts of urine. DI may be due to the discoordination of the bladder musculature. "I feel the urge and I cannot make it to the toilet," is the usual complaint.

Overflow incontinence, usually related to a neurogenic bladder, occurs when the bladder fills to capacity and overflows at random times. Diabetes and other neurological diseases and pelvic or gynecological surgery can be the causes.

If the woman cannot sense the urge to urinate or cannot make it to the toilet independently, she is *mechanically incontinent*. Altered states of consciousness, dementia, coma, paralysis, severe arthritis, and immobility can all cause incontinence

Treatment
Using a variety of methods, most women will find significant improvement in urinary incontinence. Treatment includes behavioral and lifestyle changes and

Table 21.5 Non-surgical therapy for urinary incontinence

Type	Behavioral therapy	Pharmocotherapy
Stress incontinence	Pelvic Muscle Exercises* Biofeedback* Super tampon or pessary in certain circumstances	Estrogen vaginal cream Imipramine (5–50 mg bid)**
Detrusor instability	Bladder training Electrostimulation	Oxybutinin (2.5–5.0 mg qd to qid** or long-acting (5–15 mg every morning) Tolterodine 1–2 mg bid** Estrogen vaginal cream Imipramine (5–50 mg bid)** Other antidepressants, e.g. doxepine 50–75 mg qhs** Calcium channel blocker, e.g. nifedipine sustained release 30 mg qd**
Overflow incontinence	Intermittent catheterization	Bethanecol 5–25 mg bid to qid

*Judged effective by Clinical Evidence. **Reported by RCTs.

pharmocotherapy based on the definition or diagnosis of the type of incontinence (Table 21.5). Using these methods, many women can have significant improvement.

There is a wide variety of mechanical, electrical, and magnetic therapies, with little good evidence supporting their use. No criteria for their use have been developed. Many studies have examined only a very few patients. In most studies, placebo groups have a response rate of 50% or more. Simply studying and paying attention to incontinence improves the problem in many individuals.

There has been a great deal written on, and many investigations of, the various forms of surgical therapy, but no criteria have been developed for their use over other forms of therapy. There have been no studies specifically comparing lifestyle changes, pharmocotherapy, and electrical treatment with surgical treatment, and no guidelines or criteria have been developed for proper indications for surgical treatment. Thus, non-surgical treatment should be the first step.

There has been a moderate amount of analysis assessing the strength of evidence towards the treatment of UI. Clinical Evidence (CE), the Cochrane Group (C), and the Agency for Healthcare Research and Quality (AHRQ) have assessed the evidence, and the recommendations that follow in this chapter will be identified by their source.

Table 21.6 Medications that affect bladder control adversely

Drug	Note
Alcohol	May cause sedation, immobility, diuresis
Anticholinergic/Antispasmodic drugs	Anticholinergic effect may cause urinary retention and overflow incontinence
Antihypertensives: alpha-adrenergic sympatholytics (prazosin, terazosin), beta-adrenergic agents	Increase urethral tones; may cause stress incontinence to become symptomatic
Antipsychotics/antidepressants	Anticholinergic effect may cause urinary retention and overflow incontinence; antipsychotics may cause sedation and immobility
Antiparkinson drugs	Anticholinergic effect may cause urinary retention and overflow incontinence
Caffeine	Diuretic effects
Calcium-channel blockers	Reduce smooth-muscle contractility and cause overflow incontinence
Diuretics	May induce or worsen UI
Sedative hypnotics	May cause sedation and immobility

Using a variety of methods, most women will find significant if not complete improvement in urinary incontinence. A recent study found that general practitioners in the UK, using a variety of methods, including pelvic floor exercises, estrogen, electrostimulation, anticholinergic drugs, and bladder training, helped 70% (69/99) of the women to improve their urinary control significantly.[28]

Immediate treatment

Urinary incontinence, especially if recent or short-term, may be caused or worsened by infections or medications. Treatment for urinary-tract infections with antibiotics or elimination of an unneeded medication may resolve or improve UI. A review of medications to reduce or change those that may worsen urinary control may also improve UI (Table 21.6).

Effective non-surgical treatment for stress urinary incontinence does exist.

Lifestyle changes

Good evidence from RCTs suggest that pelvic floor muscle exercises (PFME) are effective in reducing symptoms and are more effective than placebo or the use of vaginal cones, although most of the studies have concentrated on young women who were mostly postpartum.[29,30] Although a meta-analysis of a few studies showed improvement with biofeedback, the addition of biofeedback to PFME showed no added improvement.[9]

Medication

One systematic review on various forms of estrogen found that while un-controlled trials suggested that estrogen improved SUI, three RCTs found no improvement in the amount of urine lost or the number of incontinence episodes.[31] In women with atrophic vaginitis, and in menopausal women with no contraindications to estrogen creams, this may be a useful additional ther-apy. In women who are taking oral estrogen, additional intravaginal estrogen cream may be of additional efficacy. In addition, in women who cannot take oral estrogen, the estrogen ring (Estring™) can be used because it has almost no systemic absorption.

In a few small RCTs, oral antidepressants such as imipramine have been shown to be effective in improving episodes of wetness.

Mechanical/electrical

There is conflicting evidence about the efficacy of pelvic floor electrical stimu-lation on improvement of SUI. The methods of delivery of the electrical stim-ulation were not comparable in several studies. One study found that the cure rate with electrical stimulation was no better than with no treatment.[32] Studies examining electrical stimulation of the abdomen wall, vagina, perineum, and rectum, and magnetic stimulation of the pelvis, have been published, but they included only small numbers of women, and without placebo.

There are no criteria for which women may profit from surgical treatment instead of medical treatment.

Surgical

Since SUI is the most common form of UI, most surgery has been done for this type of incontinence. Whether surgical and non-surgical methods of treatment have ever been compared could not be determined. Criteria for suggesting surgical treatment instead of medication, exercise, or behavioral therapy have not been developed.

Anterior vaginal repair has been the standard surgical treatment for SUI.[33] A Cochrane review of nine trials found that anterior repair was less effective than abdominal retropubic suspension. Failure rates as high as 29% were reported, with 3–4% subsequent prolapse after surgery. The review concluded that there were not enough data to compare surgical therapies adequately. Review of the use of suburethral sling operations found that there were too few trials to determine whether these were better or worse than other therapies.[34]

Urge incontinence or detrusor instability

Lifestyle modification definitely can improve symptoms and wetness caused by DI. Bladder training, the practice of timed visits to the toilet, is strongly recommended to reduce UI in nursing-home residents.[35] However, in community-dwelling adults, a review found only tentative evidence of improvement in seven trials and insufficient comparison with drug and electrical therapy.[36]

Several medications have some effect on UI, although side effects may limit their use. Oxybutinin and tolterodine are both marketed primarily for DI. A meta-analysis found similar efficacy at reducing episodes of wetness but found tolterodine was tolerated better.[37] Other drugs can be used for their side effects of urinary retention, including antidepressants and calcium channel blockers.

Overflow incontinence

If urinary incontinence is caused by obstruction, then surgical treatment for the cause of the obstruction is necessary. Tumors, especially rectal and ovarian carcinomas, can lead to local spread or metastases that cause obstruction. For those patients for whom surgery is not an option, intermittent catheterization is suggested, although there is no strong evidence to support this.

In patients in whom overflow incontinence is a result of bladder malfunction caused by neurological disease or diabetic neuropathy, treatment of the underlying condition, if possible, may improve bladder control. Use of bethanecol (5–25 mg two to four times daily) may also help. Intermittent catherization rather than an in-dwelling catheter is recommended.

Mixed incontinence

Using a variety of methods can improve the incontinence of women with mixed symptoms. Behavioral therapy, drug treatment, or both, have been found in an RCT to improve the symptoms.[38]

Conclusions

UI is a very frequent but often hidden symptom. A variety of pharmacological and behavioral methods can produce improvement.

Urinary tract infections

Between 20 and 60% of women will have at least one UTI during their lives, and 20% will have several recurrences.[39] The incidence of UTIs in sexually active women is 0.5–0.7 infections per person per year.[40] While diagnosis and treatment of a solitary UTI is not difficult, recurrent UTIs must be rigorously diagnosed, followed, and treated. Even though chronic UTIs are no longer a common cause of renal failure, they should not be a factor in illness.

Risk factors

Risk factors for UTIs include variations in sexual behaviors, antibiotic use, and use of diaphragms or condoms for contraception.[41] Intermittent sex or the sudden start or restart of sexual relationships may lead to a UTI. Anatomically abnormal urinary tract and kidney stones also predispose to UTIs. Anything that causes stasis – stones, extrinsic tumors such as very large uteruses or ovarian tumors, pregnancy, or poorly working collecting systems – will predispose to UTIs.

Symptoms

The symptoms of UTI are well known, distinctive, and often diagnostic – polyuria, nocturia, dysuria, and frequency in urination. This may have occurred for hours to days before the woman approaches the physician. There may be costovertebral angle (CVA), flank, and/or suprapubic pain and tenderness. The urine may be dark, cloudy, or bloody. The symptoms are so distinctive that women who have had a previous UTI are very accurate in diagnosing a second or recurrent UTI in themselves.[42]

Severe back and flank pain, fever, chills, nausea, and vomiting may accompany an episode of pyelonephritis and would suggest a systemic infection that needs more aggressive treatment. Although microscopic hematuria often accompanies a UTI, painless or painful macroscopic hematuria, especially if there are clots, may signal a bladder lesion, polyp, or cancer, and cystoscopy is needed soon.

Evaluation

Physical examination may be totally normal. Suprapubic or CVA tenderness may be found. Fever and tachycardia may suggest pyelonephritis.

Laboratory evaluation of urine is the primary diagnostic tool. Dipstick evaluation of urine will show positive leukocyte esterase tests and will be positive for nitrites. However, leukocyte esterase tests have a sensitivity of only 57% and a negative predictive value of 68%, and nitrites have a sensitivity of only 27% and a negative predictive value of 87% for UTI defined by culture.[43]

Pyuria defined as more than five white blood cells per high-power field of spun urine and bacteriuria will occur in UTIs. Hematuria can occur. Casts are not usual.

A urine culture is usually performed. However, to reduce the cost of UTIs, some experts have used only a urine analysis for a simple or first UTI, with a repeat analysis after antibiotic therapy. Although UTI from a clean catch urine is defined as more than 10^5 organisms of a single type, a lower number may indicate a UTI if the woman is pregnant or symptomatic or if this was not a first morning urine. Antibiotic sensitivities of the organism should be reported.

Escherichia Coli, especially in first, simple, or occasional UTIs, causes 80% of UTIs. *Staphylococcus saphrophyticus* causes approximately 10% of UTIs.

Table 21.7 Treatment for simple urinary tract infection

Drug	Dose(mg)	Times a day	Duration (days)
Amoxicillin	250–500	3	3–14
Cephalexin	250–500	3	3–14
Ciprofloxacin	250–500	2	3–5
Nitrofurantoin	50–100	2–4	3–5
Norfloxacin	400	2	3–5
Trimethoprim	100	2	3–5
Trimethoprim/sulfa	1 DS tablet	2	3–5

Diagnosis

In one review of several studies, a woman who presented with any one of the symptoms of dysuria, hematuria, back pain, and CVA tenderness had a 50% chance of a positive urine culture. Two symptoms increased the likelihood to 90%. Self-diagnosis also increased the probability of a UTI.[44]

Women with a history of UTIs can accurately diagnose repeat UTIs. Eighty-eight women with recurrent UTIs accurately diagnosed another UTI 84% of the time.[33]

Radiologic evaluation

For a first or occasional UTI, no radiological evaluation is needed.

In a woman with recurrent UTIs or pyelonephritis, further evaluation is essential after the UTI is cleared and the urine is proven sterile. In retrospective studies of women in urology clinics, between 5 and 21% of women with recurrent UTIs had abnormal urinary tracts.[45] In one retrospective study of radiological studies in women with pyelonephritis severe enough to require hospitalization, more than 20% had abnormal urinary tracts or previously undiagnosed kidney stones.[46]

A renal ultrasound to find kidney stones or dilation suspicious for obstruction is necessary. A voiding cystourethrogram may be a good second test, especially if hydroureter or hydronephrosis occurs or if reflux is suspected. An intravenous pyelogram (IVP) or renal scan is probably indicated to define function.

Treatment

For symptoms consistent with a simple UTI, a three-day course of trimethoprim/sulfa or a fluoroquinolone is acceptable treament.

Simple or first infection

Once a UTI is suspected, the treatment is an empiric course of antibiotics. The length of treatment has shortened from ten days to one to five days (Table 21.7).

Table 21.8 Single-dose treatment for simple urinary tract infection

Drug	Dose
Amoxicillin	3 g
Cefuroxime	1000 mg
Cephalexin	3 gm
Ciprofloxacin	1 g
Nitrofurantoin	400 mg
Norfloxacin	400 or 800 mg
Sulfisoxasole	2 g
Trimethoprim	400 or 600 mg
Trimethoprim/sulfa	2 DS tablets

One-day treatment has been suggested (Table 21.8), but this is less effective than 10–14-day treatment. Three-day treatment is usually effective in curing simple UTIs.

Some experts believe that the standard of therapy for treatment is trimethoprim/sulfa for three days.[47] However, the number of E. coli isolates that are resistant to ampicillin, carbenecillin, tetracycline, and trimethoprim/sulfa varies from area to area, but is increasing, so that medication choice may be affected. Fluoroquinolone resistance is still less than 5% in most E. coli populations.[48] Instead of trimethoprim/sulfa or ampicillin as a first choice, a fluoroquinone, nitrofurantoin, or cephalosporin may be a better first choice.

For severe pain, pyridium (100–200 mg three times daily, orally) may be used as an adjuvant for one to two days. Pyridium is a bladder anesthetic and relieves the dysuria immediately. However, it should not be given to patients with renal failure or for more than two days. Patients should be reminded to continue to take the antibiotic, even if the pain is gone. Patients should be advised that pyridium turns urine, and sometimes even sweat, bright orange.

Repeat culture or at least a urine analysis is wise, two to three weeks after infection, to prove sterility and cure.

Recurrent infection

Approximately one-quarter of women will have a second UTI within six months of their first UTI. Most immediate recurrences are reinfections, so a different antibiotic should be used.[49]

First, the present UTI must be treated with antibiotics. Because the woman (and her bacteria) have already seen one antibiotic, a different antibiotic or one chosen after obtaining sensitivities should be used. Antibiotics should be used for 10–14 days.

Table 21.9 Antibiotic doses for prophylaxis of recurrent urinary tract infections

Antibiotic	Dose for daily use	Dose for postcoital use
Cephalexin	250 mg	250 mg
Nitrofurantoin	50–100 mg	50 mg
Sulfamethoxazole	500 mg	500 mg
Trimethoprim/sulfa	½ DS tablet	½ DS tablet
Ciprofloxacin	250 mg	

Prevention of recurrent infections

There is a variety of methods with a variety of strength of evidence suggested for the prevention of recurrent UTIs. Clinical Evidence (IV) found no systematic reviews on prevention of recurrent UTIs.

Low-dose continuous daily or nightly antibiotic use has been suggested for prophylaxis. Several RCTs found lower rates of infection with antibiotic use.[50,51] Various antibiotics, including nitrourantoin, ciprofloxacin, norfloxacin, and trimethoprim/sulfa, were used and had similar lower rates of reinfection than placebo. Post-intercourse antibiotic use was as effective as nightly use in one study (Table 21.9).[32]

Other methods include dietary, hormonal, and mechanical treatments.

Ingestion of more water, *Lactobacillus* juice, and cranberry or other juices has been suggested for the prevention of recurrent UTIs. One RCT of 150 women found that 50 ml of cranberry-ligonberry concentrate reduced recurrences by approximately 50% while ingestion of *Lactobacillus* GG juice had no effect.[30]

In menopausal women, supposed urethral and periurethral tissue laxity has been treated with topical and oral estrogens. These hormones are supposed to increase the strength and tone of the urethral tissues, promoting more effective bladder emptying. Estrogen vaginal cream has been used two to three times a week. A small RCT found that women with recurrent UTIs who used the Estring, the vaginal estrogen-embedded ring with no systemic absorption, prolonged the time until the next occurrence and more than doubled the number of women who had no further UTIs when used for 36 weeks.[52]

Mechanical treatments include bladder retraining – reminders to urinate every two hours – and intermittent catheterization for women with overflow incontinence.

Indications of upper tract disease and need for hospitalization

Although dysuria, polyuria, and nocturia are primarily symptoms of lower tract disease, they can also occur with upper tract infection or pyelonephritis. CVA or flank tenderness can occur in both, but fever, chills, nausea, and vomiting are more likely to occur in pyelonephritis. In women with pyelonephritis, the white blood cell (WBC) count is likely to be elevated. WBC casts are diagnostic for pyelonephritis but are rarely seen.

There is no test that determines or detects upper tract versus lower tract disease. If symptoms of pyelonephritis occur or a woman with a simple UTI does not improve with three- or five-day therapy, then 10–14-day therapy is indicated.

Indications for hospitalization and intravenous antibiotic medication include dehydration, vomiting, inability to take oral medication, and severe pain. Women with diabetes or abnormal urinary tract are more likely to need intravenous antibiotics and hospitalization.

REFERENCES

1 Browning, SM. Office management of common anorectal problems. *Prim. Care* 1999; **26**:113–21.
2 Feldman, J. H. Epidemidogy. In *Feldman, Sleisenger and Fordtran's Gastrointestinal and Liver Disease*, 6th edition. Philadelphia: WB Saunders; 1998. p. 692.
3 Talley, N. J., O'Keefe, E. A., Zinsmeister, A. R. and Melton, L. J., III. Prevalence of gastrointestinal symptoms in the elderly: a population-based study. *Gastroenterology* 1992; **102**:895–901.
4 Fine, K. D. and Schiller, L. R. AGA technical review on the evaluation and management of chronic diarrhea. *Gastroenterology* 1999; **116**:6.
5 Talan, D. A., Moran, G. J., Ong, S., *et al.* Prevalence of *E. coli* O157:H7 and other enteropathogens among patients presenting to US emergency departments with bloody diarrhea. In Abstracts of the International Conference on Emerging Infectious Diseases (Atlanta), 8–11 March 1998.
6 Guerrant, R. L., Van Gilder, T., and Steiner, T. S. Practice guidelines for the management of infectious diarrhea. *Clin. Infect. Dis.* 2001; **32**:1001.
7 DuPont, H. L. Guidelines on acute infectious diarrhea in adults. The Practice Parameters Committee of the American College of Gastroenterology. *Am. J. Gastroenterol.* 1997; **92**:1962–75.
8 Khan, W. A., Seas, C., Dhar, U., Salam, M. A. and Bennish, M. L. Treatment of shigellosis: V. Comparison of azithromycin and ciprofloxacin. A double blind, randomized, controlled trial. *Ann. Intern. Med.* 1997; **126**:697–703.
9 Thompson, W. G. The irritable bowel. *Gut* 1984; **25**:305–11.
10 Mitchell, C. M. and Drossman, D. A. Survey of the AGA membership relating to patients with functional gastrointestinal disorders. *Gastroenterology* 1987; **92**:1282–9.
11 Saito, Y. A., Schoenfeld, P. and Locke, F. R., 3rd. The epidemiology of iritable bowel syndrome in North America. A systemic review. *Am. J. Gastroenterol.* 2002; **97**:1910–15.
12 Borum, M. L. Irritable bowel syndrome. *Prim. Care.* 2001; **28**:147–62.
13 Gupt, V., Sheffield, D. and Verne, G. N. Evidence for autonomic dysregulation in the irritable bowel syndrome. *Dig. Dis. Sci.* 2002; **47**:1716–22.
14 Abrahamsson, J. Gastrointestinal motility in patients with the irritable bowel syndrome. *Scan. J. Gastroenterol. Suppl.* 1987; **130**:21–9.
15 Everhart, J. E. and Renault, P. F. Irritable bowel syndrome in office based practice in the United States. *Gastroenterology* 1991; **100**:998–1003.

16 Walling, M. K., O'Hara, M. W., Reiter, R. C., *et al.* Abuse history and chronic pain in women II: a multivariate analysis of abuse and psychological morbidity. *Obstet. Gynecol.* 1994; **84**:200–206.

17 Lièvre, M. Alosetron for irritable bowel syndrome. *Br. Med. J.* 2002; **325**:555.

18 Tougas, G., Snape, W. J.,Otten, M. H., *et al.* Long term safey of tegaserod in patients with constipation predominant irritable bowel syndrome. *Aliment. Pharmocol. Ther.* 2002; **16**:1701–8.

19 Morganroth, J., Ruegg, P. C., Dunger-Baldauf, C., *et al.* Tegaserod, a 5-hydroxytryptamine type 4 receptor partial agonist, is devoid of electrocardiographic effects. *Am. J. Gastroenterol.* 2002; **97**:2321–7.

20 Rekers, H., Drogendijk, A. C., Valkenburg, H. and Riphagen, F. Urinary incontinence in women from 35 to 79 years of age: prevalence and consequences. *Eur. J. Obstet. Gynecol. Reprod. Biol.* 1992; **43**:229–34.

21 Burgio, K. L., Matthews, K. A. and Engel, B. T. Prevalence, incidence and correlates of urinary incontinence in healthy, middle-aged women. *J. Urol.* 1991; **146**: 1255–9.

22 Grimby, A., Milsom, I., Molander, U., Wiklund, I. and Ekelund, P. The influence of urinary incontinence on the quality of life of elderly women. *Age Ageing* 1993 **22**:82–9.

23 Simeonova, Z., Milsom, I., Kullendorff, A. M., Molander, U. and Bengtsson, C. The prevalence of urinary incontinence and its influence on the quality of life in women from an urban Swedish population. *Acta Obstet. Gynecol. Scand.* 1999; **78**:546–51.

24 Seim, A., Sandvik, H., Hermstad, R. and Hunskaar, S. Female urinary incontinence – consultation behaviour and patient experiences: an epidemiological survey in a Norwegian community. *Fam. Pract.* 1995; **12**:18–21.

25 Brown, J. S., Grad, D., Ouslander, J. G., *et al.* Prevalence of urinary incontinence and associated risk factors in postmenopausal women. *Obstet. Gynecol.* 1999; **94**:66–70.

26 Chiarelli, P. and Cockburn, J. Promoting urinary continence in women after delivery: randomised controlled trial. *Br. Med. J.* 2002; **324**:1241.

27 Gladzener, C. M. A., Lang, G., Wilson, P. D., *et al.* Postnatal incontinence: a multicenter randomised controlled trial of conservative treatment. *Br. J. Obstet. Gynaecol.* 1998; **105**:47.

28 Seim, A., Eriksen, B. C. and Hunskaar, S. Treatment of urinary incontinence in women in general practice: observational study. *Br. Med. J.* 1996; **312**:1459–62.

29 (CE-4) Berghmans, L. C. M., Hendriks, H. J. M., Bo, K. *et al.* Conservative treatment of stress urinary incontinence in women: a systematic review of randomised trial *Br. J. Urol.* 1998; **82**:181–91.

30 (C) Hay-Smith, E. J. C., Bo, K., Berghmans, L. C. M., *et al.* Pelvic floor muscle training for urinary incontinence in women. In *The Cochrane Library*, issue 2. Oxford: Update Software; 2002.

31 Fantl, J. A., Cordozo, L. K., Ekberg, J., *et al.* Estrogen therapy in the management of urinary incontinence in postmenopausal women: a meta analysis. *Obstet. Gyencol.* 1994; **83**:12–18.

32 (CE-4) Bo, K., Talseth, T. and Home, I. Single blind randomised controlled trial of pelvic floor exercise, electronical stimulation, vaginal cones and no treatment in the mangement of genuine stress incontinence. *Br. Med. J.* 1999; **318**:4487–93.

33 (C) Glazener, C. M. A. and Cooper, K. Anterior vaginal repair for urinary incontinence in women. In *The Cochrane Library*, issue 2. Oxford: Update Software; 2002.

34 (C) Bezerra, C. A. and Bruschini, H. Suburethral sling operations for urinary incontinence in women. In *The Cochrane Library*, issue 2. Oxford: Update Software; 2002. www.update-software.com/abstracts/ab001754.htm

35 (AHRQ – A recommendation) Burgio, L. D., McCormick, K. A., Scheve, A. S., *et al.* The effects of changing prompted voiding schedules in the treatment of incontinence in nursing home residents. *J. Am. Geriatr. Soc.* 1994; **42**:315–20.

36 (C) Roe, B., Williams, K. and Palmer, M. Bladder training for urinary incontinence in adults. In *The Cochrane Library*, issue 2. Oxford: Update Software; 2002.

37 Harvey, M. A. Tolterodine versus oxybutynin in the treatment of urge urinary incontinence: a meta-analysis. *Am. J. Obstet. Gynecol.* 2001; **185**:56–61.

38 Burgio, K. L., Locher, J. L., Goode, P. S., *et al.* Behvioral vs. drug treatment for urge urinary incontinence in older women. *J. Am. Med. Assoc.* 1998; **280**:1995–2001.

39 Kontiokari, T., Sundquist, K., Nuutinene, M., *et al.* Randomised trial of cranberry ligonberry juice and Lactobacillus GG drink for the prevention of urinary tract infections in women. *Br. Med. J.* 2001; **322**:1571.

40 Hooton, T. M., Scholes, D., Hughes, J. P., *et al.* A prospective study of risk factor for urinary tract infection in young women. *N. Engl. J. Med.* 1996; **335**:468–74.

41 Handley, M. A., Reingold, A. L., Shiboski, S. and Padian, N. S. Incidence of acute urinary tract infection in young women and use of male condoms with and without nonosynol-9 spermicides. *Epidemiology* 2002; **13**:431–6.

42 Gupta, K., Hooton, T. M., Roberts, P. L. and Stamm, W. E. Patient-initiated treatment of uncomplicated recurrent urinary tract infections in young women. *Ann. Intern. Med.* 2001; **135**:51–2.

43 Saman, S., Borremans, A., Verhaegen, J., *et al.* Disappointing dipstick screening for urinary tract infection in hospital inpatients. *J. Clin. Pathol.* 1998; **51**:471–2.

44 Bent, S., Nallamothus, B. K., Simel, D. L., Fihn, S. D. and Saint, S. Does this woman have an uncomplicated urinary tract infection. *J. Am. Med. Assoc.* 2002; **287**:2701–10.

45 Nickel, J. C., Wilson, J., Morales, A. and Heaton, J. Value of urological investigation in a targeted group of women with recurrent urinary tracts. *Can. J. Surg.* 1991; **34**:591–4.

46 Rosenfeld, J. A. Radiological abnormalities in women admitted with pyelonephritis. *Del. Med. J.* 1987; **59**:717–19.

47 Garrison, J. and Hooton, T. M. Fluoroguinolones in the treatment of acute uncomplicated urinary tract infections in adult women. *Expert Opin. Pharmacother.* 2001; **2**:1227–37.

48 Dyer, I. E., Sankary, T. M. and Dawson, J. A. Antibiotic resistence in bacterial urinary tract infections 1991 to 1997. *West. J. Med.* 1998; **169**:265–8.

49 Foxman, B. Recurring urinary tract infection: incidence and risk factors. *Am. J. Publ. Health* 1990; **80**:331.

50 Stamm, W. E., Counts, G. W., Wagner, K. F., *et al.* Antimicrobial prophylaxis of recurrent urinary tract infections: a double blind placebo controlled trial. *Ann. Intern. Med.* 1980; **92**:770–75.

51 Melekos, M. D., Asbach, H. W., Gerharz, E., *et al.* Post intercourse versus daily ciprofloxin prophylaxis for recurrent urinary tract infections in premenopausal women. *J. Urol.* 1997; **157**:935–9.

52 Eriksen, B. A randomized open, parallel-group study on the preventive effect of an estradiol releasing vaginal ring (Estring) on recurrent urinary tract infections in postmenopausal women. *Am. J. Obstet. Gynecol.* 1999; **180**:1072–9.

Index

Page numbers in *italics* refer to figures and tables.

Printed in the United States
by Baker & Taylor Publisher Services

Printed in the United States
by Baker & Taylor Publisher Services